Gynaecological Ultrasou

Scanning

Kamal Ojha
Department of Obstetrics and Gynaecology, St George's University Hospital, London, UK

Sonal Panchal
Dr. Nagori's Institute for Infertility and IVF, Ahmedabad, India

Lukasz Polanski
Assisted Conception Unit, Guy's Hospital, Great Maze Pond, London, UK

Shama Puri
Department of Radiology, Royal Derby Hospital, Derby, UK

Sheila Radhakrishnan
Department of Gynaecology, Royal Free London NHS Foundation Trust, London, UK

Sotirios H. Saravelos
IVF Unit, Hammersmith Hospital, Imperial College, London, UK

Francisco Sellers López
Instituto Bernabeu, Centre for Assisted Reproduction and Gynaecology, Alicante, Spain

Thierry Van den Bosch
Department of Obstetrics and Gynaecology, University Hospitals Leuven, Leuven, Belgium

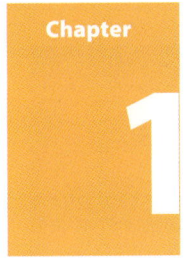

Get to Know Your Machine and Scanning Environment

Kamal Ojha

The aim of this chapter is to explain the basic principles of gynaecology ultrasound for all those who are beginning to learn to perform scans, especially transvaginal ultrasound. These same principles will also benefit those who are keen to improve their scanning skills. In this chapter, we shall focus initially on the ultrasound machine itself and then on the scanning techniques, which will help you either as a beginner or to improve your scanning capability. Chapter 3 will focus on awkward or difficult clinical scenarios.

Adopting a systematic approach to gynaecology scanning (pelvic scan) is essential. One could start scanning in the longitudinal view and then move to a transverse view. Anatomically, scanning the uterus first makes most sense, followed by the right and then the left ovary and adnexa. It is not uncommon that one, especially in the initial stages of training, may focus on an obvious pathology, e.g. a large ovarian cyst that is evident at the start of examination, and subsequently may become distracted and forget to scan other pelvic structures. A systematic approach to scanning will avoid such unnecessary omissions in scanning structures that form part of routine examination.

Ultrasound Equipment Used in Gynaecological Scanning

Machine and Keyboard

Knowledge of your machine, both for a beginner and an experienced scanner using a new machine before starting to scan, is an essential step in getting the best out of your equipment. Switching on modern machines is a bit like switching on a laptop or a computer, whereas if you have an older machine you will see an on/off switch on the side of the machine. Once the machine has been switched on, it may take one or two minutes to boot-up, as it is generally based on a Windows* environment. This gives you a good opportunity to have a look at the machine's keyboard and screen. The keyboard can be daunting for beginners; it is advisable to initially identify a few important buttons (Figure 1.1a) before one starts scanning, such as:

1. freeze, to capture an image once obtained;
2. frequency;
3. measurement and set button (allowing one to obtain additional measurements);
4. greyscale/gain;
5. depth;
6. focus;
7. left/right and up/down screen display buttons;
8. save and print options; and
9. Doppler and 3D scanning functions.

Some ultrasound machines, in addition to having a keyboard, may have an interactive touch screen (see Figures 1.1b and 1.2). It is important to understand that these touch screens are dynamic, so the display will show options for each function. For example, *frequency* display, on tapping the screen, will show three options: normal, resolution and penetrative mode. The penetrative mode is a lower-frequency setting and hence allows us to see deeper structures such as large fibroids. Higher frequency is generally good for smaller structures but specifically designed probes have made it easier to select the correct frequency. Hence, knowledge of potential options for each function is useful to ensure best use of the equipment. Those who have already achieved basic scanning skills may wish, in addition, to familiarize themselves with the Doppler and 3D scanning functions on the keyboard. It may be helpful to have a skilled scanner or systems specialist to demonstrate these functions. Some machines allow you to save individual frequently used settings, displayed as a personalized option to select before one starts scanning, especially where there are multiple users of the same machine. Machines may also have organ-specific settings – for example uterus, endometrium or the

(a)

(b)

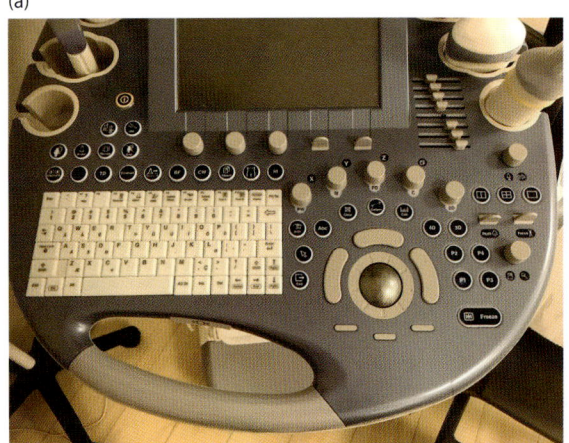
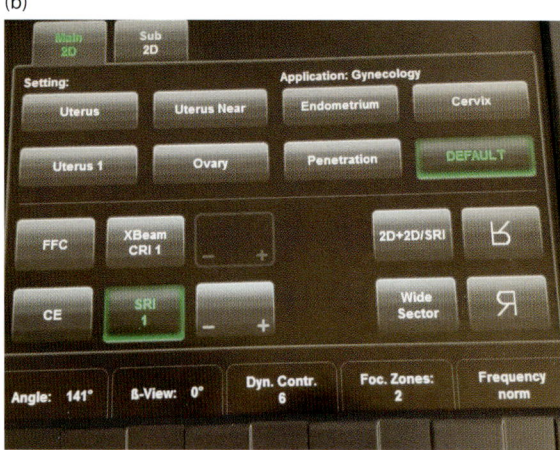

Figure 1.1 (a) Keyboard of an ultrasound machine with a dynamic touch screen. (b) A touch screen giving options to select ultrasound settings for different organs. Frequency, angle, focal zone, up/down and right/left modes of scanning are among the basic functions which will be useful for a beginner. The touch screen is dynamic and hence selection of the options allows one to choose appropriate settings while scanning.

ovary in gynaecology and similar options for obstetrics – which may save time when commencing the scan. Software on all ultrasound machines provides an arrow or a cursor, which is quite useful when explaining the scan findings on the screen to the patient. The tracker ball serves as a computer mouse and helps move the cursor or the measuring point.

Technique and Steps for Ultrasound Examination

It is useful to understand the movement of the transducer while performing the ultrasound examination. The probe needs to be moved from left to right, or the reverse, for longitudinal scan, and up and down for a transverse scan. Ensure that while the probe is moving the organ being scanned is kept in the centre of the field of view, otherwise the organ will move on the screen without the scan being completed. The probe needs to move from one end of the organ being scanned to the other end, and go beyond the structure so that the structure is completely lost on the screen. Repeat this process for transverse examination to avoid missing uterine malformations and subserosal fibroids.

Imagine that your palm with the fingers is the ultrasound transducer and the thumb indicates the direction. When the thumb is facing upwards, the probe is held in a longitudinal mode, and when the thumb is pointing to the right side of the patient, this constitutes the transverse mode of scanning (Figures 1.3 and 1.4). Once the structure is identified

and good contact is maintained, the movement of the probe resembles the movement of the palm at the wrist joint from right to left, and the reverse, until you have completely scanned the structure in the longitudinal/sagittal plane. In the transverse mode, the palm moves at the wrist with up-and-down motions. Please note that any axial movement (rotation) of the probe will make identification of the true axis of the structure difficult and is a common mistake made by those learning to scan (an exception is scanning foetal long bones, when axial rotation of the transducer allows identification of the actual length of the bone).

In summary, the structure being scanned should be identified clearly, good contact with the tissue should be maintained while the scan is performed to acquire a good-quality image, and the probe should move very slowly for a thorough examination of the structure being scanned. Failure to identify the structure, or lack of good contact and axial rotation, are generally the main reasons why most beginners initially struggle to acquire good-quality images.

Transvaginal Probe and Scanning (TVS)

Once the machine has been switched on, the next step is to identify the probes attached to the machine. On the keyboard, or the panel, there will be a sign for probe selection, which will display the transducers available for use. Almost all machines will have a two-dimensional (2D) transvaginal and a 2D abdominal transducer for gynaecology scanning. Three-dimensional (3D) probes

(a) (b)

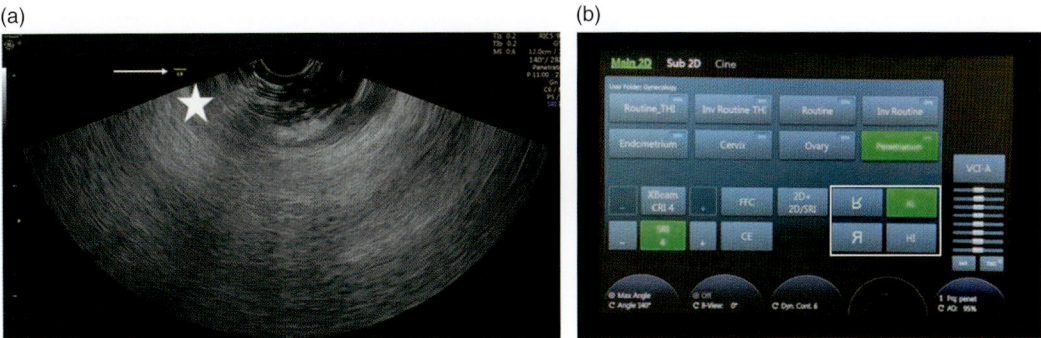

Figure 1.2(a,b) (a) displays the mark on the left side of the screen (arrow) and the corresponding markers indicating the direction of scanning are inactive (rectangle on (b)). This is the preferred way of scanning and most of the images in this book are displayed this way. The * indicates where the bladder would be in each of the orientations.

(c) (d)

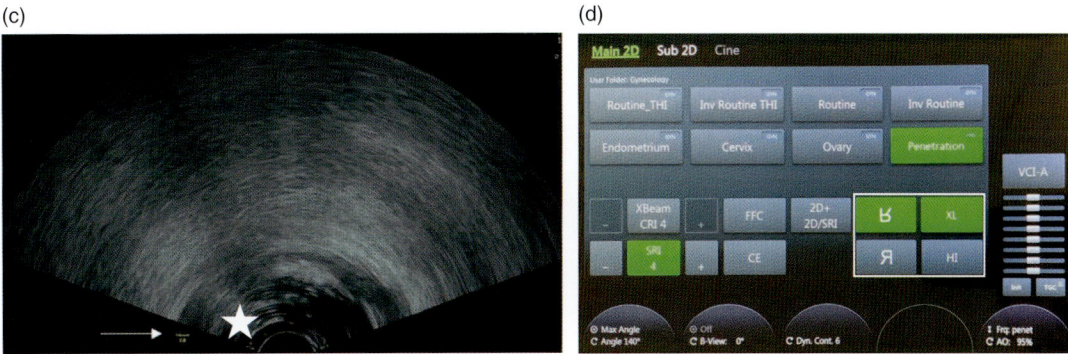

Figure 1.2(c,d) Activating one of the buttons (highlighted green in (d), within the white box) flips the image displayed on the screen by 180 degrees. Notice the mark on the bottom left side of the screen (arrow in (c)).

(e) (f)

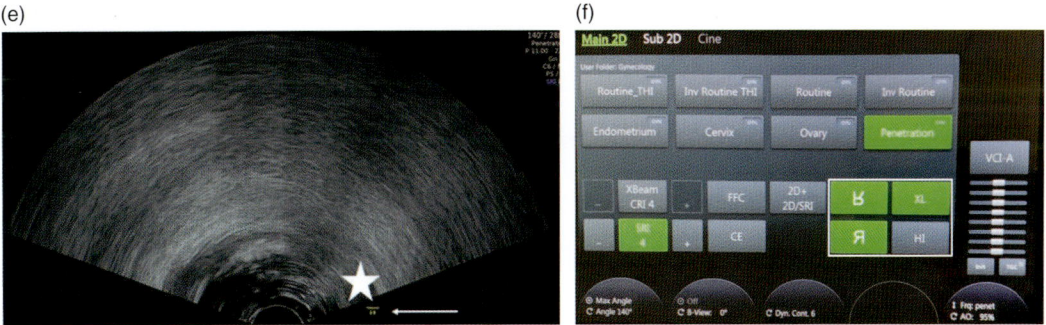

Figure 1.2(e,f) Activating both markers (green within the box) flips the display by 180 degrees and changes right for left. Notice the mark on the screen (arrow in (e)).

are provided separately and are much bulkier in appearance, especially the abdominal transducer. When changing probes, it may be necessary to press the freeze button to activate the transducer. If selecting the transvaginal probe, a semicircle image will appear on the screen. This semicircle is the active part of a TVS image measuring to an angle of up to 180 degrees

(scanning angle), which can be adjusted. A wider angle allows for an overview of the structures of interest and the surrounding tissues, whereas a narrow angle allows one to focus on a specific area. This is especially important when assessing moving objects, particularly the foetal heartbeat in early gestation, as a wide angle has a low screen refresh rate (measured in hertz (Hz) and

(a)   (b)

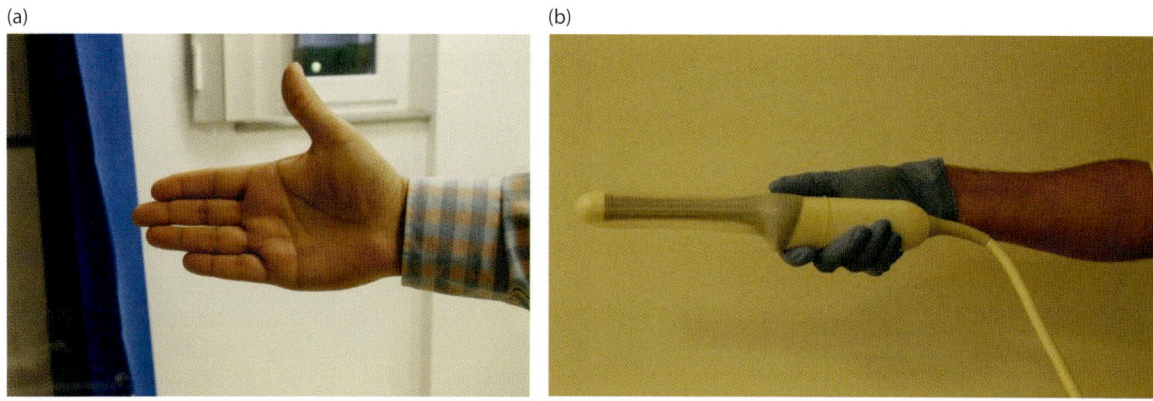

Figure 1.3 (a) The palm with the thumb upwards representing the probe in a longitudinal axis; the movement of the probe is sideways at the wrist joint. (b) Probe held correctly for a longitudinal image with thumb facing upwards.

(a)   (b)

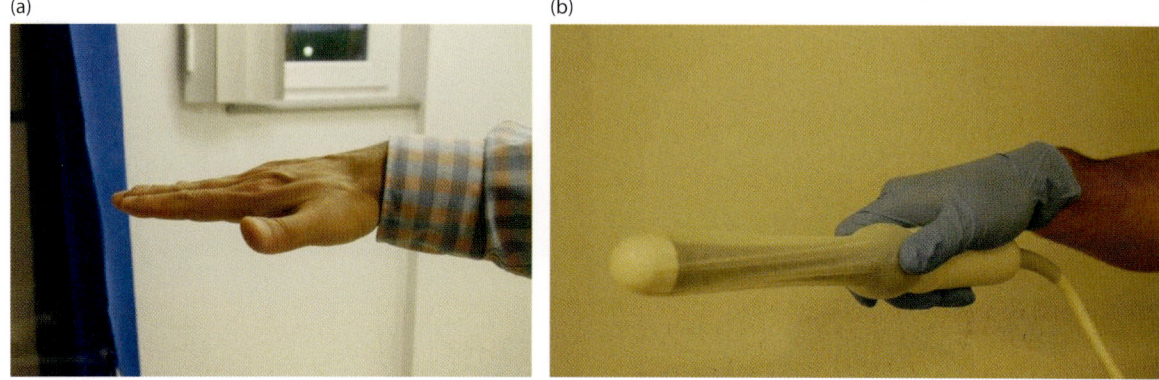

Figure 1.4 (a) Palm with thumb pointing towards the right side of the patient for a transverse scan, with movement at right angles up and down. (b) Probe held correctly for a transverse image with the thumb facing the right side of the patient.

displayed on the screen); narrowing the angle allows for a faster screen refresh and better identification of foetal heartbeat. An abdominal probe has a curvilinear image appearance with a slight curvature representing the probe surface. Thus, by just looking at the screen one can identify which probe is being used, and probes may be changed as appropriate.

Holding the Probe

The first step to correctly hold the probe is to identify either a groove or a depression on the probe handle. While doing a TVS, the thumb should be placed on the depression or the groove of the transducer (Figure 1.5). Holding the probe correctly while scanning is an important step. Scanning with the thumb facing upwards allows you to perform longitudinal imaging

(Figure 1.3) and with the thumb placed to the right of the patient allows transverse imaging of the structure being scanned (Figure 1.4). Scanning with the thumb facing to the left of the patient or downward may lead to mistakes related to location of structures (Figure 1.6). Aligning the top and bottom and the right and left sides of the image on the screen is the next important step. The image on the screen shows a mark (this could be the logo of the scan machine company) identifying the 'right' in a *transversely* held probe and 'top' in a *longitudinally* held probe (Figure 1.7). This mark can be reversed or inverted by pressing appropriate buttons on the keyboard (Figure 1.2). A very important point to remember for all who are learning to scan is to follow one particular system while scanning. Ensure the mark is in the same position on every occasion that one

(a)

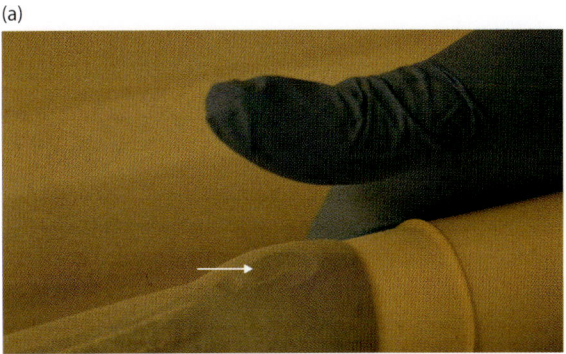

(b)

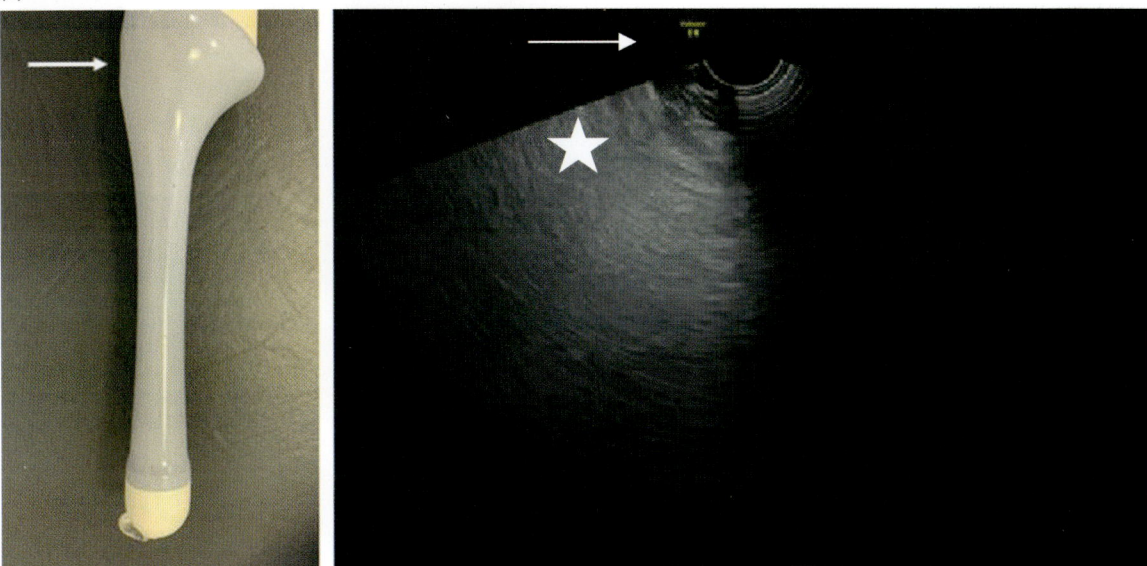

Figure 1.5 (a) The thumb should be placed on the groove (arrow) of the TVS probe. (b) When ultrasound gel is applied to the surface of the transducer on the side where the groove is (arrow), the corresponding image displayed on the screen displays the mark on the left side of the screen. This is the preferred way of scanning and most of the images in this book are displayed in this way. The * indicates where the bladder would be in each of the orientations.

performs scans by making appropriate adjustments on the keyboard with the invert and right/left buttons. For consistency, all descriptions in this chapter assume the mark to be on the top and the left side of the screen (Figure 1.2a). Whatever the preferred settings are, these need to be changed accordingly before scanning is commenced.

In the image on the screen, the right and top are aligned with the patient's (and not the scanner's) right; making a note of this is very useful to avoid a basic error of sides and position (right- or left-sided ovarian cyst or a breech/cephalic presentation in an abdominal scan). A good way of demonstrating this is to hold the probe as in a longitudinal scan (thumb is placed up as in Figure 1.2) and then if you place a small amount of gel on the top of the probe before the probe is inserted into the vagina the screen will show the structure; in this situation 'the gel' is on the left side of the screen (Figure 1.5). Any part of the scanned organ that appears on the left side of the screen in a longitudinal view is cranial in an abdominal scan and top (anterior) in a transvaginal scan, and on the right half of the screen is caudal (posterior in a TVS). For example, in an anteverted uterus on a longitudinal scan the fundus will be on the left side when looking at the screen and the cervix on the right when looking at the screen,

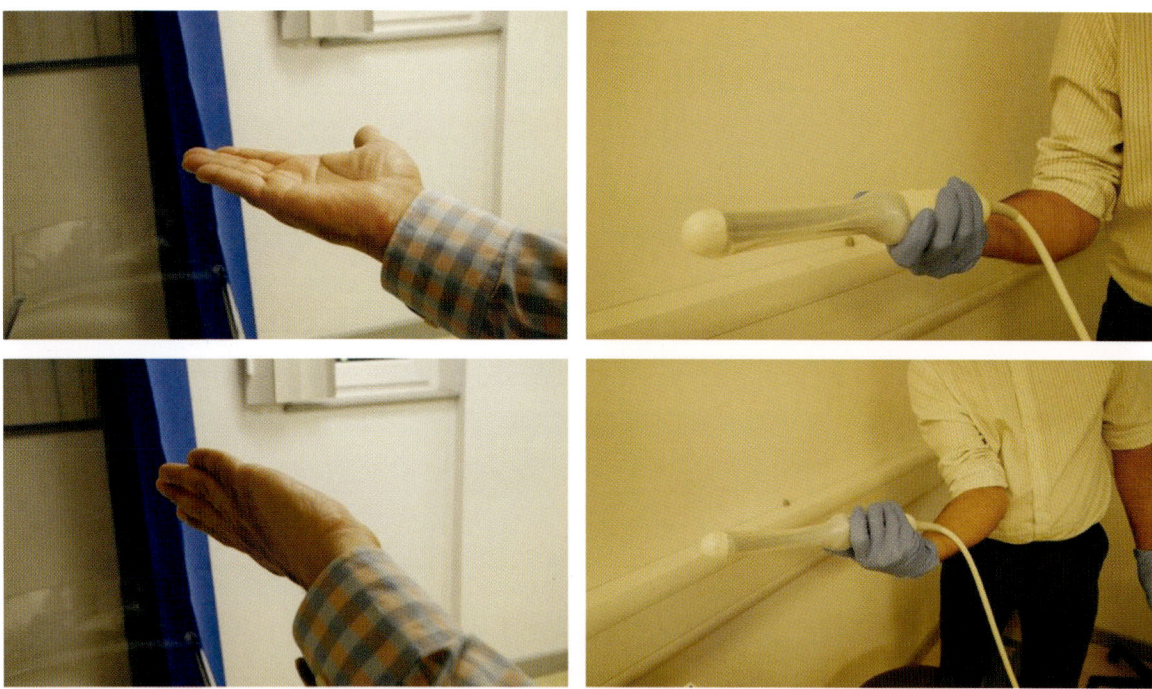

Figure 1.6 Thumb facing the left side or downwards should never be the position of the probe while doing TVS scanning.

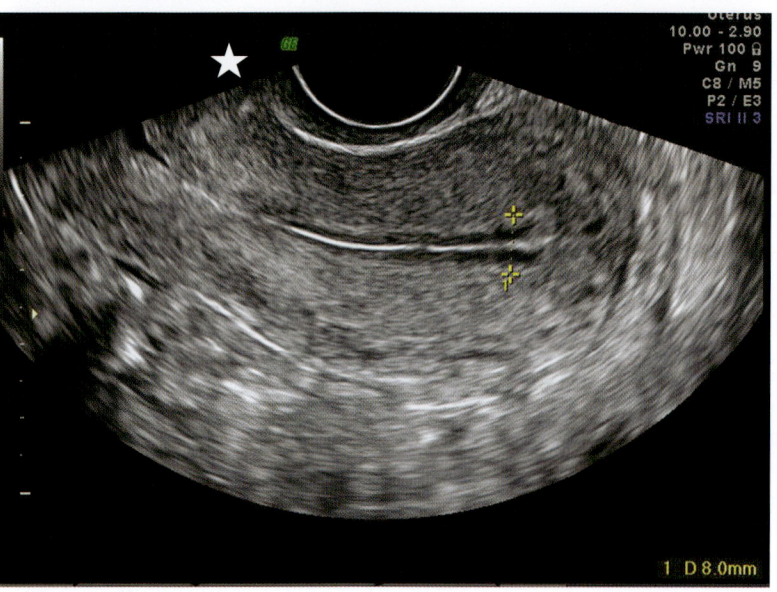

Figure 1.7 TVS scan showing marker on the left of the screen (*) with a retroverted uterus. The cervix appears on the left of the screen and the fundus appears on the right of the screen on a longitudinal scan.

whereas in a retroverted uterus it is the reverse, i.e. the cervix appears on the left side of the screen and the fundus on the right (Figure 1.7).

In terms of ultrasound physics, the ultrasound transducer contains piezo-electric crystals, which both emit and receive ultrasound waves. These waves are emitted into the tissues that are scanned and then are reflected back towards the transducer, where they are received by the piezo-electric crystals. On receiving these sound signals, the ultrasound waves are converted to electrical energy, which is transmitted through the cable fibres to the machine, where the software converts these inputs into an image displayed on the screen. The degree of reflection and penetration of the sound waves varies according to the density of the structures. The soft tissue allows the ultrasound waves to penetrate through the structure and beyond, as well as reflect them back in a small fraction. However, more dense structures, like bone, do not allow the ultrasound waves to traverse, reflecting or scattering them all and hence producing an acoustic shadow beyond. Amniotic fluid or urine allow ultrasound waves to traverse freely, creating a perfect window to scan the foetus in early pregnancy, or the uterus and ovaries during a gynaecological transabdominal scan, respectively. A full bladder is not required for a transvaginal examination; in fact, an empty bladder is recommended. A full bladder during TVS will cause discomfort to the patient and may displace the uterus to an axial position, making assessment of fine endometrial or fundal details difficult.

During a scan, the ultrasound waves are continuously transmitted and the movement of the probe results in multiple images of tissues being received and displayed on the screen, allowing us to view the scan as a real-time, 2D image series. This principle is important to understand when scanning. Hence, slowly moving the probe while scanning is essential to allow time for the machine to emit and receive ultrasound waves, as each image represents a slice of the organ being scanned. This also allows the scanner time to see and comprehend these images. Fast movement, besides causing pain or discomfort to the patient, may also make it difficult for the probe to send and receive the sound waves of the organ being scanned. The increased speed of the images received due to rapid movement of the probe may result in difficulty interpreting the images, or result in missing a fine pathology. The clear message here is: *slow scanning of the tissues has two advantages, one, being gentle to the patient (who thus allows you to do an intimate examination even when structures are tender and difficult to see) and two, allowing time for one to correctly interpret the images appearing on the screen.* While scanning moving structures and observing a real-time 2D examination, such as a moving foetus or foetal heart, observing blood flow or bowel movement, or contrast dye, the probe needs to remain static and directed at the moving structure.

Scanning Principles

Longitudinal Image

For systematic scanning, start the pelvic examination with a longitudinal assessment followed by a transverse examination. The probe cover is applied with ultrasound gel on the inside and the outside; the one inside is necessary to obtain good ultrasound images as it allows ultrasound waves to be transmitted uninterrupted from the transducer to the tissues. Absence of gel or air bubbles may create a poor-quality image or no image at all. The gel on the outside of the probe is used to help introduce the probe easily, especially when the patient finds the examination uncomfortable. Holding the TVS transducer as described above, with the thumb placed on the groove and facing upwards, the probe is introduced into the vagina. When the probe is just beyond the introitus, it is important to start looking at the screen and not advance it further blindly (this is similar to endoscopic surgery, where the camera identifies the landmarks which help to guide the next movement). At this point, important landmarks such as the urethra (anteriorly) and the bowel (posteriorly) will become apparent (Figure 1.8). Similarly, a track with air bubbles will become visible, which represents the two vaginal walls opposing each other with air in between. At some point the bladder will also appear. Aiming the transducer in the direction of the track will lead to a grey tissue area representing the cervix (Figures 1.8 and 1.9). At this point follow the length of the cervix; with an anteverted uterus, your hand will be going downwards with the tip of the transducer pointing upwards to identify the uterine body. In a retroverted uterus the reverse is true; the forearm goes upwards with the tip of the transducer pointing downwards. *Not following a systematic approach, one may fail to notice the landmarks such as the cervix or the uterovesical fold, and the probe may go beyond the cervix, pointing at the pouch of Douglas, showing bowel instead of the uterus* (Figure 1.9). If this does happen it is best to withdraw the probe towards the introitus and start again, as described above. When scanning any organ, good contact with the organ results in very good image quality. Conversely, poor contact with the tissue produces a blurred image. Good contact and a wide angle will allow a good image of the uterus. Once the midline of the uterus is identified in the longitudinal plane, moving the probe sideways in both directions helps to complete the longitudinal examination of the uterus.

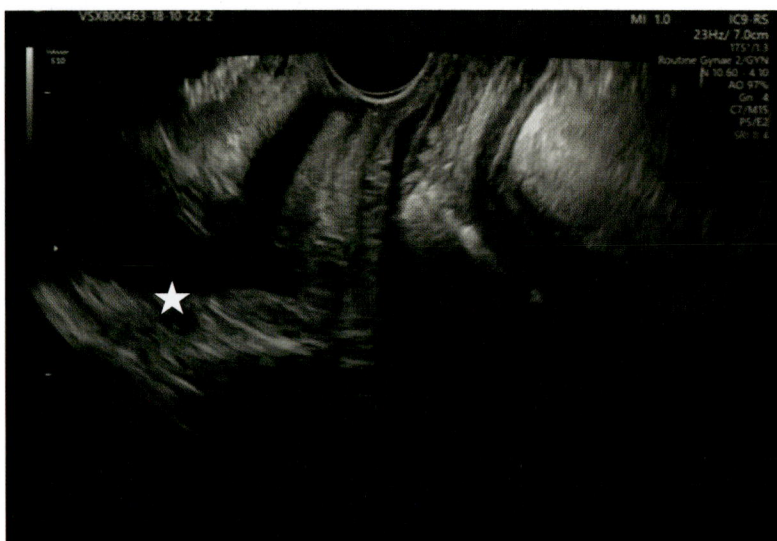

Figure 1.8 Image with probe at the introitus showing the urethra and bladder (*) in the front, rectum in the back, and in the midline is a tract showing the vagina. The tract in the vagina is generally the direction the probe needs to progress anterior to the cervix, eventually coming in close contact with it just below the uterovesical junction.

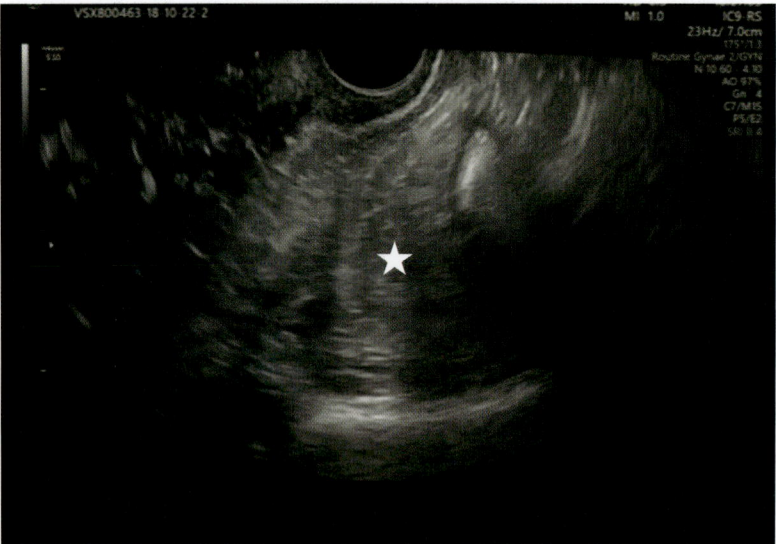

Figure 1.9 Probe wrongly beyond the cervix in the posterior fornix showing bowel in the POD (*). If this is the case it is best to withdraw the probe and restart the scan from just beyond the introitus, looking for the landmarks as described in the text.

When scanning as described (thumb pointing upwards), a longitudinal scan will help identify an anteverted or retroverted uterus, whereas a transverse scan will identify whether a lesion is on the right or the left. Transverse scanning is most useful for fibroid mapping.

Transverse Images

Scanning transversely is ideal for identifying the ovary. Finding the ovaries can be daunting for beginners; however, following some basic steps will help in most cases. While completing the longitudinal examination and maintaining good contact with the uterus, the probe is rotated at the level just below the fundus, with the thumb pointing to the right side of the patient. Thus, the transverse examination is started. The examination of the uterus is completed from fundus to the cervix. This step is particularly useful for mapping fibroids and identifying uterine malformations such as a septate or a bicornuate uterus.

The first landmark when looking for the ovaries is to start just below the fundus of the uterus, where the interstitial part of the fallopian tubes can be seen (see Figure 1.11). Moving the probe in the same plane

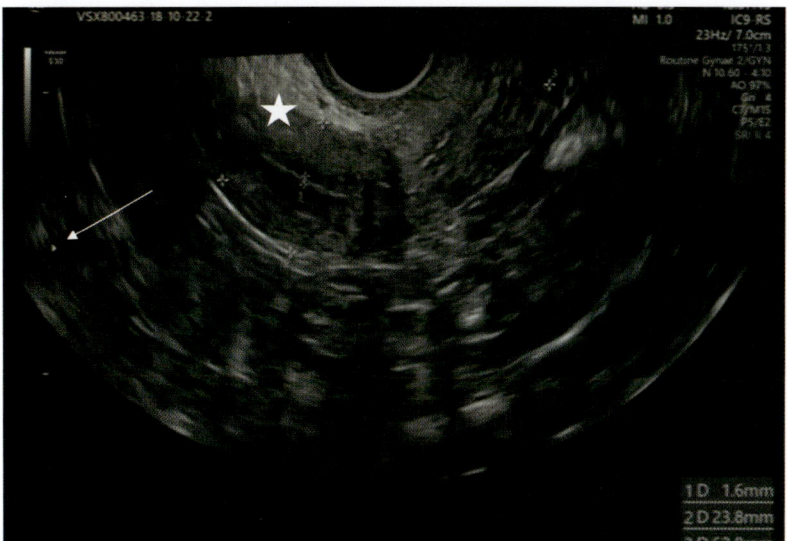

Figure 1.10 TVS probe placed in contact with the cervix just below the uterovesical (*) fold of the peritoneum in a post-menopausal woman with atrophic uterus and thin endometrium. The focal point is seen on the middle of the left side of the screen image (arrow).

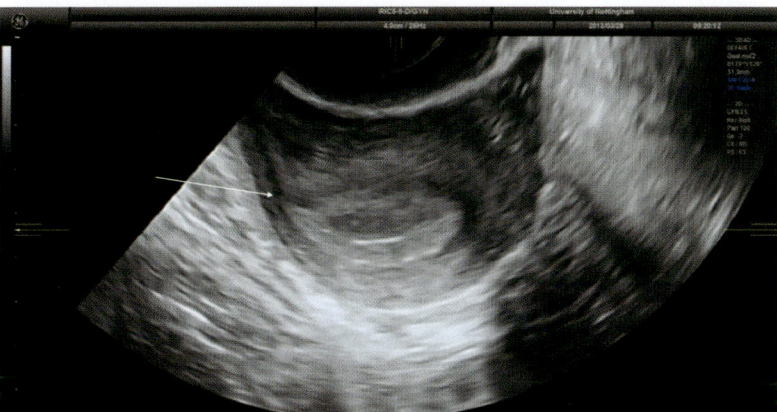

Figure 1.11 Interstitial portion of the tube (arrow) leaving the endometrial complex (top image). Following the blood vessels originating from the lateral aspect of the uterus laterally provides the best plane to follow sideways (to the patient's right side) in order to identify the right ovary.

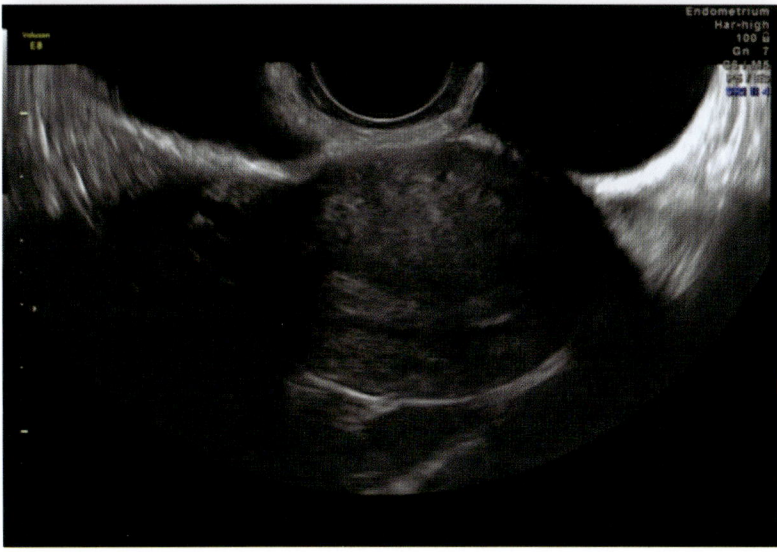

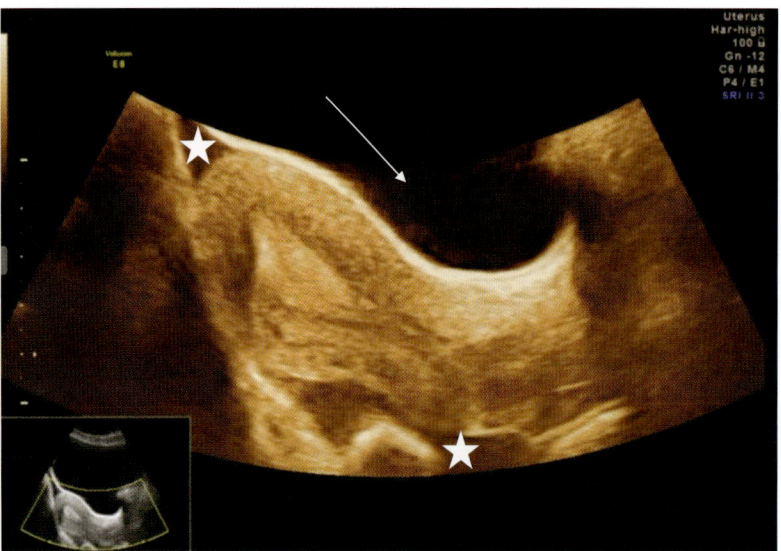

Figure 1.12 Transabdominal image of an anteverted uterus. The E8 mark is on the left side of the screen (as is the fundus). The distended bladder (arrows) allows for a detailed view of the endometrium. Some free fluid is noted in the pouch of Douglas and above the uterine fundus (*). The image is part of a larger image seen on the bottom left-hand corner. The zoom box functionality allows for this kind of magnification.

towards the right adnexum should visualize at least part of the ovary; slow up-and-down movements of the probe will help visualizing the ovaries in their entirety in most cases. The second landmarks that may be helpful are the common iliac vessels located on the pelvic sidewall, which are easily identified by their pulsation and abundant Doppler signal. Normally the ovaries are at the ovarian fossae, which are located below and medial to the bifurcation of the common iliac vessels into external and internal iliac vessels. The ovary may be at times surrounded by bowel and sometimes gentle pressure by holding the probe steady for a short while helps to move the bowel away and facilitates visualization of the ovary. Holding the probe steady over the bowel also demonstrates peristalsis, whereas the ovary and any structures originating from it remain static. This helps to differentiate between bowel and ovary, and especially ovarian masses such as dermoid cysts, which may have a mixed echogenic content. Bimanual examination with the left hand on the patient's abdomen and the TVS probe in the right fornix will help to move the bowel away and make the examination of the ovary easier in some cases. Once the ovary is identified, the image is magnified and slow up-and-down movements are used to complete a thorough examination of the ovary. This process is repeated on the left side. While examining the contralateral ovary, it is important to start again as described above from the point just below the uterine fundus, directing the transducer along the same plane to the left adnexum. The probe is held in the same position, i.e. with the thumb pointing to the right side of the patient. This is important as it helps to identify the correct side of the ovary (or any pathology within the ovary). It may be useful while saving images to label them as right or left ovary for future reference. While moving the probe to the left adnexum it is useful to ease off the pressure on the transducer to allow it to slide over the uterus without causing too much discomfort while keeping it at the same level (or plane). Often the contralateral ovary is at the same level and thus, having identified one ovary, identification of the second one should be easier.

More information on systematic scanning of the uterus may be found in Chapter 14.

Abdominal Probe and Ultrasound Images

An important tip is to apply gel to the abdominal probe and move this with your finger before you start scanning, as this helps to see the top and bottom in a longitudinal scan, and right and left on a transverse scan. The principles are the same as for TVS. A full bladder in this case creates a fluid medium for sound waves to traverse and provides good views of underlying structures (Figure 1.12). In a longitudinal scan, the bladder appears as a triangle with its apex on the right side of the screen, whereas in a transverse scan the bladder becomes almost rectangular in shape. The abdominal probe should have complete contact with the abdominal wall. Loss of contact with the abdominal wall produces dark shadows. Gently pressing the probe onto the abdominal wall helps to minimize or avoid

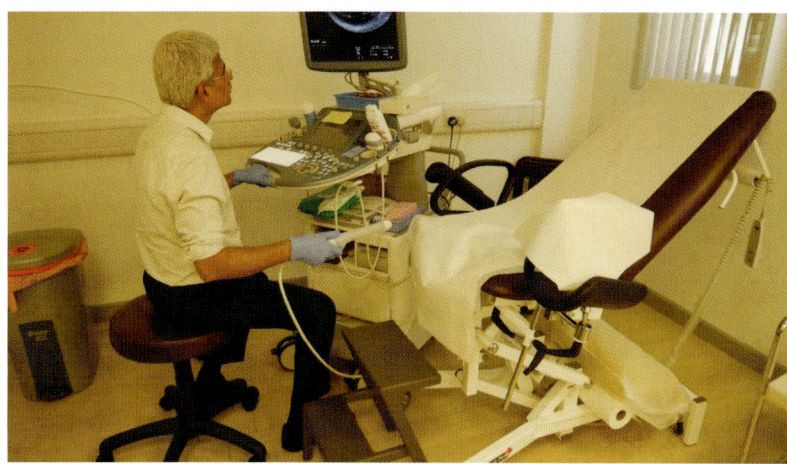

Figure 1.13 Position of the scanner with the machine on the left and the patient's couch on the right. The height of the bed, machine and stool should be adjusted to avoid unnecessary strain.

the loss of contact and improves the image. Initially, the probe is placed vertically on the abdomen in the midline, just above the *symphysis pubis*. The uterus is in the pelvis, unless it is enlarged, hence the probe should be pointing downwards. Keeping the midline as your axis plane, the probe is tilted, not moved, to the right and then to the left. This may be sufficient to complete the whole examination of the pelvis, including the uterus and adnexa, with a transverse placement of the probe only occasionally needed. The probe very rarely may need to be moved from the midline axis, unless the structures observed are large or very laterally placed. While doing an abdominal scan, one should follow the same systematic approach as for TV scans. In obstetrics, an abdominal longitudinal scan will help identify the location of the foetal head to exclude a breech presentation and allow for localization of the placenta to exclude *placenta praevia*. During transverse abdominal examination, rotate the probe so that the thumb is pointing to the right side of the patient.

Ergonomics

Once a good image is obtained on live scanning, 'freezing' it will capture the image. Here, ergonomics of scanning are briefly explained. Most scanners have to be ambidextrous and able to use both hands. It is important to keep the machine close, so that the left hand can use the keyboard without leaning towards the machine and to minimize the movement of the right hand, which is holding the transducer. This will minimize the strain on the back and shoulder muscles and ensure the captured image is not lost. Most scanners prefer to be sitting, so ensure you adjust the height of the machine, the height of the patient's couch or the clinician's stool. A gas lift stool with wheels and an

adjustable height option is useful. In relation to where to sit while scanning, some operators prefer to be on the side of the patient close to the machine or in between the legs while the patient is lying in a semi-lithotomy position (Figure 1.13). Once an image is obtained and you are completing your measurements, ensure that the right hand relaxes, thus releasing the tension in the arm and the shoulder muscles. Adjustment of the distance between the couch and the machine, appropriate height of the couch and relaxation of the right hand, as described above, will help in the long term to reduce work-related injuries (especially in a busy unit). Common ultrasound-related injuries in operators with a heavy workload include musculoskeletal injuries to the back, neck and forearm. The preferred position of the machine is on the left and the patient on the right.

Measurements and Calculations

The freeze button helps to capture the optimal image and then to complete the measurements. Generally, there are two types of calliper buttons. There is a simple distance measurement from A to B, and another that is organ specific, e.g. when measuring the dimensions of the ovary or the uterus. This will be indicated by three measurements leading on to an area or a volume. A typical example will be looking at an ovarian cyst or ovarian volume. You would take three measurements, which include length (maximum longitudinal diameter in a longitudinal plane), breadth (maximum antero-posterior diameter in a longitudinal plane) and width (transverse diameter in transverse plane) (Figure 1.14), and the machine will calculate the volume automatically. Similarly, when doing an early pregnancy scan to determine the gestational age, most ultrasound machine software is equipped with

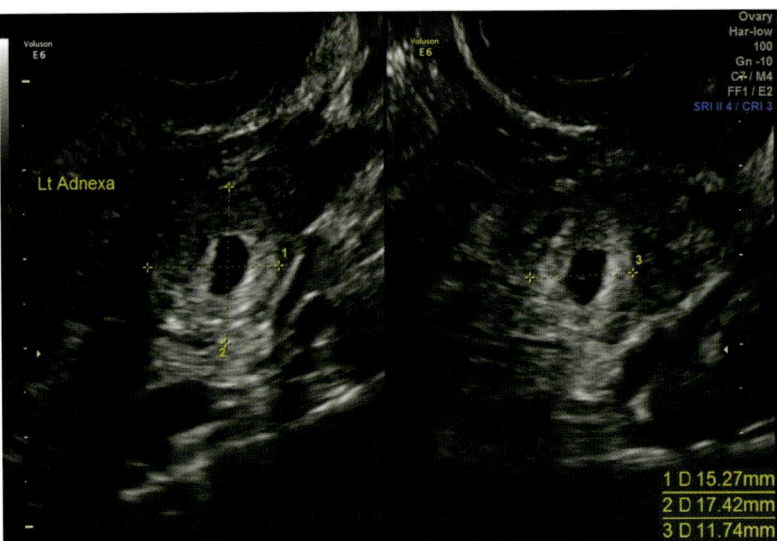

Figure 1.14 Measurement of a left tubal ectopic pregnancy. Measurements are carried out in three orthogonal planes, each with an assigned number from 1 to 3.

a predefined measuring mode used to determine crown–rump length (CRL) (callipers placed on the crown and the rump) that will determine the distance between these points and compare it with inbuilt nomograms for gestational age. This will be described in more detail in the subsequent chapters.

Depth

It is advisable to adjust the depth of the field of vision to ensure that the organ of interest occupies the majority of the screen. This may be done by appropriate toggles or knobs on the dashboard of the machine. This is an important tool to ensure good-quality images and appropriate assessment of fine details. Large depth of vision may be used initially to identify the surrounding structures, which then should be decreased to encompass the organ of interest. Too shallow a depth will lead to an incomplete assessment of the tissues or organs and missing pathology (Figure 1.15). The zoom function serves a similar purpose and allows enlarging the entire image or a selected portion of it to obtain appropriate assessment (Figure 1.12). This is used most often when measuring the nuchal fold in early pregnancy.

Focal Points

This refers to the situation when the ultrasound waves produce the best resolution by adjusting the focal point depth with appropriate toggles on the dashboard. Most commonly, this is represented by a triangle on the side of the screen (Figure 1.10). There is an option of at most three focal points

being added, but this does not improve the overall image resolution and should be discouraged. The focal point should be placed at or just below the level of the area of interest for the best results.

Greyscale

Adjusting the greyscale can change the appearance of the image. Most ultrasound images are either a lighter or darker shade of grey. Each person has their own particular degree of greyscale that they prefer. The greyscale can be adjusted by turning the 2D knob for the whole image (Figure 1.16), or individual parts of the screen can also be altered (Figure 1.17) with a slider on the dashboard (time–depth gain sliders). It is a matter of personal choice how dark or light the image appears; however, in general, a darker image allows for better appreciation of the contrast of different structures reflected on scanning. When using a contrast medium to check for tubal patency (i.e. hystero-contrast sono-salpingography, or HyCoSy), a slightly darker image may provide more useful information. Adjusting the gain while performing a 3D scan will be useful; however, the settings can be changed to an extent after a 3D volume has been obtained. This is also relevant with 3D power Doppler scans, as Doppler in general is sensitive to alterations of the gain.

Frequency

The frequency of a probe is the rate per second of vibrations emitted by the transducer (expressed in

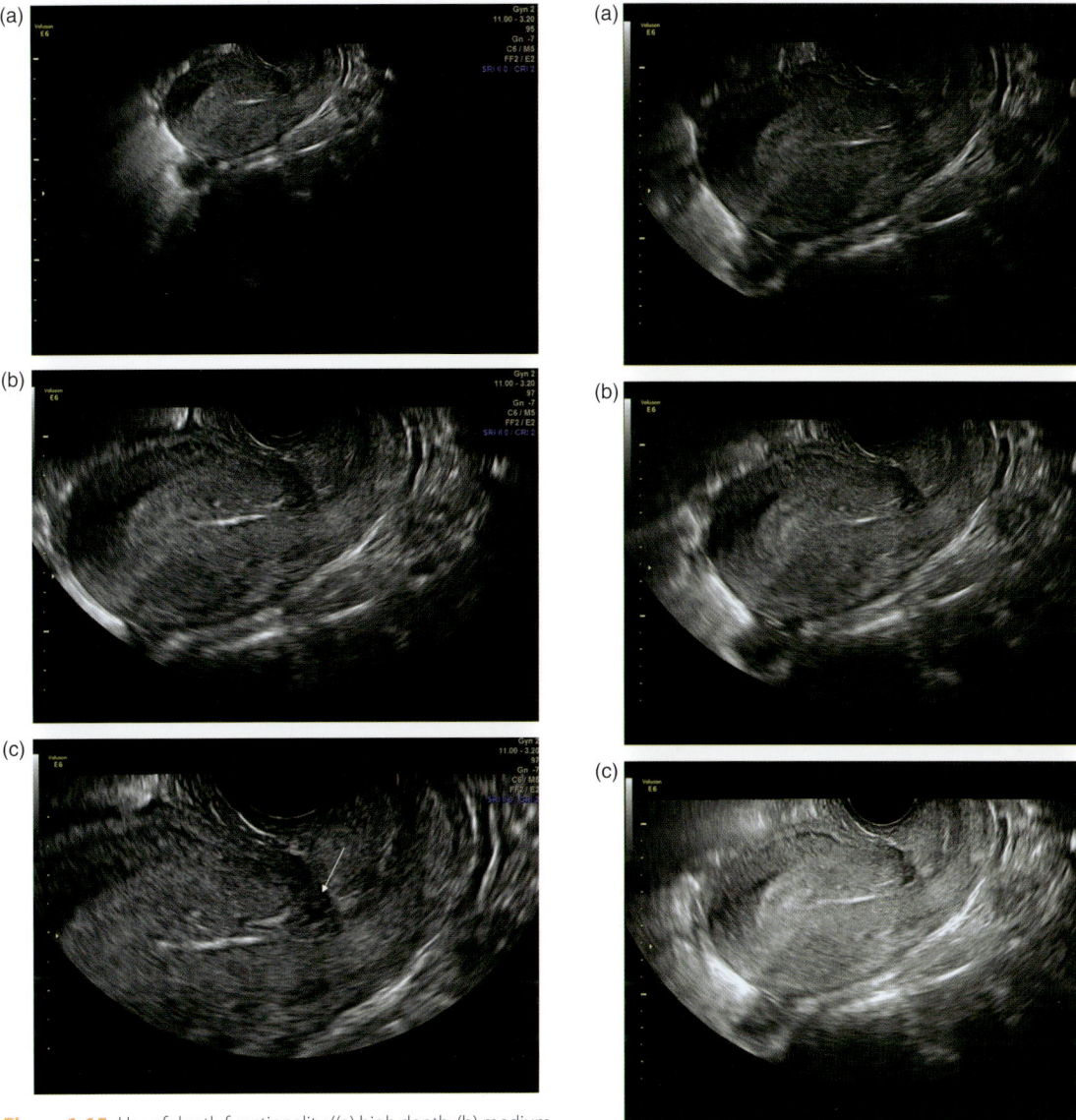

Figure 1.15 Use of depth functionality ((a) high depth; (b) medium depth; (c) shallow depth). The uterus in (a) occupies a fraction of the screen space and, as such, fine details are difficult to assess. It does, however, allow for assessment of the surrounding structures and the relation of the uterus to these. (c) The depth is set too low and as such a part of the fundus is missing. This may fail to identify any fundal pathology (e.g. fundal fibroid). (b) This image focuses on the uterus and as such provides an excellent example of how to adjust depth to fit the scanned organ in question. An arrow indicates a Caesarean section scar.

Figure 1.16 Different gain settings and the corresponding brightness/darkness of the image of the uterus on the screen ((a) low gain; (b) medium gain; (c) high gain). Very bright gain settings (c) cause loss of definition of the endometrio-myometrial junction.

hertz (Hz)). There are three predefined frequency modes: normal, penetration and resolution. In general, the frequency for transvaginal ultrasound is higher (5–8 MHz or even 11 MHz, allowing for better resolution) than for an abdominal transducer, as the structures observed with transvaginal probes are small and close to the emitter. The 'penetration mode' utilizes the lower frequency of the transducer spectrum. This is particularly useful when an organ is bigger, the patient is obese, or multiple fibroids are present in an enlarged uterus. Lower-frequency ultrasound waves have an ability to travel further, but the resolution of

13

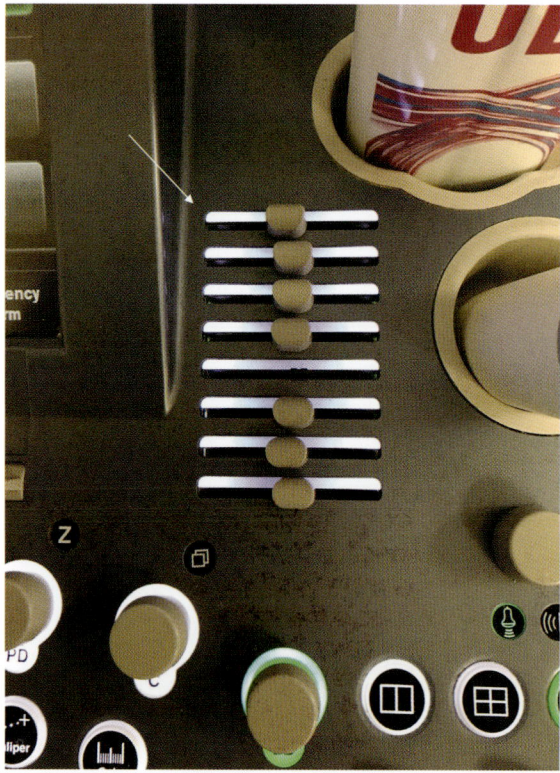

Figure 1.17 Gain settings on the dashboard for individual aspects of the screen can be controlled by sliding (arrow). The overall gain that is commonly used is controlled by rotating the 2D knob to increase or decrease the gain.

the image is poor. The 'resolution mode' utilizes the higher end of the spectrum emitted by the transducer and, as such, produces excellent-resolution images of structures close to the surface of the transducer. Structures more distant are poorly visible. The 'normal mode' is somewhere in between the two and is useful for general gynaecological scanning.

Other Useful Settings

Activation of the colour, power Doppler and M mode modalities utilizes the Doppler effect of ultrasound waves, allowing for a detailed study of blood flow and vascular resistance in organs. This is further explained in subsequent chapters.

The 3D/4D mode, if available, is accompanied by a special transvaginal and abdominal probe, which is much bulkier than the corresponding standard 2D probe. During a 3D scan, the mobile piezo-electric sensor array within the head of the probe sweeps through a predefined angle while emitting and receiving ultrasound data. This way, the longitudinal and transverse planes are scanned simultaneously, with the ultrasound machine software reconstructing and displaying the coronal plane (third dimension) as a static image. A 4D scan utilizes 3D principles but in real time, allowing for visualization of a (mobile) 3D structure in real time. An important aspect to remember while doing 3D scans is to remain as still as possible during the 3D acquisition. This applies both to the operator and to the patient. Motion artefacts may significantly distort the image. More details on 3D ultrasound in gynaecology may be found in Chapter 5.

One of the other important factors to be aware of while scanning is to save the derived images. This is very useful for future review or for reporting purposes. Before commencing the scan, inputting and checking the correct patient details into the scanning software allows for easy traceability and identification of images, which then can be saved on the machine or transferred to an online reporting system. It is recommended to save the image digitally, with a printed copy provided to the patient if they wish. If there are no facilities for digital storage of images, these need to be printed and stored in patients' paper records. The buttons for printing and saving images differ on ultrasound machines, but are generally separate or customizable.

Once you acquire the basic skills of operating the ultrasound machine, you are ready to start scanning. There are other aspects that you may need to know, but what has already been explained will put you in a good starting position.

Infection Control

In order to minimize the risk of infectious agent transmission through the transducers, basic infection control principles should be followed, including handwashing and wearing gloves. The ultrasound scan probe should be wiped with antiseptic wipes between cases or a cleansing solution spray suitable for use on ultrasound machines (e.g. Tristel Duo) should be applied. Before application of the cleaning solution, it is recommended to wipe the coupling gel from the transducer surface. The solution should be applied directly onto the transducer, ensuring coverage of the entire surface. Afterwards, the transducer may be wiped dry with tissue towel or allowed to air-dry.

Tristel Duo ULT is sporicidal, mycobactericidal, viricidal, fungicidal and bactericidal in 30 seconds. Chlorine dioxide has been tested in accredited laboratories worldwide and is proven effective against microorganisms of concern in ultrasound, such as:

- *Acanthamoeba castellanii*
- Polyomavirus SV40 (surrogate of HPV)
- *Candida albicans*
- *Gardnerella vaginalis*
- *Neisseria gonorrhoeae*
- Adenovirus
- *Staphylococcus aureus*
- *Streptococcus agalactiae*
- human immunodeficiency virus (HIV)
- hepatitis B virus
- hepatitis C virus
- herpes simplex virus.

Ultrasound Scan Probe in Procedure Room and Embryo Transfer Theatre

If visibly contaminated, the probe is washed and dried as above. The ultrasound scan probe is wiped with a hand towel sprayed with 'O safe' antiseptic, which is not toxic in the laboratory area.

Purchasing Ultrasound Equipment

When purchasing an ultrasound machine, the key aspects to be kept in mind include:

1. What is the main purpose of the scanner?
2. What is the professional expertise of those who are going to use the scanner?

A 3D ultrasound machine should not be purchased unless there is a need and the expertise to use the software exists. Most modern 'basic' ultrasound machines are very good for the daily running of early pregnancy and emergency gynaecology units. Cost should also be factored into the equation when making a purchase.

Tips and Tricks

1. Get to know your machine before the first scan. Not being familiar with your equipment causes unnecessary anxiety for the operator and the patient.

2. Utilize your equipment to produce the best-quality image.
3. Develop your own pathway for scanning and always follow it. That way you will be systematic and never miss a step.
4. Orientate yourself first: place a finger on the probe to correlate with what you are seeing on the screen.
5. For vaginal scanning: always start with your thumb (and the corresponding groove) facing upwards. For abdominal scanning: the groove should be facing towards the patient's head.
6. Gentle and small movements are all that is needed for transvaginal scanning.
7. When scanning any organ (e.g. uterus, ovaries) always scan through its entirety so that it disappears from view on the longitudinal and transverse planes.
8. Be comfortable when scanning. Relax when the image is frozen and measurements are obtained. This minimizes the risk of repetitive strain injury.
9. Adjust depth so that the majority of the screen is occupied by the area of interest; also use zoom to achieve this.
10. Place the focal points at or just below the area of interest for the best resolution.
11. Adjust frequency to what you are scanning: for tissues very close to the transducer, use high-frequency modes; for tissues far away, use low-frequency modes.
12. Doppler modality will help to differentiate a blood vessel from other tortuous, tubular structures.
13. Always adhere to infection control principles: clean the transducer and your hands between every scan.

Bibliography

1. Abramowicz JS, Evans DH, Fowlkes BJ, Maršal K, terHaar G. Guidelines for cleaning transvaginal ultrasound transducers between patients on behalf of the WFUMB Safety Committee. *Ultrasound* 2017;**43**:1076–9.

2. Society and College of Radiographers and British Medical Ultrasound Society, *BMUS Guidelines for Professional Ultrasound Practice*, Revision 2, December 2017.

Baseline Sonographic Assessment of the Female Pelvis

Lukasz Polanski and Kanna Jayaprakasan

Introduction

Ultrasound remains one of the most routinely performed medical investigations and a mainstay of clinical decision-making rests upon the obtained results. Due to the relative proximity of the pelvic organs to the abdominal surface and easy access via the vaginal route, gynaecological scanning should be in the armamentarium of every gynaecologist. As with every gynaecological assessment, and procedures of an intimate nature, explanation to alleviate anxiety and obtain informed consent is essential. The woman should feel safe and comfortable when the procedure is performed, which relates to the equipment in the scan room, presence of a chaperone and the security of the scan room. In this chapter, we will discuss the principles of sonographic assessment of the normal female pelvis.

Indication for Scanning

As with every investigation, a clear clinical question must be asked. Ad hoc investigations often lead to incidental findings of clinically insignificant lesions, which increase the patient's anxiety and lead to unnecessary interventions. Conversely, one could argue that such a finding could save lives due to early detection of insidiously developing malignant changes (i.e. ovarian cancer). Yearly gynaecological check-ups could serve this purpose, provided the healthcare system can support this practice.

In the UK, a great majority of gynaecological ultrasound is performed to investigate pre-existing gynaecological or surgical symptoms. Clear clinical indication for the ultrasound assessment is therefore provided. This approach allows for symptom-focused scanning. When scanning, however, the sonographer cannot only focus on the issue at hand, but must perform a thorough and complete pelvic organ assessment.

In most cases, an abdominal and transvaginal (TV) ultrasound should be performed for completion. This allows for exclusion of large masses that have developed or migrated above the pelvic brim and, due to their position, would be missed with only TV scanning.

Initialization of Transvaginal Scanning

As described in the previous chapter, this examination should be performed in a secure environment with a chaperone and after the woman has provided consent. Allergy or sensitivity to latex should be checked and accordingly a latex or non-latex probe cover is to be used. Appropriate infection control measures are taken by ensuring the probe is cleaned with disinfectant wipes. Following application of an adequate amount of sonographic gel to the probe cover, some water-based lubricant should be applied on top of the probe cover. Good amounts of lubricant allow for excellent ultrasound transduction and minimize signal loss before it reaches the tissues. Once the probe is placed at the vaginal introitus, the screen should be observed in order to determine the direction of the vaginal canal (Figure 2.1). The probe should be introduced along the vaginal canal until the fornix is reached. This allows for a smooth and pain-free introduction of the transducer. Initial optimal positioning of the tip of the transducer is the anterior fornix. If this cannot be achieved at the beginning of the examination, the probe should be withdrawn a few centimetres and, aiming upwards, reintroduced until the fornix is reached. A systematic approach with observation of appropriate landmarks, like the urethra leading to the bladder base, anterior fornix and cervix and cervical canal, with each and every scan will help to achieve smooth and accurate scanning.

The Uterus

Once the transducer is in the anterior vaginal fornix, the cervix should come into view. Using small rotational and angling movements of the transducer, the cervical canal should be visualized, allowing for

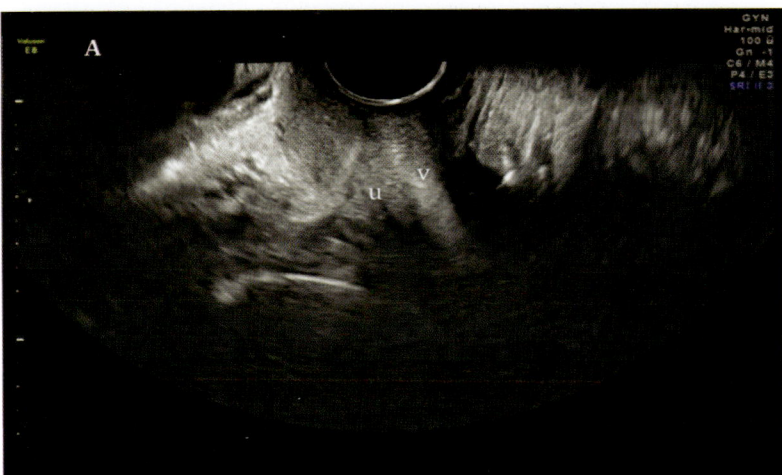

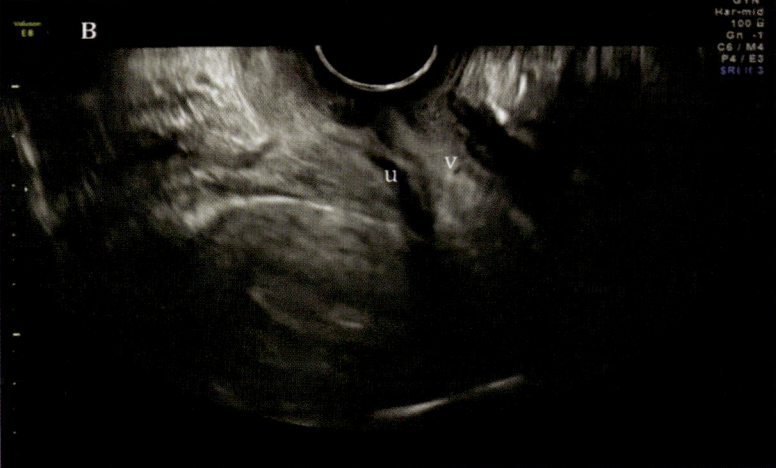

Figure 2.1 Probe at the introitus (a) showing vagina (v) with linear echogenic shadow due to presence of air. Urethra (u) linear echoic shadow due to presence of some residual urine. Probe is advanced further in the vagina (b), getting close to the cervix in the anterior fornix.

identification of the sagittal cross-section of the uterus. Good contact between the tissues and the ultrasound transducer should always be achieved. The uterus should then be positioned in the middle of the screen. The image should be enlarged to minimize the amount of noise, i.e. bowel and adipose tissue located in the pouch of Douglas (POD), and optimize the view for analysis and description (Figure 2.2).

Uterine measurements should include the length of the cervix and measurements of the uterine corpus in three dimensions. The cervical muscular layer should appear homogeneous and isoechoic, with myometrial appearance. Within the endocervical canal, depending on the stage of the cycle, hyperechoic normal glandular lining may be visualized. In the proliferative phase of the cycle, hypoechoic watery mucous within the endocervical canal can be visualized. In nulliparous women, the total uterine length is approximately 7 cm, with an increase to over 9 cm in multiparous women. In the same populations of women, the cervical length measures approximately 2.9 ($\pm$0.5) and 3.7 ($\pm$0.6) cm, respectively [1] (Figure 2.3).

Anterior and posterior uterine walls should be similar in diameter and should have a similar and homogeneous echotexture. Doppler signal should show uniformly distributed blood vessels traversing from the myometrium to the endometrium (Figure 2.4). Application of gentle pressure allows demonstrating the sliding sign and allows for identification of significant pelvic adhesions.

Once the endometrial cavity is in view, the uterus occupies approximately two-thirds of the screen. The endometrium should be measured where the upper one-third and lower two-thirds of the cavity meet, or at the thickest part. The callipers should be placed at the edges of the endometrium and should be perpendicular

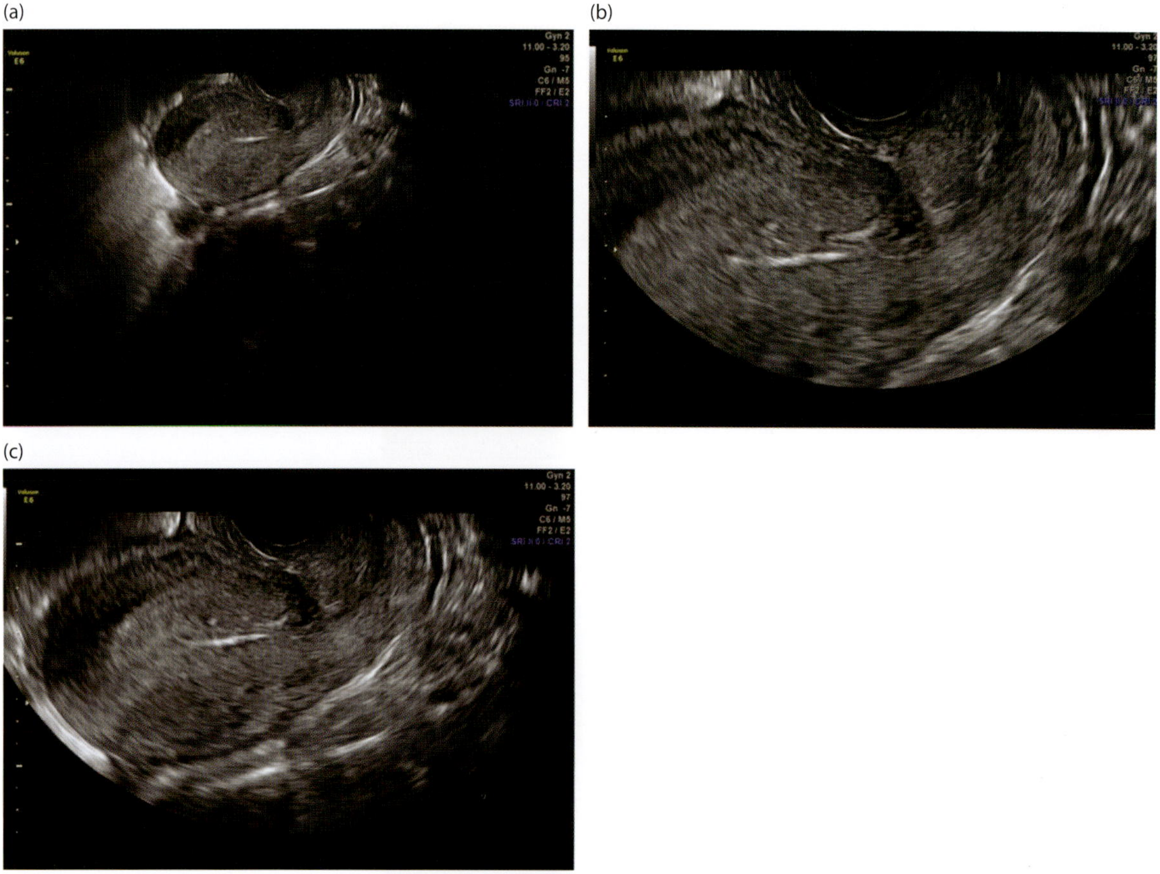

(a)

(b)

(c)

Figure 2.2 Optimization of image: (a) uterus occupies one-third of the screen and any details are difficult to detect; (b) the image is too enlarged, cutting off part of the uterine fundus and thus not allowing for assessment of the entire organ; (c) the image is optimized, with the uterus occupying the majority of the screen and the pouch of Douglas still visible.

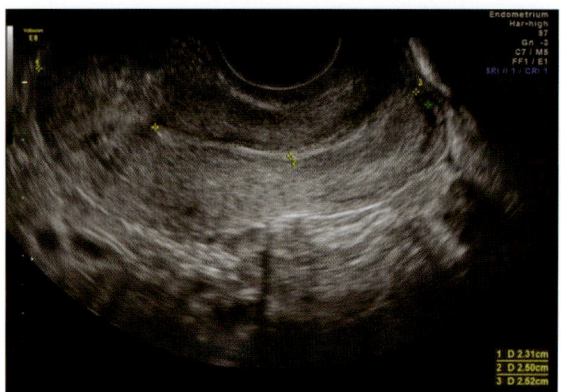

Figure 2.3 Sagittal view of the uterus with measurements of the cervix, endometrial cavity and fundus. Note the irregular appearance of the fundal portion of the myometrium, with linear striations (shadows) suggesting adenomyotic changes.

to the long axis of the uterus (Figure 2.5). Once the measurement is done, a comment on the endometrial pattern should be made. Endometrial pattern corresponds to the stage of the menstrual cycle, and in the context of assisted reproduction provides important information regarding endometrial receptivity.

Endometrial Physiology Recap

- Endometrium is composed of two layers, the *zona basalis* and *zona functionalis*.
- The *zona functionalis* is shed during menstruation.
- During endometrial proliferation, the endometrial glands grow in length and become increasingly tortuous.
- Spiral arteries increase in number and undergo remodelling in the second half of the menstrual cycle.

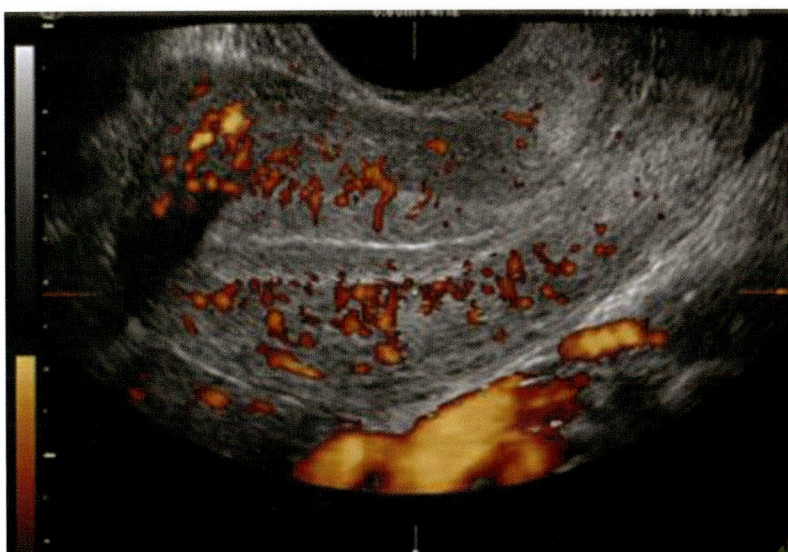

Figure 2.4 Doppler signals within the uterus showing blood vessel distribution.

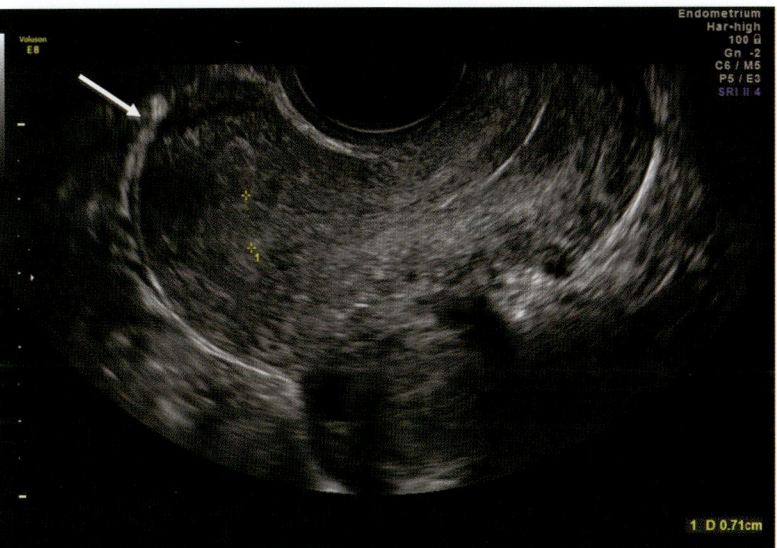

Figure 2.5 Measurement of endometrial thickness with callipers positioned in the thickest part of the endometrium. Note the irregular endo-myometrial junction with mixed echogenic myometrium (small arrow) suggestive of adenomyosis. There is a large posterior wall subserosal fibroid (large arrow).

- Endometrial growth is driven by oestrogen.
- Secretory changes are caused by progesterone and lead to accumulation of intracellular glycogen.
- Endometrial thickness varies from 2 mm to 20 mm throughout the menstrual cycle.
- Optimal endometrial receptivity in the ART cycle has been associated with endometrial thickness of >6–8 mm and a volume of >2 cm³.

During menstruation, the endometrium is thin (<5 mm) and hyperechoic compared to the myometrium, and represents the *zona basalis* (Figure 2.6). Blood and sloughed endometrium may be visible within the endometrial cavity. Close and static observation of the cavity may reveal active endo-myometrial contractions and associated movement of the content, which aids to expel the content. The menstrual content can be differentiated from acquired uterine anomalies with the use of power Doppler.

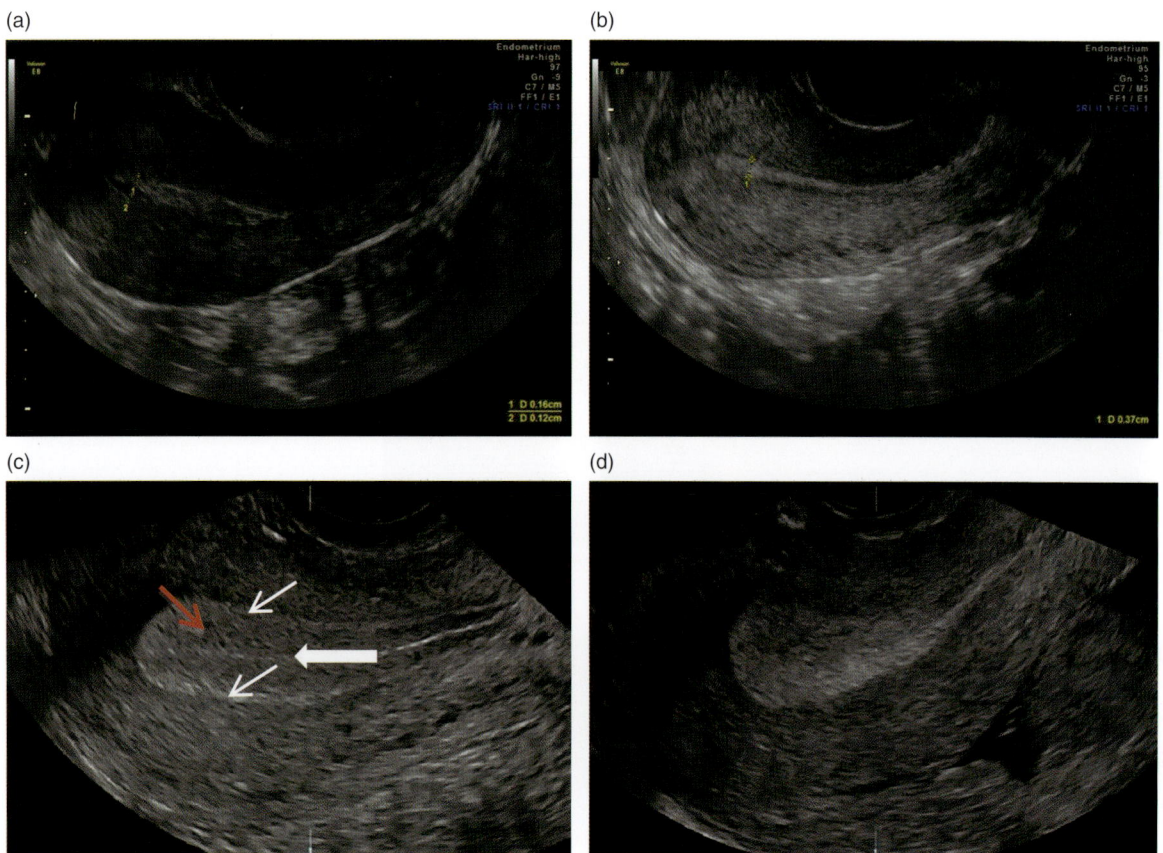

Figure 2.6 Various appearances of the endometrium during different phases of the menstrual cycle. (a) Menstrual endometrium: hyperechoic endometrial stripe encompasses the mixed echogenicity cellular debris and anechoic (black) fluid most likely representing menstrual blood. (b) Early follicular phase endometrium with a visible isoechoic stripe of endometrium. (c) Triple-layer appearance of peri-ovulatory endometrium; small arrow = hyperechoic zona basalis; red arrow = zona functionalis; large arrow = interface between the two endometrial surfaces. (d) Hyperechoic appearance of luteal phase endometrium.

When a fibroid or polyp is present, Doppler signal will be present within the lesion; on the other hand, menstrual debris will be devoid of vascular patterns (Figure 2.7).

When menstruation ceases, the endometrium grows in thickness and becomes more isoechoic compared to the myometrium. At around day 8 of a 28-day cycle, a thin hyperechoic line appears at the apposition of the anterior and posterior leaf of the endometrium. This becomes more distinct as time passes. The two basal layers of the endometrium and the midline echo are hyperechoic and encompass hypoechoic *zona functionalis*, giving the endometrium a triple-layer appearance around the time of ovulation (Figure 2.6c) [2]. Increasing levels of progesterone shortly after ovulation cause secretory changes within the endometrium. Changes related to

increasing intracellular glycogen storage cause the endometrium to gradually become hyperechoic, starting from the outside and progressing inwards towards the midline [3,4]. Hyperechoic decidual change is complete around day 19 of the cycle. Withdrawal of progesterone in non-conception cycles causes temporary spasm and dilation of spiral arteries and apoptosis of the oestrogen-dependent stromal cells [5]. This occasionally can be visualized around cycle day 26–27 on ultrasound and appears as hypoechoic irregular patches within the otherwise hyperechoic endometrium.

Throughout the menstrual cycle, the vascular patterns within the subendometrium remain constant in appearance and are homogeneously spread throughout the anterior and posterior walls of the uterus. The

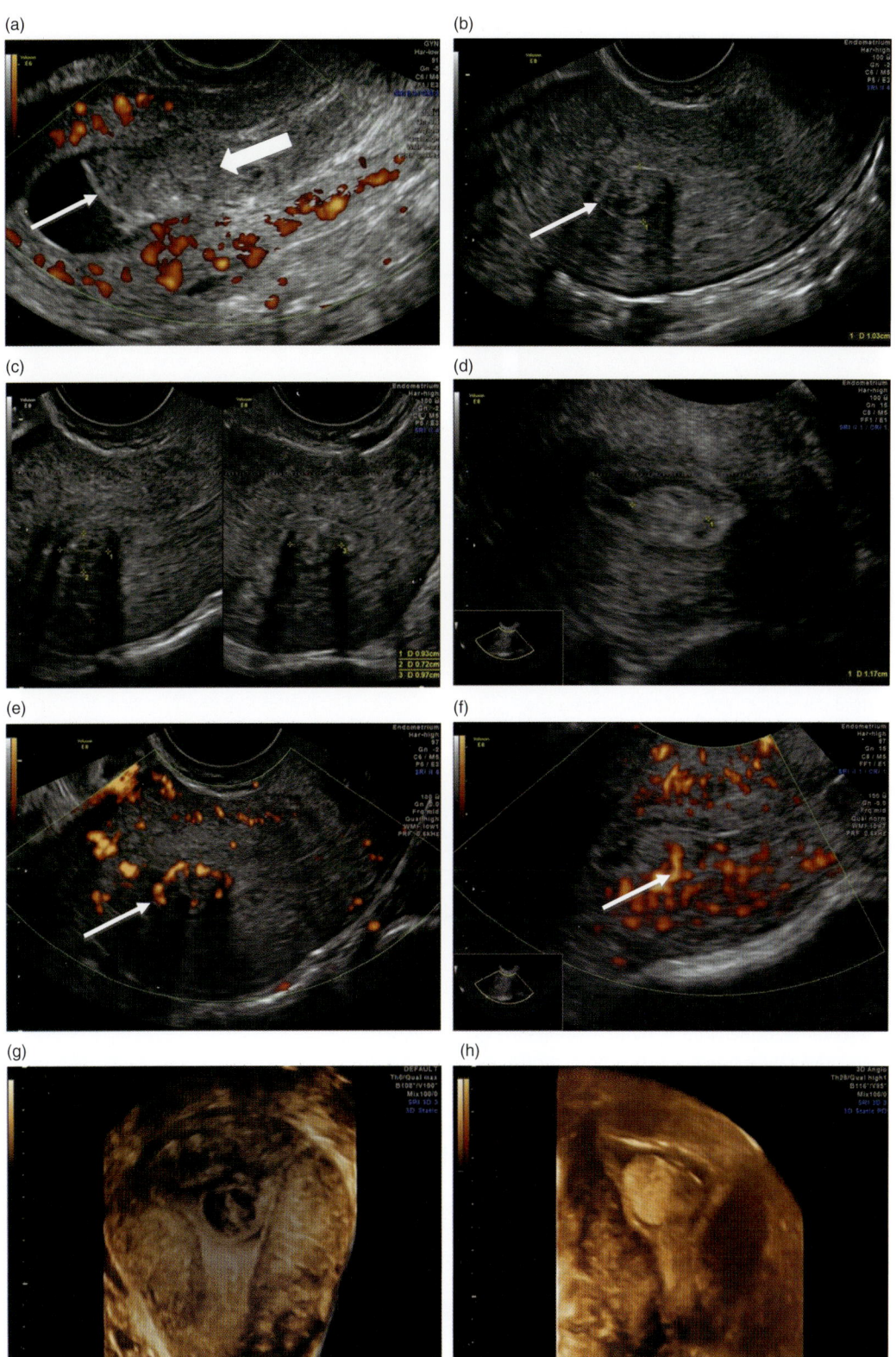

Figure 2.7 Acquired and congenital changes within the endometrial cavity. (a) Blood clot and products of conception during a miscarriage in progress. Note the fluid level within the endometrial cavity (thin arrow) and the absence of Doppler signal within the content of the

(a)　(b)

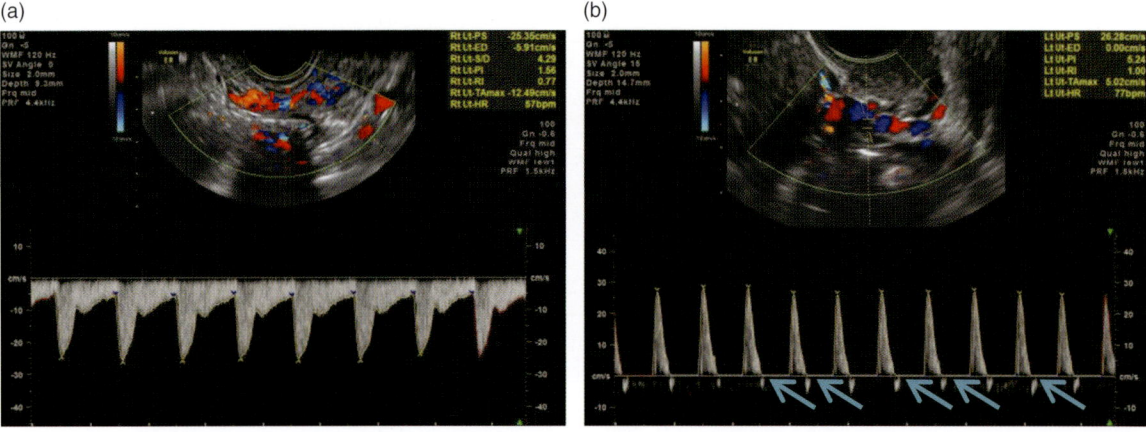

Figure 2.8 Uterine artery Doppler velocimetry: (a) normal, low-resistance uterine artery blood flow pattern; (b) high-resistance uterine artery blood flow with absent and reversed diastolic flow (arrows).

presence of Doppler signal within the endometrium is a good prognostic feature for pregnancy success following assisted reproductive technology (ART), as absence of vascularity observed with colour Doppler has been associated with reduced or absent pregnancies [6,7]. Observed 3D power Doppler vascularity changes throughout the cycle suggest a gradual increase in perfusion towards ovulation, with a nadir at the time of presumed window of implantation followed by a rise in Doppler signal [8]. Uterine artery Doppler assessment can be carried out as well to assess the resistance in the vascular beds and attempt to predict the chances of conception and possible pregnancy complications (Figure 2.8).

In order to achieve the optimal measurements of blood flow parameters using pulsed wave Doppler, the ultrasound transducer should be placed in the vaginal fornix. The internal cervical os should be visualized and the beam aimed to the parametrium. Colour Doppler should be activated and a pulsating ascending branch of the uterine artery should be identified. The pulse wave Doppler gate should be displayed and adjusted so that the box fits within the lumen of the uterine artery

(usually 2 mm) and the angle of insonation should be no more than 30 degrees [9]. At least two representations of cardiac cycle should be identified in order to accurately represent the blood flow parameters with no interference from other vessels [10]. The predictive values of vascularity indices for pregnancy outcomes are presented in Chapter 11.

The Tube and Ovary

Identification of the ovary can be the most challenging step during TV scanning. This is related to the relative mobility of the organ, its small size and interference from surrounding bowel. In the obese patient, excessive adipose tissue can preclude identification of one or both ovaries. Assessment of the ovary should include abdominal and vaginal scans. The abdominal route should be performed at the beginning of the scan session as the patient is likely to have a full bladder, which makes the assessment possible.

The bladder should be identified, with the uterus being behind it. In the sagittal plane, the probe should be angled to the right and left iliac fossa. The ovary, if visible, should be located at the edge of the bladder.

Caption for Figure 2.7 (cont.)

endometrial and cervical canal (large arrow). (b) and (c) Sagittal and transverse sections of the uterus with a small type 0 fibroid within the endometrial cavity (arrow); note the heterogeneous structure of the fibroid and the acoustic shadowing caused by the dense tissue. (d) Small endometrial polyp. Note the uniform structure and distortion of the midline echo; no acoustic shadowing is present. (e) Small type 0 fibroid with circumferential blood flow (arrow). (f) Endometrial polyp with a feeding vessel (arrow) arising from the posterior endometrial wall. (g) and (h) 3D images with a coronal plane of the endometrial cavity with a type 0 fibroid (g) and polyp (h). Note the differences in the texture between these lesions.

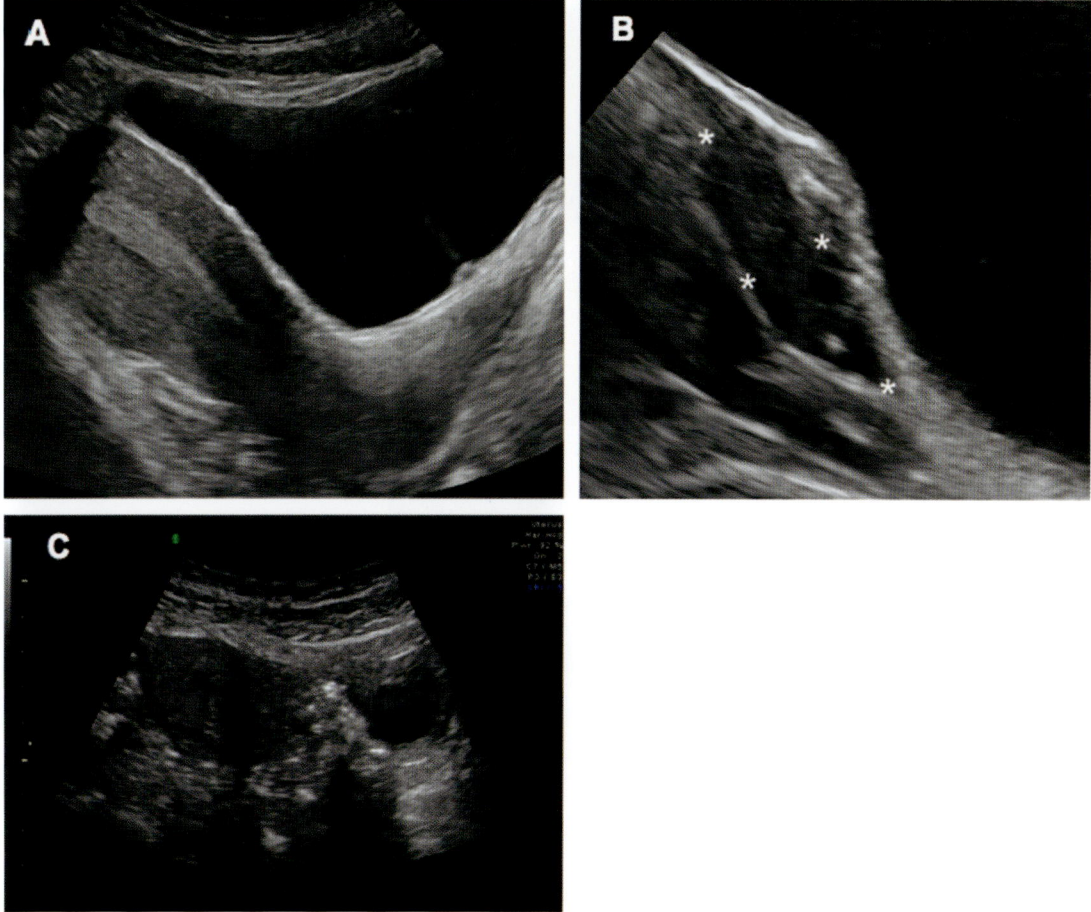

Figure 2.9 Transabdominal ultrasound assessment of the female pelvis. Uterus is displayed in the sagittal plane (a). The probe is then angled (not slid) laterally towards the iliac fossa to visualize the ovary (b). The bladder is empty (c), with the uterus displayed in transverse plane with the left ovary displaying a follicle.

Assessment should include the size of the ovary, presence of any lesions and overall appearance (Figure 2.9).

A TV scan should follow to allow close assessment. Once the uterus has been assessed, the fundus of the uterus should be identified in the transverse section. The interstitial portion of the fallopian tube is located in this area ('shoulder' of the uterus) (Figure 2.10). A normal tube is usually not visible in an unenhanced ultrasound scan; however, any dilation of the tube should be noticeable [11]. Once the area adjacent to the uterus has been screened, in order to identify the ovary, the transducer should be moved laterally and follow the tubo-ovarian pedicle along with the parametrial blood vessels leaving the uterus towards the pelvic sidewall (Figure 2.11). The ovary should normally be located in the ovarian fossa medial to the iliac vessels (Figure 2.12). As this is not always the case, tracing the ovarian and parametrial vessels with Doppler helps to locate the ovary.

When the ovary still cannot be identified despite thorough assessment of the pelvic sidewall, the pouch of Douglas should be inspected, as well as the area caudal to the fundus. In severe endometriosis or conditions with severe pelvic adhesions, the ovary can be retracted to these locations and be outside of its normal anatomical placement. When that fails, the abdominal wall should be pressed with a free hand in order to perform a 'bimanual' examination. Pressure should be applied to the vaginal transducer, allowing for approximation of the vaginal and abdominal walls. This causes displacement of the bowel and adipose tissue and may allow visualization and assessment of the ovary. These steps should be repeated on the contralateral side. In some patients,

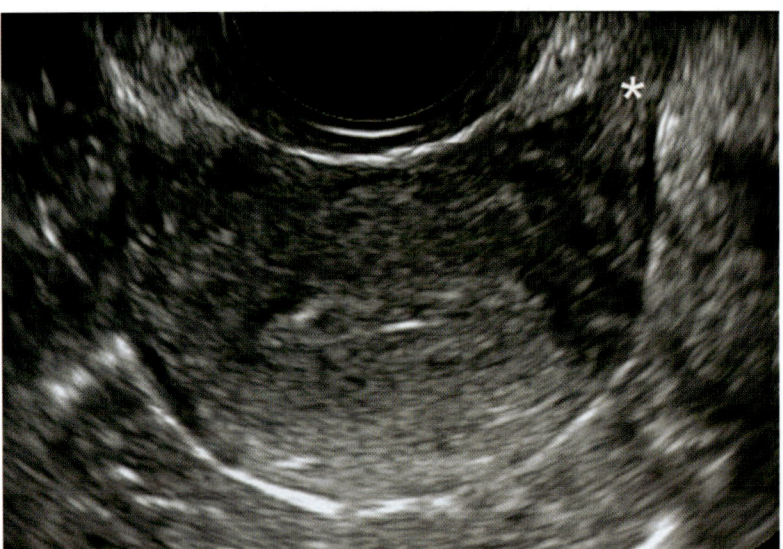

Figure 2.10 Transverse plane of the uterus showing the origin of tubo-ovarian ligament ('shoulder' of the uterus).

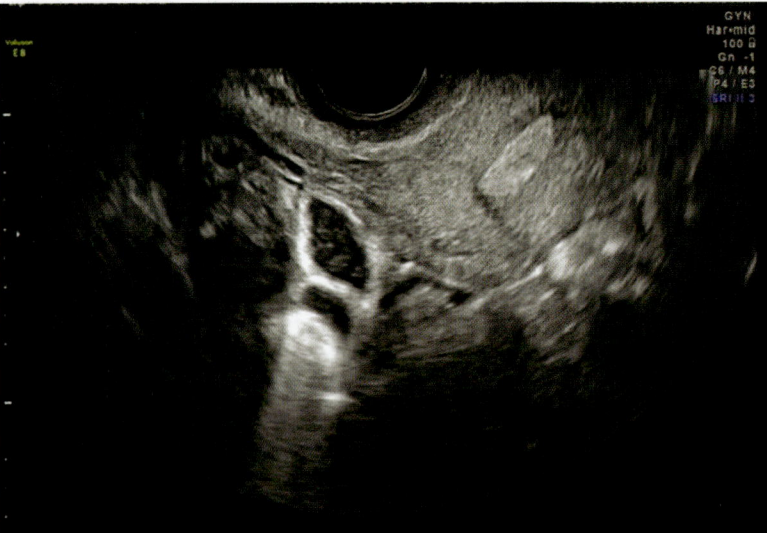

Figure 2.11 The probe is moved laterally to follow the tubo-ovarian pedicle and parametrial vessels to identify the ovary.

despite following these principles, visualization of the ovary may not be possible. If there are concerns as to the presence of cysts or malignancy, follow-up in the form of a repeat scan or magnetic resonance imaging (MRI) scan should be requested.

When the ovary has been identified, the complete assessment of the organ should include the dimensions (three orthogonal planes) (Figure 2.13), ovarian volume if the equipment allows for this (3D capability) (Figure 2.14), mobility in relation to the adjoining tissues, appearance and number of antral follicles (the antral follicle count (AFC) in the fertility work-up

setting) and presence and characteristics of ovarian lesions. Blood flow characteristics of the ovarian stromal vessels may also be established; however, this is only a research tool with no proven clinical benefit. Ovarian masses and their assessment are described in detail in Chapter 8.

The normal ovary measures approximately 4 cm in length, 2 cm in width and 8 mm in thickness [12]. Ovarian volume depends on the stage of reproductive life, with a volume of approximately 6.6 ± 0.2 cm^3 below the age of 30 and below 2.6 ± 0.01 cm^3 after menopause [13]. The ovary should slide in relation to

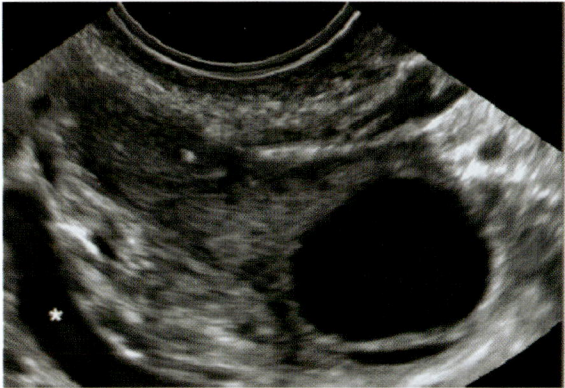

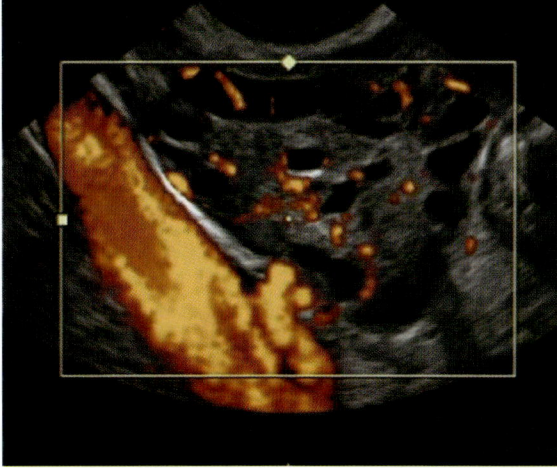

Figure 2.12 Ovary seen medial to the iliac vessel (greyscale image and Doppler image).

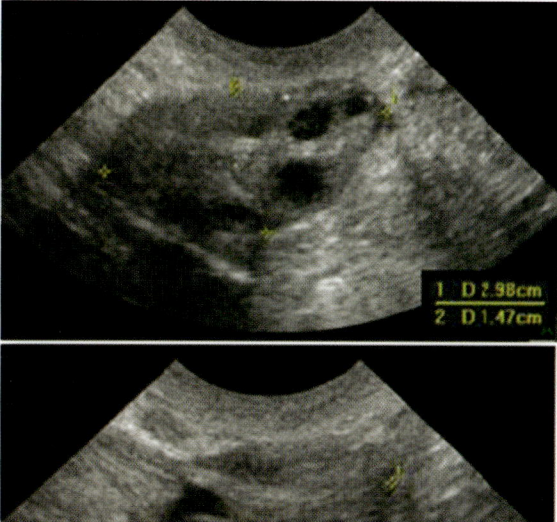

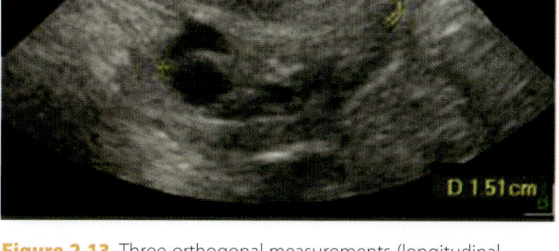

Figure 2.13 Three orthogonal measurements (longitudinal diameter, antero-posterior diameter in sagittal plane and transverse diameter in transverse plane) are made to measure ovarian volume.

the pelvic structures with gentle pressure on the transducer (positive sliding sign). According to the recent task force report from the Androgen Excess and Polycystic Ovary Syndrome Society, a cutoff for describing polycystic ovarian morphology should be ≥25 follicles of 2–10 mm per ovary, with the assessment conducted via the TV route with an 8 MHz transducer. Ovarian volume should exceed 10 cm^3 [14]. The lower reference range of follicle numbers considered as normal ovarian reserve is in the region of 5; however, when considering optimal ART outcome, a cutoff of 10 follicles should be used to predict a good treatment outcome [15]. The follicles should be evenly distributed throughout the ovary and should have different sizes, suggesting normal follicular development. Multiple follicles of similar size and with peripheral distribution are typical of polycystic ovary (PCO) (Figure 2.15). The ovarian cortex should

have a similar echogenicity as the medulla, as is the case in normal ovaries [16].

Ovarian lesions should be described in as much detail as possible. The measurements should be recorded in three orthogonal dimensions and the morphological description should include presence of septations, solid components, appearance of the fluid, and the presence of Doppler signal. The International Ovarian Tumour Analysis (IOTA) classification of ovarian lesions provides an up-to-date and detailed description of ovarian lesions, which should be followed [17].

Occasionally, oval and thin-walled cysts of varying size can be visualized next to the ovary (Figure 2.16). These most often represent fimbrial end cysts. These structures may disappear or grow. They are rarely a cause of symptoms, but with increasing size may cause pain and necessitate drainage.

Pouch of Douglas

The pouch of Douglas (POD) is a peritoneal fold located behind the uterus and vagina anteriorly and rectosigmoid colon posteriorly. As the lowest part of

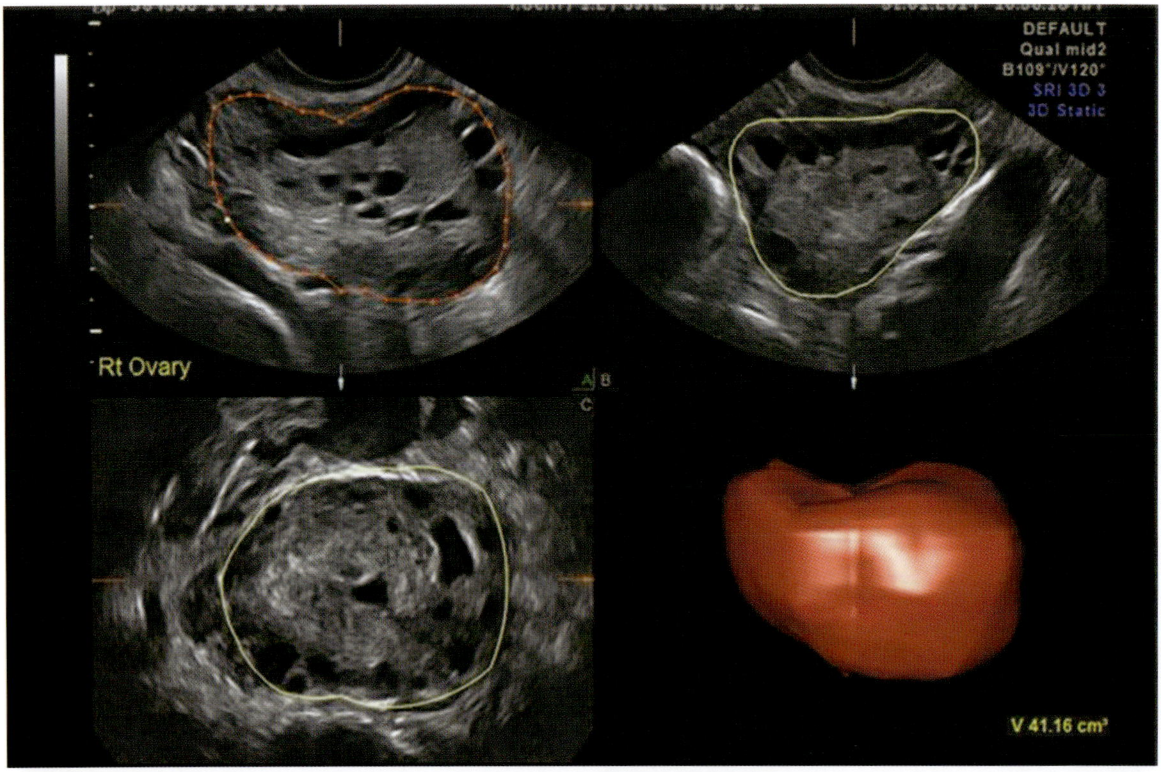

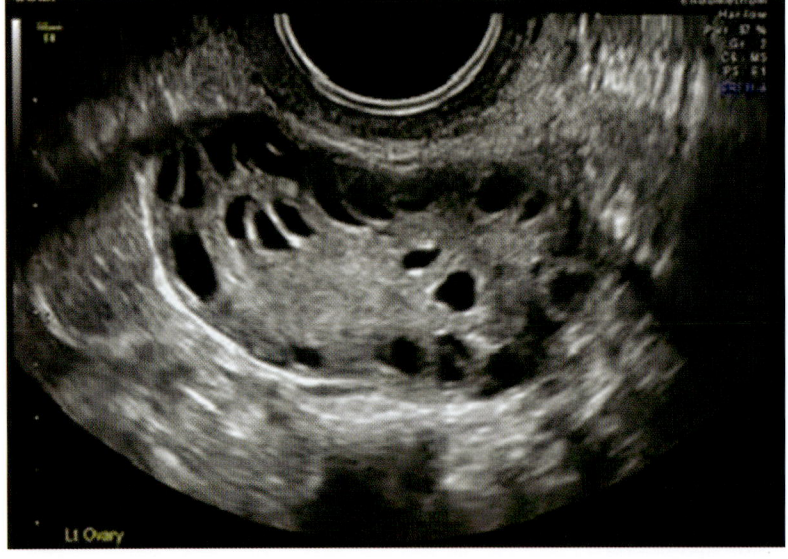

Figure 2.14 Ovarian measurement using 3D ultrasound (VOCAL software).

Figure 2.15 Ovary with polycystic appearance.

the pelvis (when erect), free abdominal fluid collects in this area and can be visualized on ultrasound. Physiological amounts of this fluid are not normally visible on ultrasound. Around the time of menstruation, retrograde menstruation may lead to accumulation of blood in the POD. At around the time of ovulation, free fluid may once again be visualized. The ovulatory fluid will be clear (non-particulate),

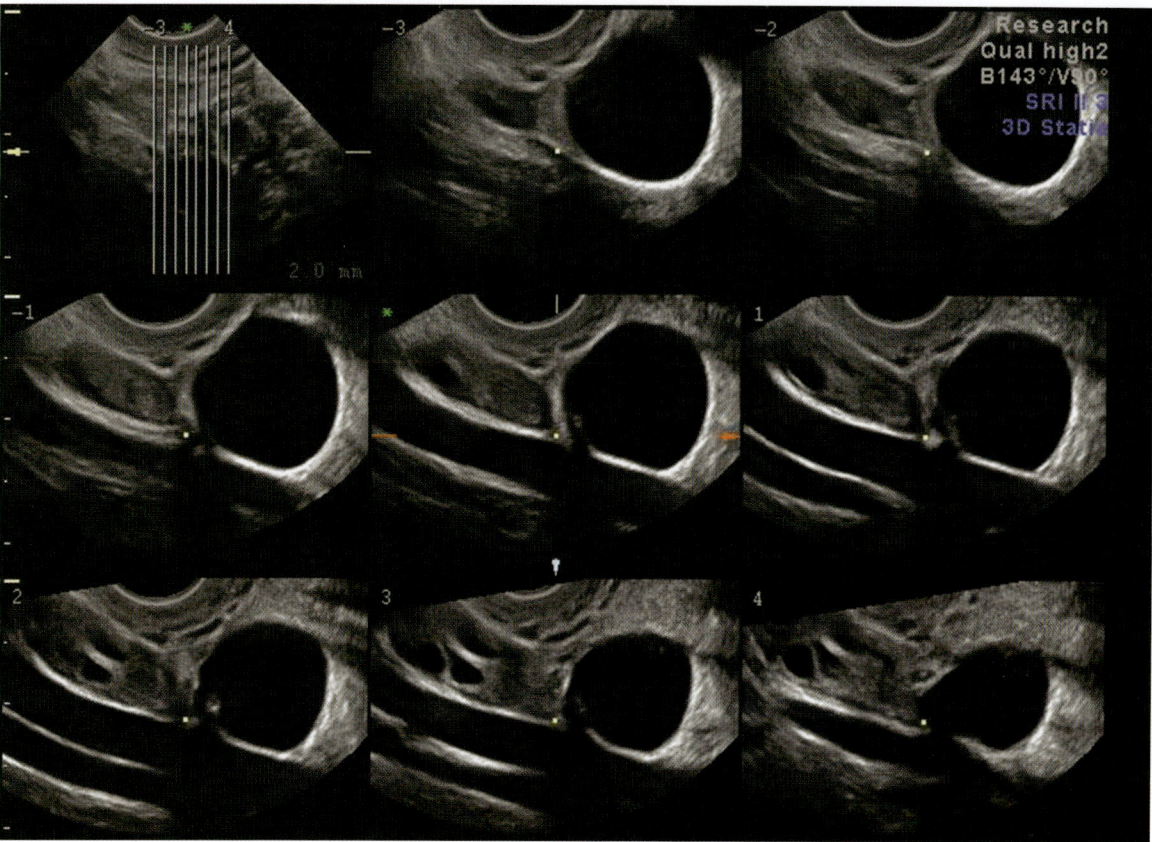

Figure 2.16 Para-tubal cyst–oval cystic structure, seen separate to the ovary. Tomographic ultrasound imaging (TUI) facility within 3D ultrasound is demonstrated here. Iliac vessels are seen just lateral to the ovary and para-tubal cyst.

whereas retrograde menstruation will appear as particulate, mixed echogenic liquid (Figure 2.17).

When assessing the woman in the context of ART, free fluid can be present in the POD during controlled ovarian hyperstimulation, following oocyte retrieval and as a feature of ovarian hyperstimulation syndrome (OHSS). In pregnancy, presence of free fluid in the POD should raise suspicion of an ectopic pregnancy, especially when an intrauterine pregnancy has not been observed. Haemorrhagic *corpus luteum* may also be accompanied by haemoperitoneum. Mixed echogenic material might represent a blood clot and may or may not be accompanied by visible free fluid in the POD. More significant amounts of fluid may cause it to extend into the upper abdomen. Visualization of free fluid in the pouch of Morrison (peritoneal space between Glisson's capsule of the liver and Gerota's fascia of the right kidney) on transabdominal scan (Figure 2.18) signifies the presence of at least 670 ml of intra-abdominal fluid [18,19].

Assessment of the POD provides some additional information apart from just the presence of free fluid. Hyperechoic, thick material in the POD in the absence of sliding organ sign indicates the possibility of adhesions, and when considering surgery, might give important information necessary to plan a difficult procedure. In the case of endometriosis, presence of hypoechoic and vascular lesions might indicate significant disease involving bowel wall and lack of sliding sign indicates POD obliteration with a very high sensitivity and specificity (83.3 per cent and 97.1 per cent, respectively) [20].

Conclusion

Transvaginal ultrasound is an important tool useful in the assessment of the female pelvis, both for physiological changes and pathological processes. Knowledge of normal sonographic anatomy of the pelvis allows for easy identification of abnormalities and appropriate management.

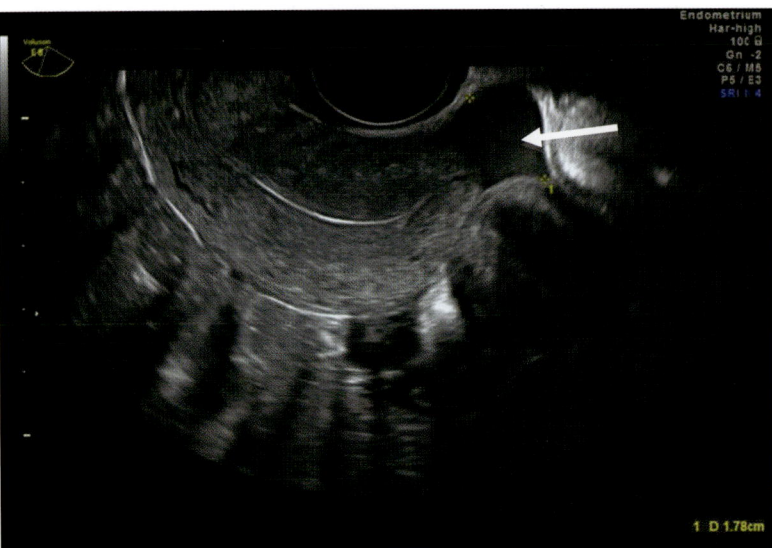

Figure 2.17 Retroverted uterus with particulate free fluid in the pouch of Douglas (arrow).

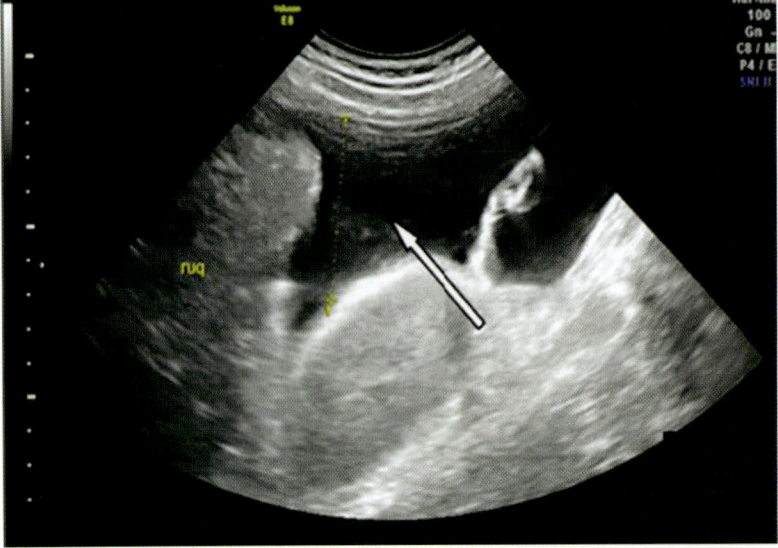

Figure 2.18 Abdominal ultrasound at the right upper quadrant demonstrating free fluid in a lady with moderate to severe OHSS.

Tips and Tricks

- Remember good scanning culture.
- Be as gentle as possible and stop when prompted.
- Maintain good contact of the transducer – abdominal and vaginal – with the assessed tissues.
- Use ample amounts of sonographic gel.
- Follow the direction of the vagina with the transducer in order to minimize discomfort.
- Sonographic appearance of the endometrium and ovary allows for identification of the stage of the menstrual cycle.
- Application of gentle pressure on the transducer allows gaining more information regarding the pelvic organs – 'ultrasound bimanual examination'.
- Use Doppler modality to get a complete pelvic organ assessment.

- Carefully assess and describe the free fluid in the POD.
- A systematic scanning approach should be adopted: uterus, ovaries, adnexa, pouch of Douglas and other pelvic organs (bladder or rectum) as appropriate.
- Inform the patient of the findings at the end of the scan – reassurance is vital!

References

1. Merz E, Miric-Tesanic D, Bahlmann F, Weber G, Wellek S. Sonographic size of uterus and ovaries in pre- and postmenopausal women. *Ultrasound Obstet Gynecol* 1996;**7**(1):38–42.

2. Sher G, Herbert C, Maassarani G, Jacobs M. Assessment of the late proliferative phase endometrium by ultrasonography in patients undergoing in-vitro fertilization and embryo transfer (IVF/ET). *Hum Reprod* 1991;**6**(2):232–7.

3. Fanchin R, Righini C, Olivennes F, et al. Computerized assessment of endometrial echogenicity: clues to the endometrial effects of premature progesterone elevation. *Fertil Steril* 1999;**71**(1):174–81.

4. Fleischer AC, Transvaginal sonography of endometrial disorders, in *Sonography in Obstetrics and Gynaecology: Principles and Practice*, A Fleischer, editor. McGraw-Hill Medical, 2011;961–78.

5. Jabbour HN, Kelly RW, Fraser HM, Critchley HO. Endocrine regulation of menstruation. *Endocr Rev* 2006;**27**(1):17–46.

6. Chien LW, Au HK, Chen PL, Xiao J, Tzeng CR. Assessment of uterine receptivity by the endometrial–subendometrial blood flow distribution pattern in women undergoing in vitro fertilization-embryo transfer. *Fertil Steril* 2002;**78**(2):245–51.

7. Yuval Y, Lipitz S, Dor J, Achiron R. The relationships between endometrial thickness, and blood flow and pregnancy rates in in-vitro fertilization. *Hum Reprod* 1999;**14**(4):1067–71.

8. Raine-Fenning NJ, Campbell BK, Kendall NR, Clewes JS, Johnson IR. Quantifying the changes in endometrial vascularity throughout the normal menstrual cycle with three-dimensional power Doppler angiography. *Hum Reprod* 2004;**19**(2):330–8.

9. Raine-Fenning NJ, Campbell BK, Kendall NR, Clewes JS, Johnson IR. Endometrial and subendometrial perfusion are impaired in women with unexplained subfertility. *Hum Reprod* 2004;**19**(11):2605–14.

10. Gill RW. Measurement of blood flow by ultrasound: accuracy and sources of error. *Ultrasound Med Biol* 1985;**11**(4):625–41.

11. Merz E, *Gynaecology*, in *Ultrasound in Obstetrics and Gynaecology*, C Benson, E Bluth, editors. Thieme, 2007.

12. Gray H, Lewis WH, *Anatomy of the Human Body*. 20th ed. Lea & Febiger, 1918.

13. Pavlik EJ, DePriest PD, Gallion HH, et al. Ovarian volume related to age. *Gynecol Oncol* 2000;**77**(3):410–12.

14. Dewailly D, Lujan ME, Carmina E, et al. Definition and significance of polycystic ovarian morphology: a task force report from the Androgen Excess and Polycystic Ovary Syndrome Society. *Hum Reprod Update* 2014;**20**(3):334–52.

15. Agarwal A, Verma A, Agarwal S, et al. Antral follicle count in normal (fertility-proven) and infertile Indian women. *Indian J Radiol Imaging* 2014;**24**(3):297–302.

16. Adams J, Franks S, Polson DW, et al. Multifollicular ovaries: clinical and endocrine features and response to pulsatile gonadotropin releasing hormone. *Lancet* 1985;**2**:1375–9.

17. Timmerman D, Ameye L, Fischerova D, et al. Simple ultrasound rules to distinguish between benign and malignant adnexal masses before surgery: prospective validation by IOTA group. *BMJ* 2010;**341**:c6839.

18. Condous G, Okaro E, Bourne T. The conservative management of early pregnancy complications: a review of the literature. *Ultrasound Obstet Gynecol* 2003;**22**(4):420–30.

19. Abrams BJ, Sukumvanich P, Seibel R, Moscati R, Jehle D. Ultrasound for the detection of intraperitoneal fluid: the role of Trendelenburg positioning. *Am J Emerg Med* 1999;**17**(2):117–20.

20. Hudelist G, Fritzer N, Staettner S, et al. Uterine sliding sign: a simple sonographic predictor for presence of deep infiltrating endometriosis of the rectum. *Ultrasound Obstet Gynecol* 2013;**41**(6):692–5.

Difficult Gynaecological Ultrasound Examination

Kamal Ojha

When performing ultrasound examination, there are times when the views are not optimal. This chapter will highlight such situations and help one to recognize them. This chapter aims to describe the findings and possible suggestions, which may help to optimize the ultrasound imaging. Following the basic principles as described in Chapters 1 and 2 will go a long way to helping with difficult cases, and these will be reinforced in each scenario described below. While reporting the findings, acknowledging the limitations of the scan findings is very important, especially as many clinicians will be managing the patients on the basis of the report only.

The Awkward Uterus

Ultrasound images of the uterus in an axial position are not optimal. In the axial position the end-on view of the body of the uterus in relation to the probe leads to image artefacts and poor image resolution, which does not allow for good-quality images. The axial uterus is more likely to be associated with the presence of a Caesarean scar, pelvic adhesions or large leiomyomas. The cervix and cervical canal will generally be easily accessible with scan and the image quality will be good, but the body of the uterus may align axially or even retroflexed, making it difficult to get good images of the body of the uterus or any endometrial details (Figure 3.1).

It is often observed that the end-on view of the endometrium in an axial uterus may give an echogenic appearance even in the follicular phase of the cycle. Bimanual manipulation with the ultrasound probe may help at times. Applying gentle pressure on the cervix with the transvaginal scanning (TVS) probe where the uterus is mobile will help to correct to an anteverted or a retroverted uterus, hence improving the image quality. At times, bimanual examination with the probe may correct an axial uterus to an anteverted or retroverted one, thus improving the

visibility. It is important to emphasize that this should be done gently, after a rapport is built up with the patient and letting her know that you are applying gentle pressure. This will minimize pain or discomfort for the patient and will allow for completion of the study. On occasion, it may be possible to alter the flexion and version of an axial uterus for the duration of the scan by asking the patient to have a full bladder. This may be uncomfortable, hence all other structures should be scanned and the patient asked to come back with a full bladder. The bladder may push the axial uterus and make it appear retroverted and retroflexed, thus allowing for an easier assessment of endometrial details. In women with uterine prolapse the correction is easy with application of gentle pressure with the ultrasound transducer. Where there is restricted mobility due to adhesions or large fibroids, any correction of uterine flexion or version may not be possible, and in such situations only slight correction may be the best one can achieve (Figure 3.2). This slight correction, along with abdominal pressure with the left hand while doing the scan with the right hand, may enable you to improve the quality of the image. An abdominal scan with an under-filled bladder may allow for a better visualization of the uterus and the endometrium, but good results can only be obtained in women with a normal BMI.

Assessment of endometrial pathology in women with very large fibroid uteri may never be possible using ultrasound. In some cases, even demonstrating the endometrial stripe is very difficult with conventional ultrasound; however, tracing the cervical canal into the cavity can be helpful (Figures 3.3–3.6). Contrast-enhanced sonography with gel or saline may allow for visualization of the endometrial cavity, relationship of the cavity to the fibroids and even assessment of fine details of the endometrium (Figure 3.7). Adjustment of depth where there are large fibroids or cysts will help in visualization of the whole lesion (Figure 3.8). Contrast-enhanced

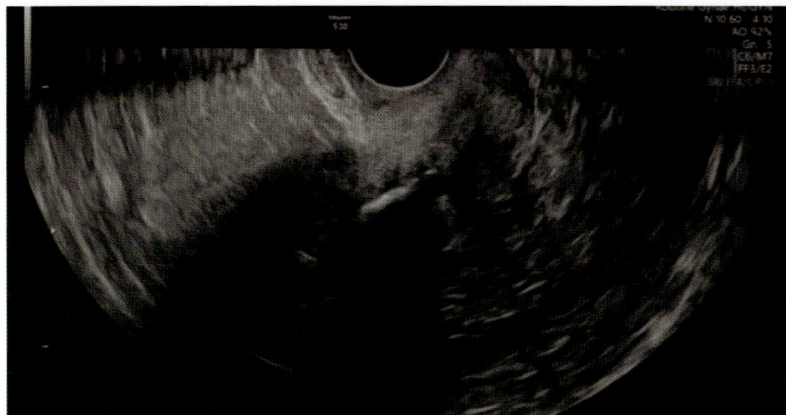

Figure 3.1 Axial uterus with previous LSCS (lower segment Caesarean section) scan with IUCD (intrauterine contraceptive device) in the uterine cavity.

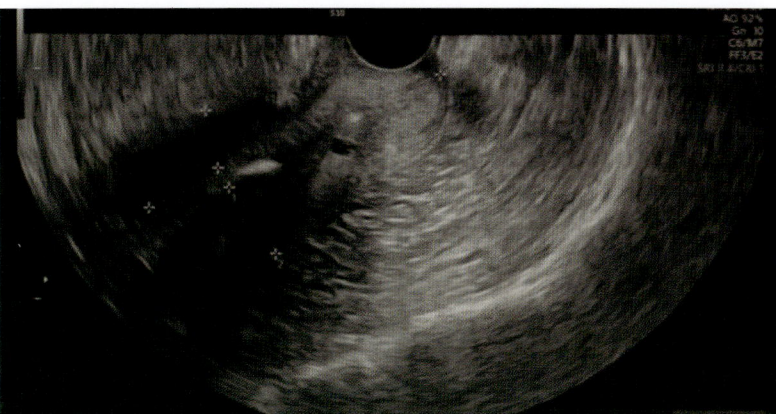

Figure 3.2 Partial correction of axial uterus with previous LSCS scan with IUCD in the uterine cavity using bimanual pressure with the TVS probe.

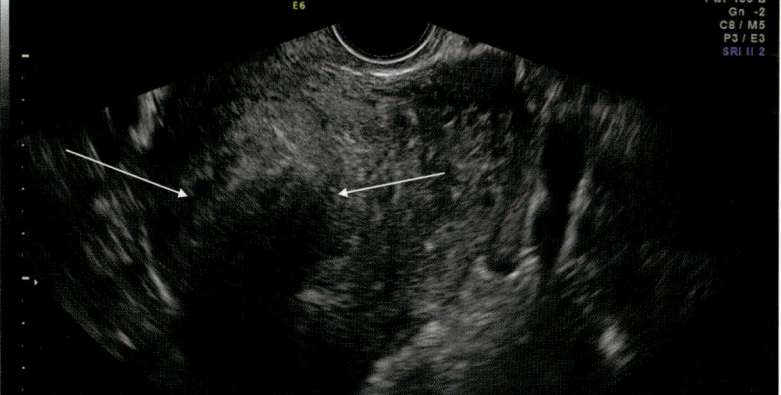

Figure 3.3 Intramural fibroid (arrows) assessed using a normal frequency setting.

ultrasound is described in detail in Chapter 6. Where ultrasound fails to demonstrate endometrial details or for fibroid mapping for larger lesions before surgery, magnetic resonance imaging (MRI) is indicated as the imaging of choice.

The Awkward Ovaries

Following basic principles as described in Chapter 1, it is easy to find ovaries, especially in the reproductive age group. For women who are postmenopausal, have had

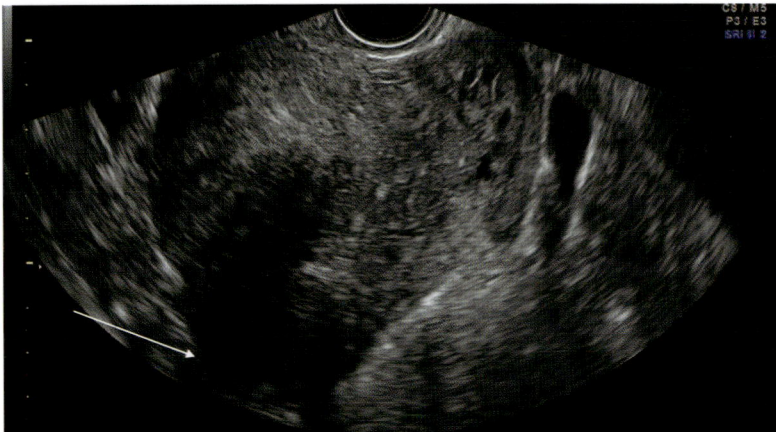

Figure 3.4 Intramural fibroid with a subserosal component (arrow) assessed using penetrative frequency.

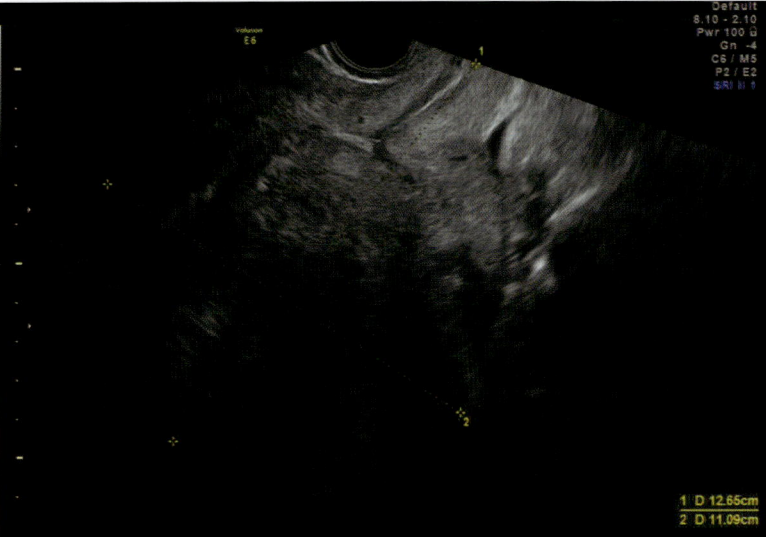

Figure 3.5 Cervical canal in a large fibroid uterus (calipers) with difficult-to-see cavity/ endometrium needing saline infusion sonography (SIS), to demonstrate details of the endometrial cavity.

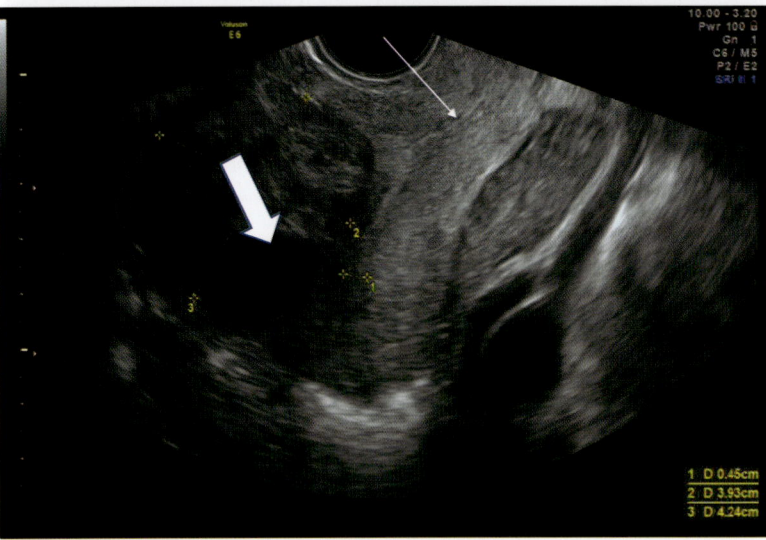

Figure 3.6 Anterior submucous fibroid (calipers) with degenerative changes (hypoechoic area; thick arrow) impinging on the endometrium.

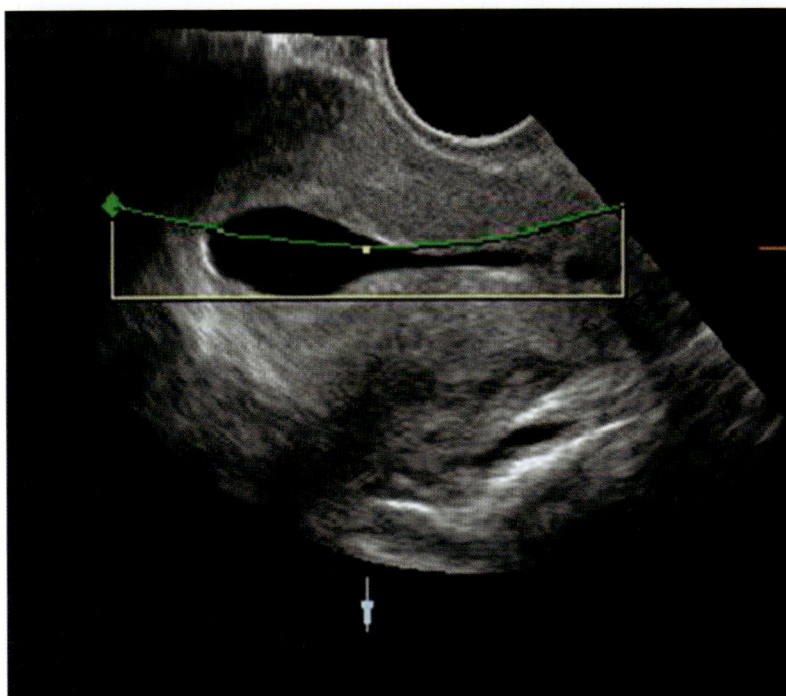

Figure 3.7 Image demonstrating endometrial cavity following instillation of saline (saline infusion sonography; SIS).

adhesions following previous surgery or pelvic infection, it may be difficult to localize the ovary. Large fibroids with calcification also can make it difficult to clearly see the ovaries due to shadowing. Following the landmarks described in Chapter 2, especially a thorough assessment of the area medial to common iliac vessels, may result in identification of the ovary. The most useful feature is bimanual examination with the left hand while scanning with the transvaginal probe. Generally, the bowel tends to be displaced and the ovary comes into view. Once the ovary is seen, by sustaining pressure the left hand can be released to increase the depth and freeze the image. At times releasing the left hand may lose the image of the ovary and in such situations an assistant is needed to freeze the image captured, or the patient is asked to press on the abdomen while the person scanning captures the image. The former is the preferred option.

Occasionally the ovary will be located behind the uterus (Figure 3.9). Increasing the depth to get a 'panoramic overview' of the pelvis will help to localize the ovary in such instances. When seen behind the uterus and if the ovary is mobile, it can be displaced laterally with gentle sustained pressure to get better images (Figures 3.10, 3.11). When mobility is restricted due to adhesions, this pressure may be associated with tenderness or discomfort (Figure 3.12). This could be worse if a myomectomy scar is present or a large lateral fibroid is obstructing the view. Using the penetrative frequency is preferred as the ovary is at a depth behind the uterus.

If the ovaries are still not seen with a TVS, a transabdominal scan has to be performed to exclude an ovarian cyst, which is probably no longer in the pelvis. If still not seen and an ovarian assessment must be carried out for clinical reasons, the patient should be referred to another experienced scanner; an MRI scan may be needed to exclude any ovarian and adnexal pathology, especially in postmenopausal women. It is important to identify the ovaries in postmenopausal women to exclude malignancy, particularly if there are clinical symptoms or raised CA-125 levels. If the ovaries are not seen, this should be clearly documented in the imaging report and tumour markers could be particularly useful for peri- and postmenopausal women.

Pedunculated fibroids may be confused with a fibroma of the ovary. Thus, it is important to see the lesion and the ovary separately, and in their entirety. A pedunculated fibroid will be arising from the surface of the uterus and generally this connection will have a vascular pedicle within, which may be observed by power Doppler

(a)

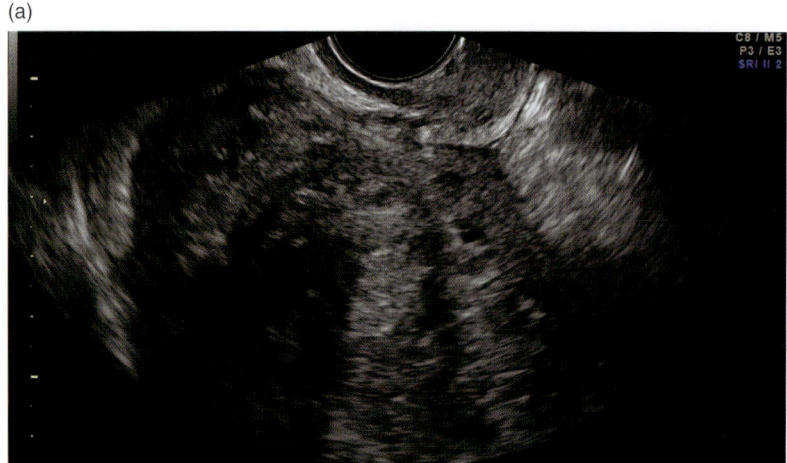

(b)

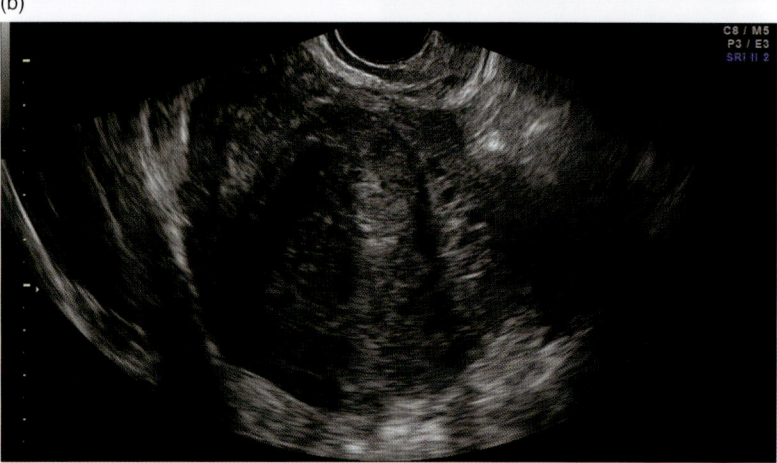

Figure 3.8 (a) Normal depth to visualize uterus with a large fibroid; in this case the depth needs to be adjusted. (b) Fibroid with depth adjusted to see the uterus completely.

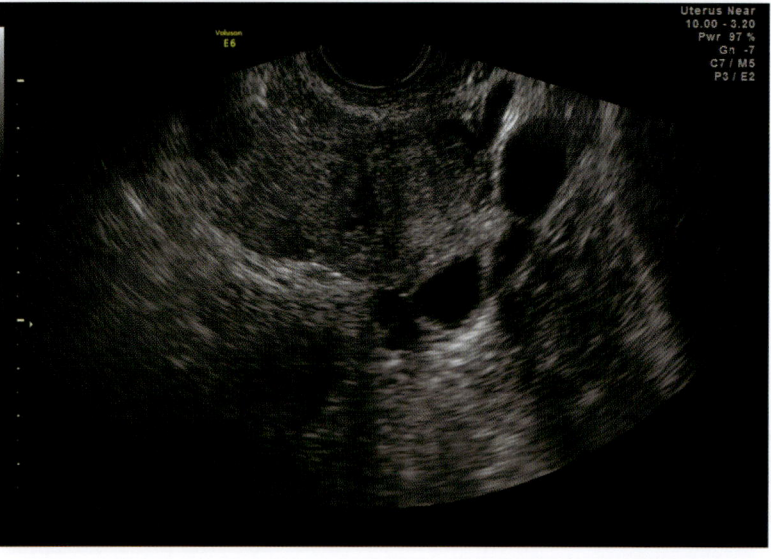

Figure 3.9 Left ovary behind the uterus with reduced mobility despite applying bimanual pressure.

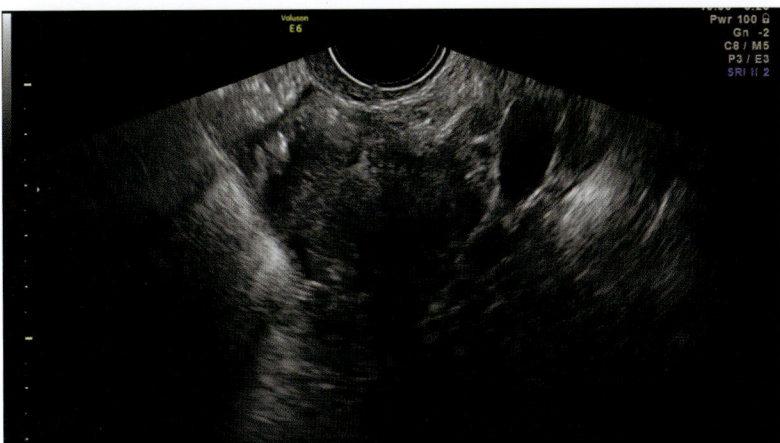

Figure 3.10 Left ovary behind the uterus on initial examination before applying abdominal pressure.

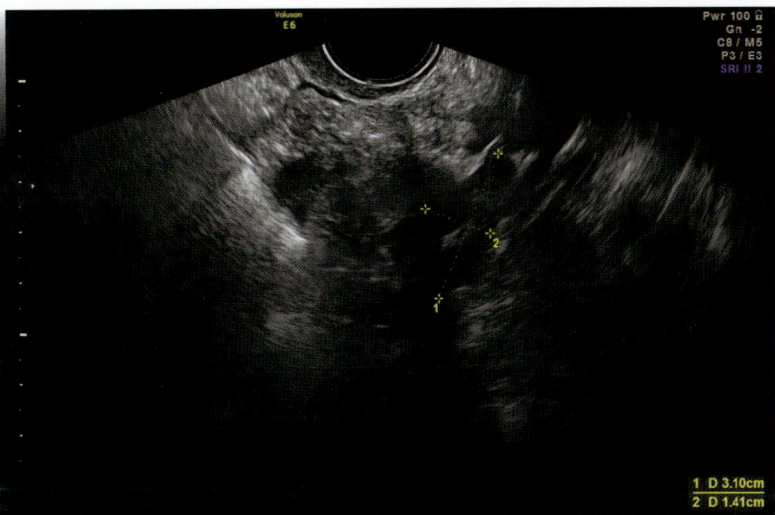

Figure 3.11 Left ovary behind the uterus on initial examination after applying abdominal pressure shows better visualization.

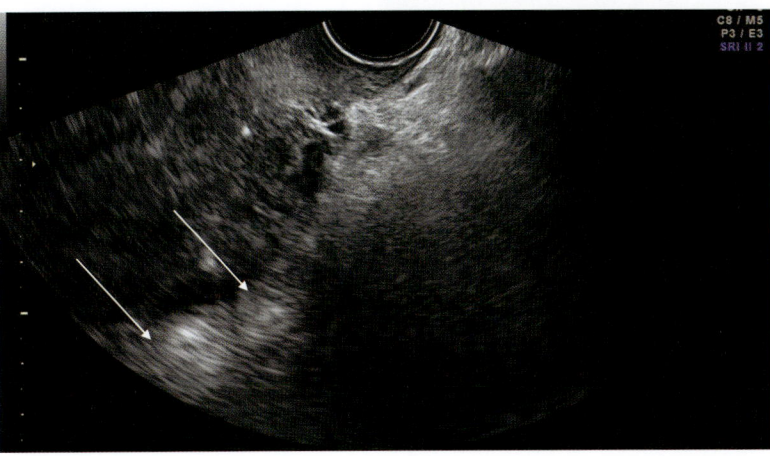

Figure 3.12 Adhesions following myomectomy (arrows).

(a)

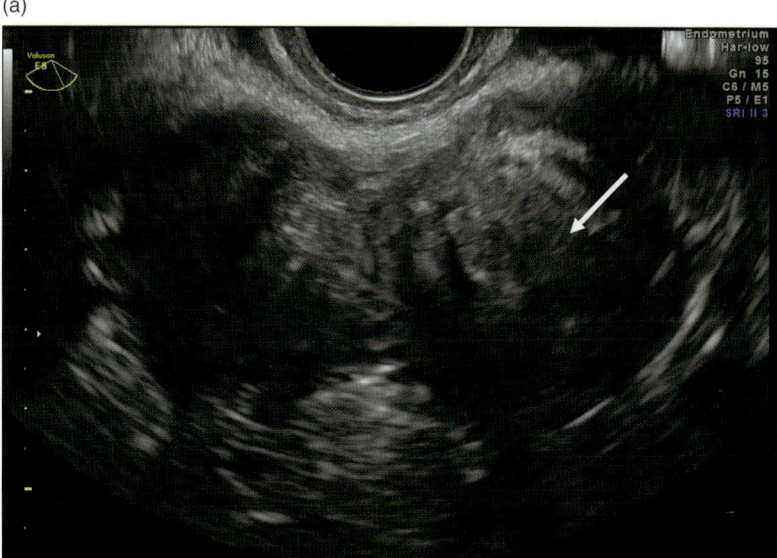

(b)

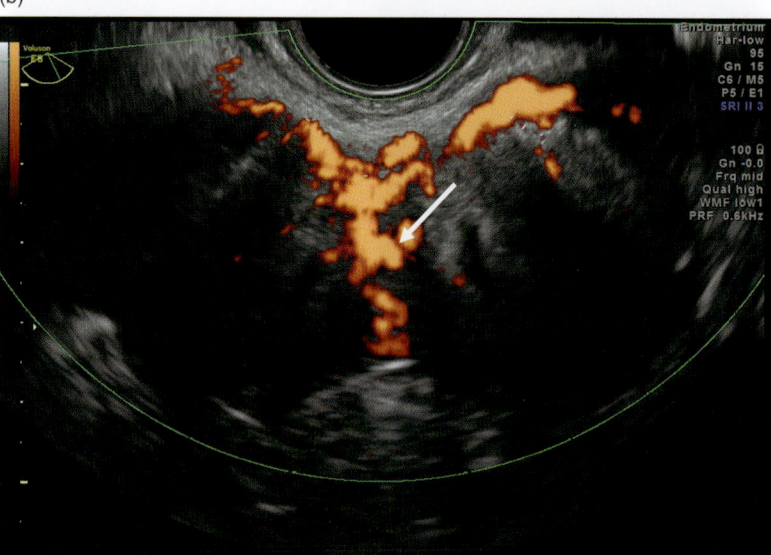

Figure 3.13 (a) Pedunculated fibroid on a transverse view at the level of the fundus of the uterus (arrow). (b) Pedunculated fibroid on a transverse view at the level of the fundus of the uterus. Doppler signal demonstrates a thick vascular pedicle (arrow).

examination (Figure 3.13). This pedicle arises from the uterus, usually somewhere different from the origin of the tube (on rare occasions, pedunculated fibroids may arise in the cornu of the uterus). A complete systematic examination of the uterus, especially in the transverse plane, should help to identify the pedunculated fibroid.

It is useful to take a medical history prior to the examination to exclude a history of oophorectomy – or even during the procedure, especially if it is not possible to localize the ovaries.

Adhesions Due to Previous Surgeries

Adhesions develop following previous pelvic surgery, such as Caesarean section, ovarian cystectomy, myomectomy, salpingectomy for ectopic pregnancy, pelvic inflammatory disease (PID) or endometriosis. These adhesions may distort the pelvic anatomy or make the visualization of structures beyond the adhesions difficult. A good history of previous surgery or PID will help you to correlate the findings. Adhesions tend to restrict mobility of structures, especially the ovary as described above. Bimanual examination with the TVS probe may help in imaging; however, dense adhesions tend to be echogenic and thus make it difficult to view organs beyond them. It may be useful to decrease the gain during the examination to overcome this issue. It is important to record tenderness during the examination as this may help in discussing management, especially when contemplating surgical intervention such as laparoscopy and adhesiolysis [1,2].

Diagnosis of adhesion by ultrasound is not generally easy to make. The key points that may help in the diagnosis of adhesions include history of surgical intervention, echogenic appearance on examination and restricted mobility with or without the presence of tenderness on ultrasound examination (Figure 3.12). The sliding sign as described below may be useful to demonstrate restricted mobility.

Endometriosis

The classical appearance of endometriosis is described in Chapter 9 and is relatively easy to identify. Minimal endometriosis and deep infiltrating endometriosis (DIE) can be difficult to diagnose with pelvic ultrasound examination. In cases of minimal endometriosis, a typical history of deep dyspareunia with cyclical pain associated with a normal scan with focal tenderness on ultrasound examination can raise suspicion. This may need to be confirmed with diagnostic laparoscopy. Demonstrating the sliding organ sign with application of gentle pressure with the ultrasound transducer on the cervix in an anteverted uterus and the fundus in a retroverted uterus may be useful to demonstrate obliteration of the pouch of Douglas with or without endometriosis (Figure 3.1) [3]. Deep endometriosis, especially of the bowel, can be demonstrated by focusing on the rectum and parametrium with visualization of the region posterior to the cervix (utero-sacral ligaments), pouch of Douglas and rectum in one plane. Complete assessment of the pelvis for DIE should also include the anterior compartment (bladder and uterovesical fold) and rectovaginal septum. Bowel preparation with an enema prior to the scan may be useful in identifying the walls of the rectum and sigmoid colon, as any lesion within can be clearly seen (Figure 3.3). DIE imaging does take time to master and has obvious limitations associated with location of the endometriotic deposits and preparation of the patient. Gel sonovaginography has been used to demonstrate posterior compartment DIE. This does require some experience and at times MRI may be a better option before considering surgery [3,4].

Appearance of Ovaries while on Combined Oral Contraceptive Pill (COCP) and Progestogen-Only Pill (POP)

Women on COCP for prolonged periods of time have suppressed ovaries with no dominant follicle. The ovaries look smaller and the antral follicle count (and anti-Mullerian hormone (AMH)) will be low or difficult to count as the ovaries are suppressed. In the pill-free week, follicular development does resume, and delay in taking the pill may result in ovulation [5]. When ovarian reserve testing is indicated, the authors feel it may be more appropriate to carry out the assessment after the onset of one or two menstrual cycles following stopping the COCP. The endometrium in women on COCP appears thin and the appearance resembles the secretory phase (hyperechogenic) throughout the cycle [5].

POP, implants and injectable. The endometrium appears thin and the ovaries tend to show simple functional cysts in 10–20 per cent of patients [6]. Patients on these contraceptives often present with intermenstrual bleeding or spotting and hence are referred to secondary care to exclude endometrial pathology, such as polyps or submucous fibroids. As they are not cycling it is difficult to correlate simple follicular cysts with stage of the menstrual cycle. Most of the time these cysts regress, and if any concerns as to the nature of the cysts are present, a second opinion should be sought or these cysts should be reimaged in 4–6 weeks to allow for resolution. Depo provera injections used for contraception are given at 12-week intervals. The ultrasound findings in these women demonstrate that ovaries continue to cycle; however, the endometrium appears thin through this period, resulting in a drug-induced secondary amenorrhoea [6].

Gonadotrophin-Releasing Hormone (GnRH) Agonists

Prolonged use of GnRH agonists induces medical menopausal hormonal status. The scan findings suggest

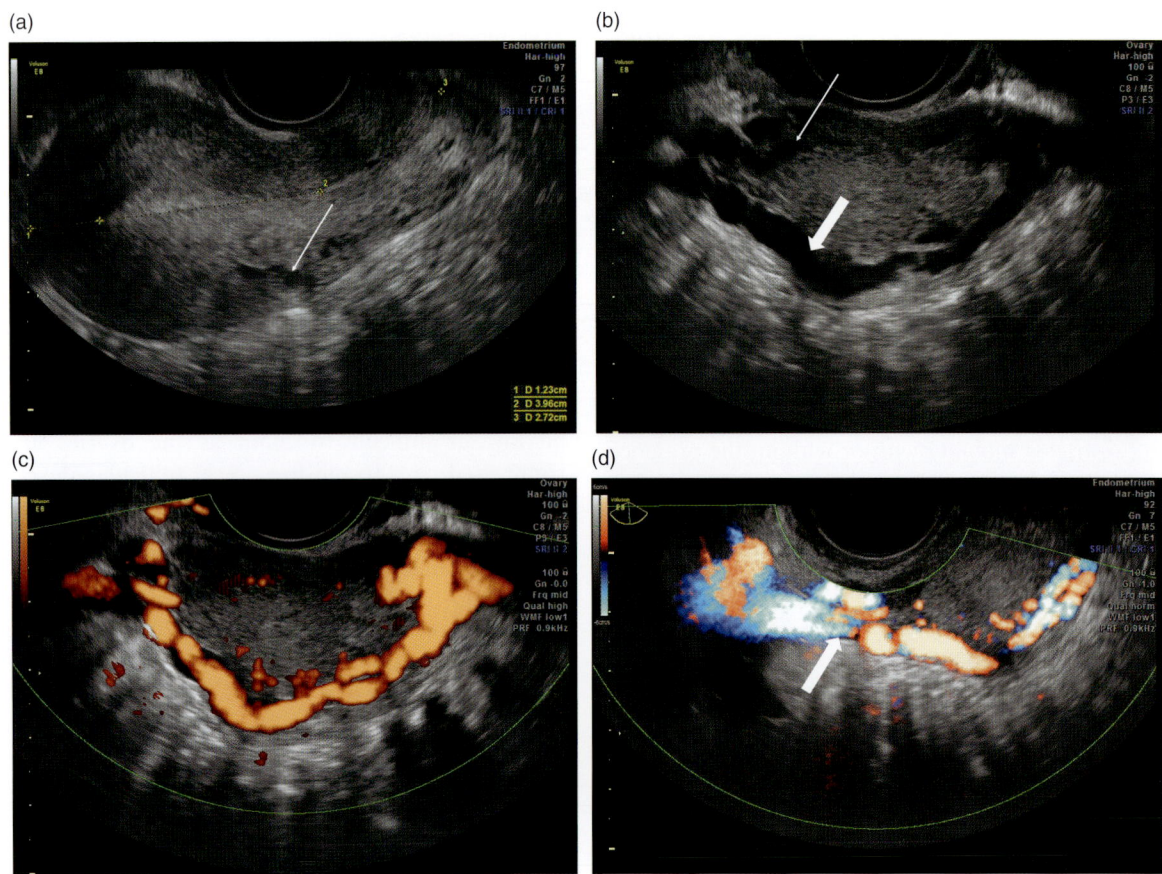

Figure 3.14 (a) Sagittal view of an anteverted uterus with multiple hypoechoic areas in the posterior wall (arrow), representing prominent blood vessels. (b) Same uterus in a transverse view. Blood vessels are visible in much more detail (thick arrow) and also encroach on the anterior uterine wall (thin arrow). (c) Application of power Doppler modality unequivocally confirms that the tortuous, tubular structures are blood vessels with marked blood flow. (d) The distended blood vessels run through the broad ligament (arrow) and extend to the pelvic sidewall. Normal ovary is lost within the colour Doppler signal arising from the congested pelvic vessels.

the ovaries are suppressed with no dominant follicle and the endometrium appears very thin. These medications are generally used in women with endometriosis following surgery to suppress the condition and provide symptomatic relief, or in women undergoing *in vitro* fertilization (IVF) treatment for down-regulation of ovaries in the long protocol regime.

Congested Pelvic Vessels, Broad Ligament Vessels

Some dilated blood vessels in the broad ligament are not uncommon. When this is severe and associated with pain and heavy periods, then review with ultrasound becomes relevant. Subserosal dilation of vessels in the uterus may also be present (Figure 3.14).

Obese Patients

Obesity provides a diagnostic challenge when assessing the pelvic organs. The adipose tissue present in the omentum and the *appendices epiploicae* causes a barrier for the ultrasound by creating additional distance between the transducer and the organ of interest, causing poor image quality. Abdominal scans are similarly difficult due to subcutaneous adipose tissue. Transvaginal scan is, however, the preferred route; it provides a far better image quality compared to abdominal scans. Mobile uterus and ovaries improve the image quality further as pressure and bimanual assessment are more likely to bring these organs into proximity to the ultrasound probe. Positioning of the patient in lithotomy and making her comfortable and relaxed during the procedure are helpful. Adjustments

(a)

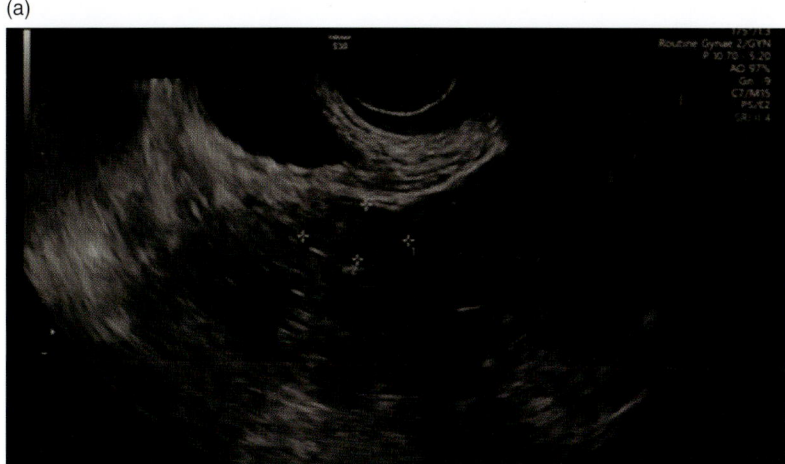

(b)

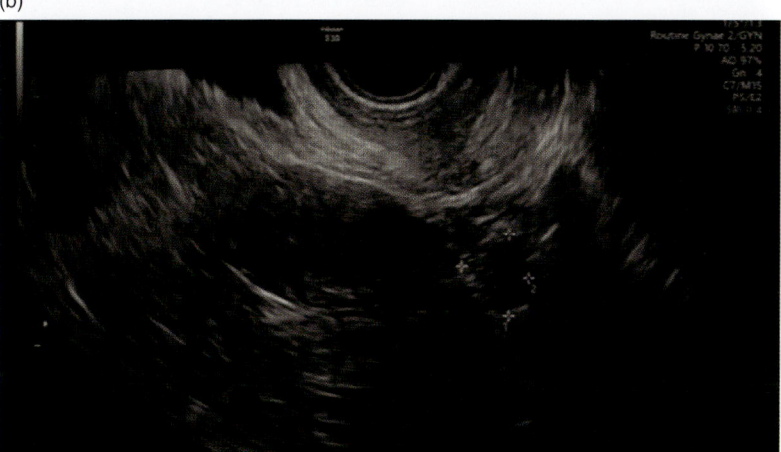

Figure 3.15 (a) Per rectal scan in a woman who refused TVS examination – longitudinal view of the uterus with the bladder in view; (b) Per rectal scan transverse view of the uterus and the left ovary with bladder in view (refused TVS examination).

of ultrasound settings such as gain, penetration and depth may be useful in some situations. In obese patients with adhesions due to previous surgery such as myomectomy or LSCS, the views will be poor despite all efforts.

Women Not Sexually Active

In women who have never been sexually active, or will not tolerate introduction of the TVS transducer due to vaginal stenosis or vaginismus, transabdominal scan may provide adequate views of the pelvic organs, especially if the bladder is full. In obese women, a transrectal scan may be carried out (Figure 3.15), but only if this is acceptable to the patient. Failure to demonstrate pelvic organs in this subgroup of women, when clinically indicated, may be an indication for an MRI scan as the only imaging modality able to assess female pelvic organs in sufficient detail.

Tips and Tricks

- Axial uterus may be better imaged using a transabdominal approach with a moderately filled bladder.
- Endometrial assessment of a bulky, fibroid uterus may be better using contrast-enhanced sonography.
- Iliac vessels provide an important landmark when looking for an ovary.
- Sliding organ sign allows for demonstration of pelvic adhesions.
- History-taking prior to ultrasound may save you the time and embarrassment of looking for an ovary that has previously been removed.
- A systematic approach to scanning is essential in difficult cases.
- A second opinion should always be considered.

- In some obese patients, adequate sonographic assessment of the pelvis despite the application of all described tricks may never be possible.

References

1. Guerriero S, Ajossa S, Lai MP, et al. Transvaginal ultrasonography in the diagnosis of pelvic adhesions. *Hum Reprod* 1997;**12**:2649–53.

2. Okaro E, Condous G, Khalid A, et al. The use of ultrasound-based 'soft markers' for the prediction of pelvic pathology in women with chronic pelvic pain: can we reduce the need for laparoscopy? *BJOG* 2006;**113**:251–6.

3. Guerriero S, Condous G, van den Bosch T, et al. Systematic approach to sonographic evaluation of the pelvis in women with suspected endometriosis, including terms, definitions and measurements: a consensus opinion from the International Deep Endometriosis Analysis (IDEA) group. *Ultrasound Obstet Gynecol* 2016;**48**:318–32.

4. Reid S, Lu C, Hardy N, et al. Office gel sonovaginography for the prediction of posterior deep infiltrating endometriosis: a multicenter prospective observational study. *Ultrasound Obstet Gynecol* 2014;**44**:710–18.

5. Killick SR, Bancroft K, Oelbaum S, Morris J, Elstein M. Extending the duration of the pill-free interval during combined oral contraception. *Adv Contracept* 1990;**6**(1):33–40.

6. Tayob Y, Adams J, Jacobs HS, Guillebaud J. Ultrasound demonstration of increased frequency of functional ovarian cysts in women using progestogen-only oral contraception. *Br J Obstet Gynaecol* 1985;**92**(10):1003–9.

Sonographic Assessment of Uterine Fibroids and Adenomyosis

Francisco Sellers López, Belén Moliner Renau and Rafael Bernabeu Pérez

Introduction

Uterine fibroids (or leiomyomas) are the most common benign gynaecological tumours, formed by smooth muscle and connective tissue. Most are asymptomatic, but sometimes may cause pain, pressure symptoms, metrorrhagia, infertility due to implantation failure, miscarriage, preterm delivery, and puerperal haemorrhage. Fibroids can be single or multiple. Their size and location vary and they may undergo benign degenerative changes: atrophic and hyaline degeneration, calcification, infection, and infarction. Malignant degeneration towards leiomyosarcoma is extremely rare, occurring in less than 0.2 per cent of cases [1].

Adenomyosis is defined as the presence of endometrial tissue with its glands and stroma, implanted in the myometrium. Dysmenorrhoea and abnormal uterine bleeding in nulliparous women are the usual presenting symptoms associated with this condition. Adenomyosis is reportedly linked to infertility; however, the exact mechanism of this negative effect is unknown [2–8]. In addition, an association between this condition and various obstetric diseases (preterm delivery, growth retardation, recurrent bleeding, etc.) has also been found [9]. Ultrasound scans – two-dimensional (2D), power Doppler (PD) angiography and three-dimensional (3D) – are often adequate to make a definitive diagnosis and plan subsequent management. These investigations are the preferred diagnostic tools due to lower cost, accessibility, patient tolerability and minimal invasiveness of the procedure compared to other modalities [10].

The aim of this chapter is to provide an overview of the ultrasound diagnosis of uterine fibroids and adenomyosis and their sonographic appearance in typical and atypical cases, and to provide guidance when pitfalls are encountered.

Uterine Fibroids

Transvaginal ultrasound with high-frequency endocavitary transducers and wide angles of acquisition constitute the best diagnostic tool for describing uterine leiomyomas. On occasion, transabdominal ultrasound may provide better details, particularly in cases of large fibroids. The lower frequency of abdominal ultrasound transducers allows assessment of structures at a greater distance, and therefore, both routes can be combined for detailed analysis (Figure 4.1). Occasionally, application of abdominal pressure with the non-scanning hand may move the fibroid closer to the transvaginal transducer, allowing better visualization of the fibroid and surrounding structures.

Modern ultrasound equipment is delivered with predefined technical settings for a gynaecological examination recommended by the manufacturer. In general, the preset parameters are very suitable and usually do not need to be modified. In 2D mode these parameters include frequency, power, gain, dynamic range and greyscale; in PD mode they include wall filter and the pulse repeated frequency (PRF); and in 3D/4D mode they include acquisition mode, volume angle, quality and various image display modalities including sectional planes and render modes. Nevertheless, in some cases these settings need to be modified depending on the patient's characteristics (body mass index, uterine position, uterine size), the particular type of examination and the preferences of the examiner. Attenuation of ultrasound waves through fibroids is common and therefore assessment in 'penetration mode' (low frequency and better depth, but at the cost of resolution) may often be needed, especially in cases of an enlarged uterus with multiple fibroids.

Myomas appear on the ultrasound as rounded or oval structures, well defined and circumscribed nodular masses, usually hypoechogenic and homogeneous with respect to the surrounding myometrium. Occasionally, these fibroids are minimally echogenic, appearing as small cystic masses in the myometrial layer (Figure 4.2). The echogenicity depends on the amount of fibrous tissue present in the smooth

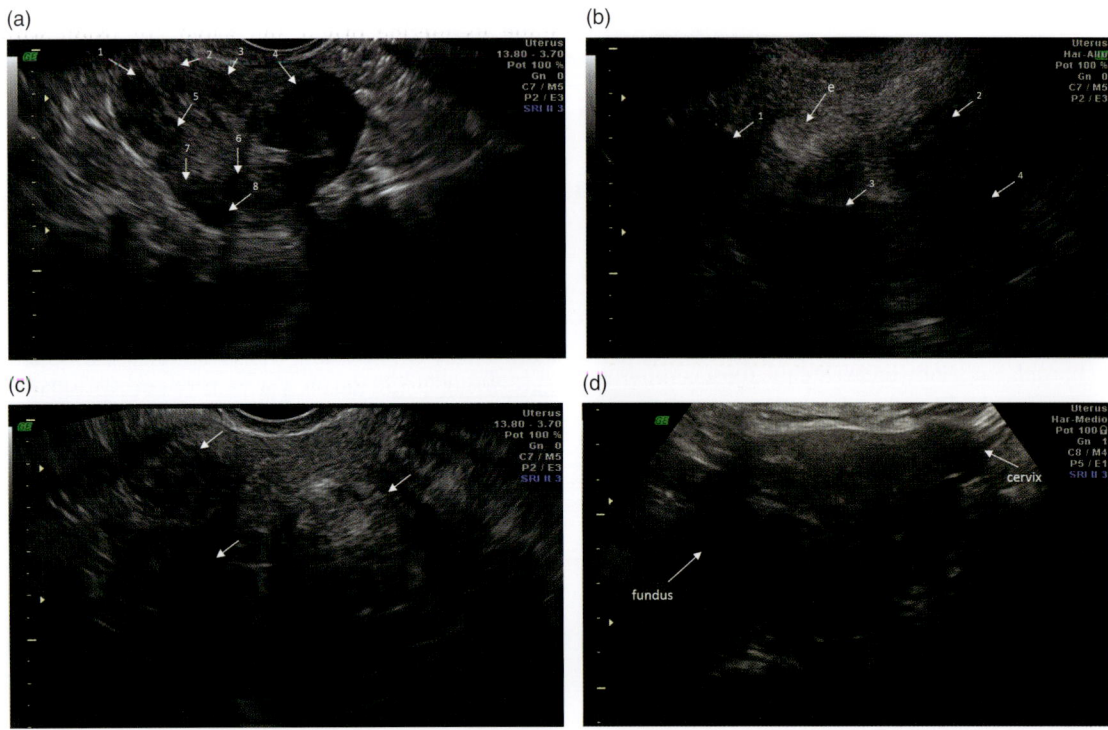

Figure 4.1 Transvaginal ultrasound showing two examples of a uterus with multiple myomas (arrows): (a) Uterus with eight fibroids. (b) Uterus with four fibroids showing endometrium (e). (c) Transvaginal ultrasound showing a large uterus with multiple myomas, partially visible. (d) Abdominal ultrasound showing the same uterus allows for complete visualization and the measurement of all its diameters.

muscle, in addition to vascular contribution and the presence of degenerative changes. Even the inner fibrous spiral architecture can sometimes be seen, since the fibres of the smooth muscle and connective tissue are arranged in a concentric pattern. It is essential to visualize the interface between the normal myometrium and the pseudocapsule surrounding the myoma, as this allows the examiner to differentiate fibroids from true adenomyosis.

Establishing the location and size of myomas [11] is necessary for a full assessment. This should be carried out in the longitudinal and transverse planes of the uterus and the fibroid location should be noted in relation to the anterior, posterior, right or left uterine walls, as well as to the endometrial cavity. This approach allows for measurement of the fibroids in three orthogonal planes. In cases of multiple fibroids and enlarged uterus, fibroid mapping can be difficult by ultrasound. Systematic scanning and identification of relevant landmarks (i.e. the bladder and cervical canal) is very helpful, especially when planning any surgical interventions. The assessment

should follow the endometrial cavity from the cervical canal to the fundus (and *vice versa*), and systematically, the mapping of fibroid location is done. Assessment should be completed by scanning the uterus from one side to the other (operator preference dictates whether the start is on the right or the left side of the uterus). When multiple fibroids are mapped, a typed report should be supplemented by a graphic representation of the exact location of the myomas.

According to the location of the myomas with respect to the uterine layers, they are classified as intramural (confined within the myometrium), sub-serosal (greater than 50 per cent of the fibroid protrudes through the serosal surface) and submucosal (distorting the endometrial cavity). Multiple types of fibroids can co-exist at any time (Figures 4.3–4.9), and intramural types, when continuing to grow, may change and indent the endometrial or serosal surfaces, thus becoming submucosal or subserosal types, respectively. Fibroids may also be intraligamentous (i.e. within the broad ligament), pedunculated, cervical or within the uterine horn (Figures 4.3–4.9).

(a)

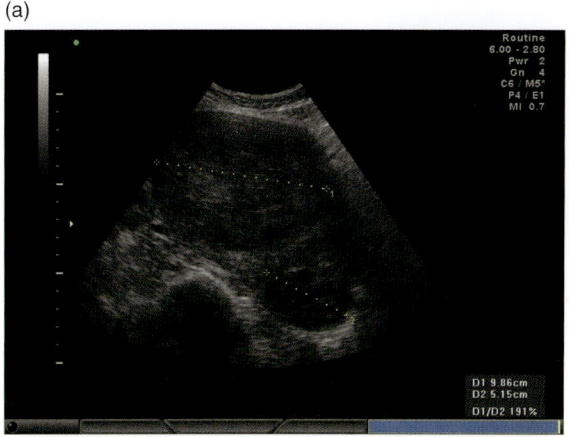

(b)

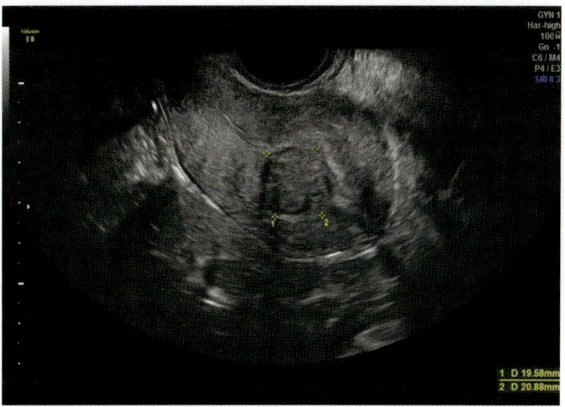

(c)

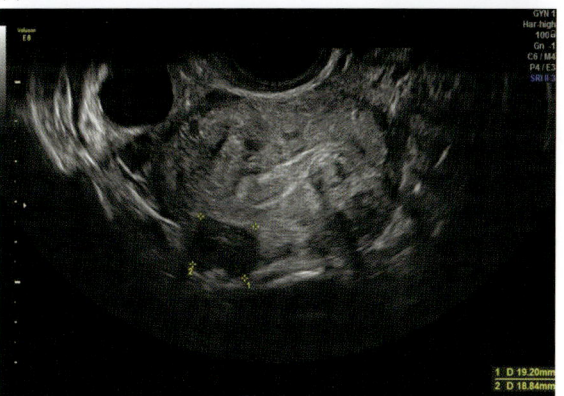

Figure 4.2 Different sonographic appearances of fibroids: (a) circumscribed nodular masses; (b) fibroid isoechogenic with respect to the surrounding myometrium; (c) small hypoechogenic masses in the thickness of the myometrium.

Subserous myomas deform the uterine contour. In the case of intraligamentous and pedunculated fibroids, locating the vascular connection with the uterus ('bridge sign') is very useful to accurately determine its uterine origin and avoid confusion with adnexal masses. Another way to determine the origin of the adnexal mass is to apply slight pressure on the fibroid with the vaginal transducer; if the mass moves with the uterus, its uterine origin is confirmed. As for intramural myomas, during a scan the normal myometrium can be clearly demonstrated surrounding the fibroid and separates them from the endometrium or the external surface of the uterus. The large leiomyomas can, however, deform the cavity or alter the uterine contour.

Submucous myomas can be confused with endometrial polyps, although polyps are usually more echogenic and most often contain one feeding vessel when visualized using Doppler sonography. It is very important, especially from the reproductive point of view, to delineate the exact relationship to the uterine cavity and to assess the degree of protrusion into it. There are several classifications, although the classical one belongs to Wamsteker and Blok and has been adopted by the European Society for Gynaecological Endoscopy (ESGE) [12], which defines them as follows: type 0 (100 per cent inside the cavity), type 1 (more than 50 per cent inside the cavity) and type 2 (less than 50 per cent inside the cavity). Other authors recently modified this classification for better management in subsequent hysteroscopy using the STEPW parameters, which include size, topography, extension of the base of the myoma, penetration of the fibroid into the myometrium, and wall [13]. Each factor is scored on a scale 0–1–2 according to predefined criteria, and in the multicenter study of 465 submucous myomas, fibroids with a score of ≤4 were resected completely and had a better sensitivity of 100 per cent (95 per cent CI 89.4–100.0 per cent) and specificity 74.1 per cent (95 per cent CI 69.7–78.1 per cent), compared to the ESGE system when using the type 1 fibroids as a cutoff (sensitivity 36.4 per cent (95 per cent CI 20.4–54.9 per cent) and specificity 84.0 per cent (95 per cent CI 80.2–87.3 per cent)) [13]. Hysterosonography or saline infusion sonography (SIS) may sometimes be very useful for reaching a definitive diagnosis of submucous myomas and to determine the extent of protrusion of the fibroid into the endometrial cavity [14] (Figure 4.10). For all types of myomas, it is essential to measure their diameter in three perpendicular planes, and for the large ones to measure at least two major perpendicular diameters (Figures 4.11–4.13).

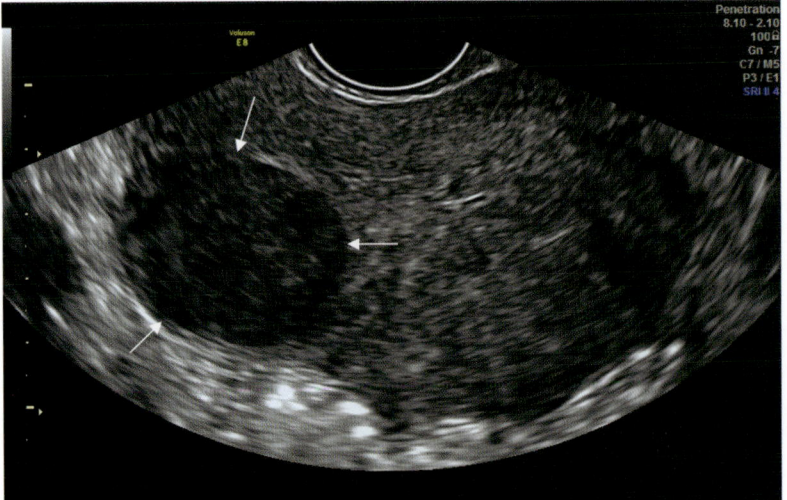

Figure 4.3 Uterus with a subserous myoma (arrows) located on the posterior wall.

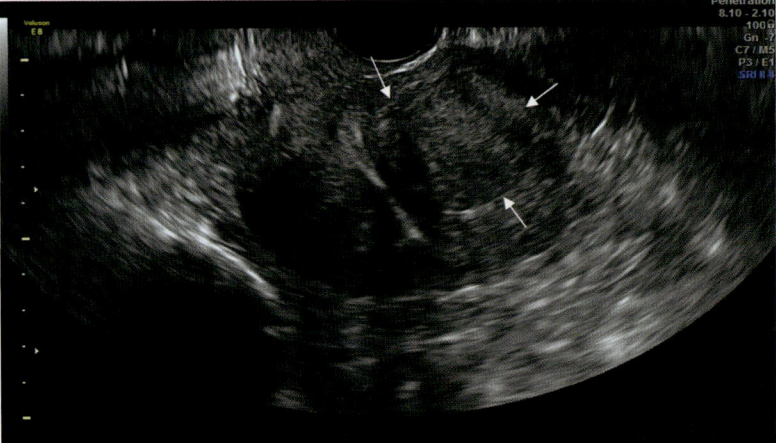

Figure 4.4 Intramural myoma (arrows) located within the myometrium, without reaching the endometrial cavity or deforming it (bright stripe below and to the left of the fibroid).

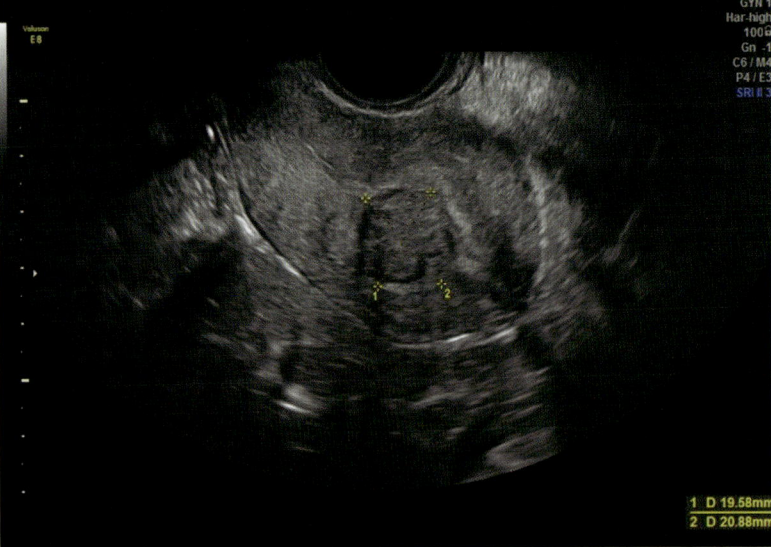

Figure 4.5 Submucous myoma easily visible and measured in two dimensions.

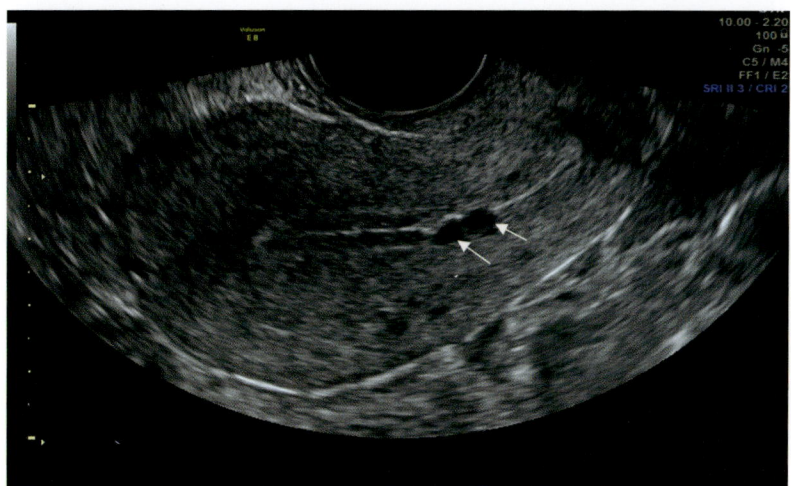

Figure 4.6 Two small submucous fibroids located near the internal cervical orifice.

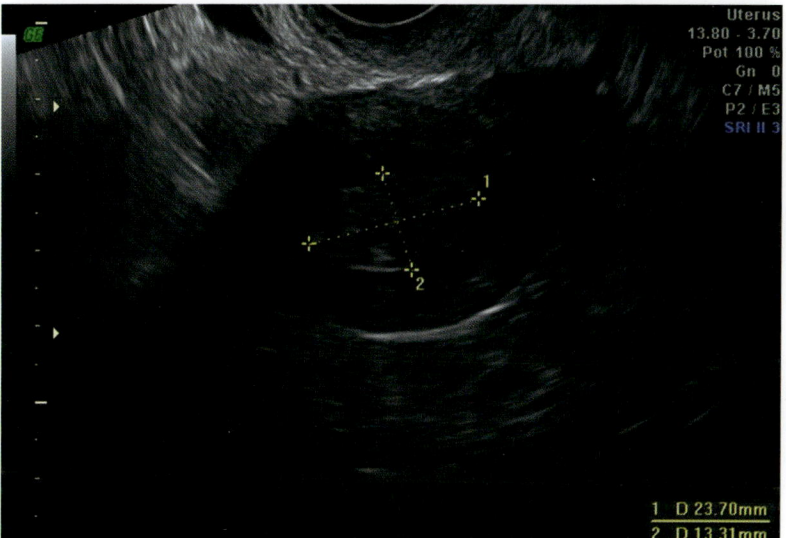

Figure 4.7 Large submucous myoma that occupies the entire endometrial cavity.

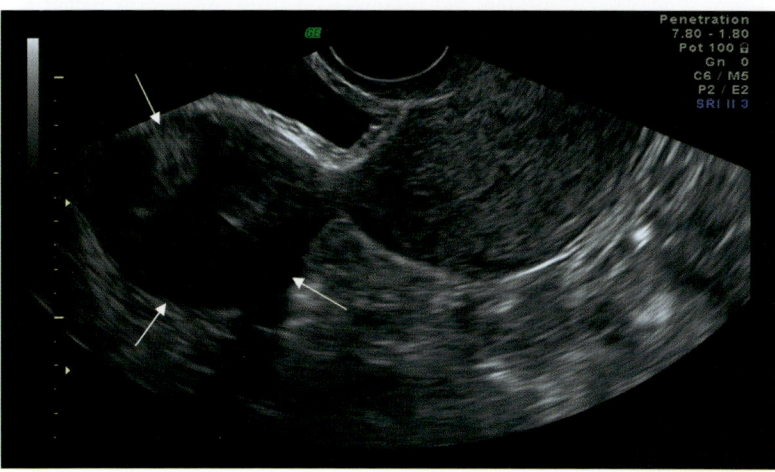

Figure 4.8 Pedunculated myoma (arrows) on the right side of the uterus.

(a)

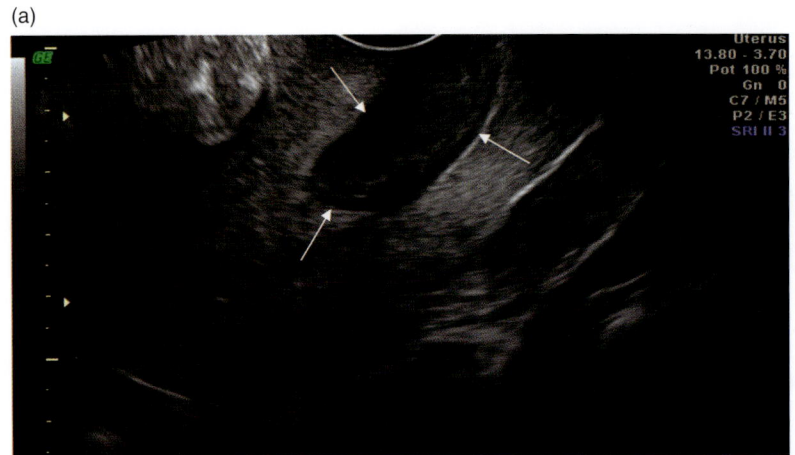

(b)

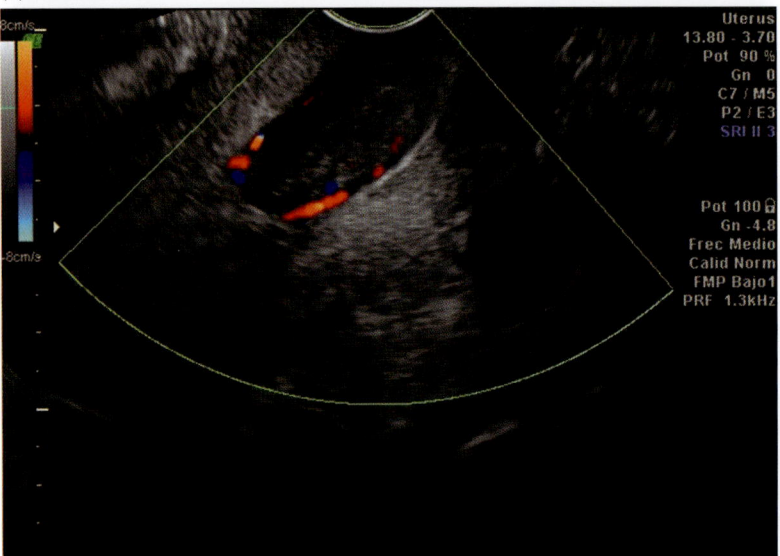

Figure 4.9 (a) A prolapsing cervical myoma (arrows) by transvaginal ultrasound; (b) colour Doppler allows for differentiation from a polyp or cervical mucus.

It should be noted that myomas can undergo degenerative phenomena so their echogenicity may change over time depending on the type of degeneration that they are undergoing. The longstanding ones may become hyperechogenic, with intense circumferential acoustic shadowing suggesting calcifications, and may be in the form of small isolated foci or a complete border surrounding the entire fibroid, with other patterns in between also being common (Figures 4.14 and 4.15).

The vascular blood supply may become insufficient to supply the entire fibroid, hence leading to vascular, ischaemic necrosis. In the beginning of pregnancy, myomas can rapidly increase in size, leading to extensive necrosis affecting the entire fibroid, with sudden and intense pain; this situation is called red degeneration. Red degeneration on ultrasound scan may appear as hypoechogenic structures that may be confused with blood vessels or adenomyotic cysts. Prior knowledge of presence and location of fibroids may be of help when making the diagnosis. Using power Doppler modality or elastography is also useful to clarify the nature of the observed structure. The presence of Doppler signal indicates a blood vessel, whereas a red contour on elastography indicates a high-density structure (i.e. fibroid). Doppler imaging in early pregnancy should only be used if absolutely necessary.

In cases when the blood supply to the fibroid is reduced gradually, its degeneration may be in the

(a)

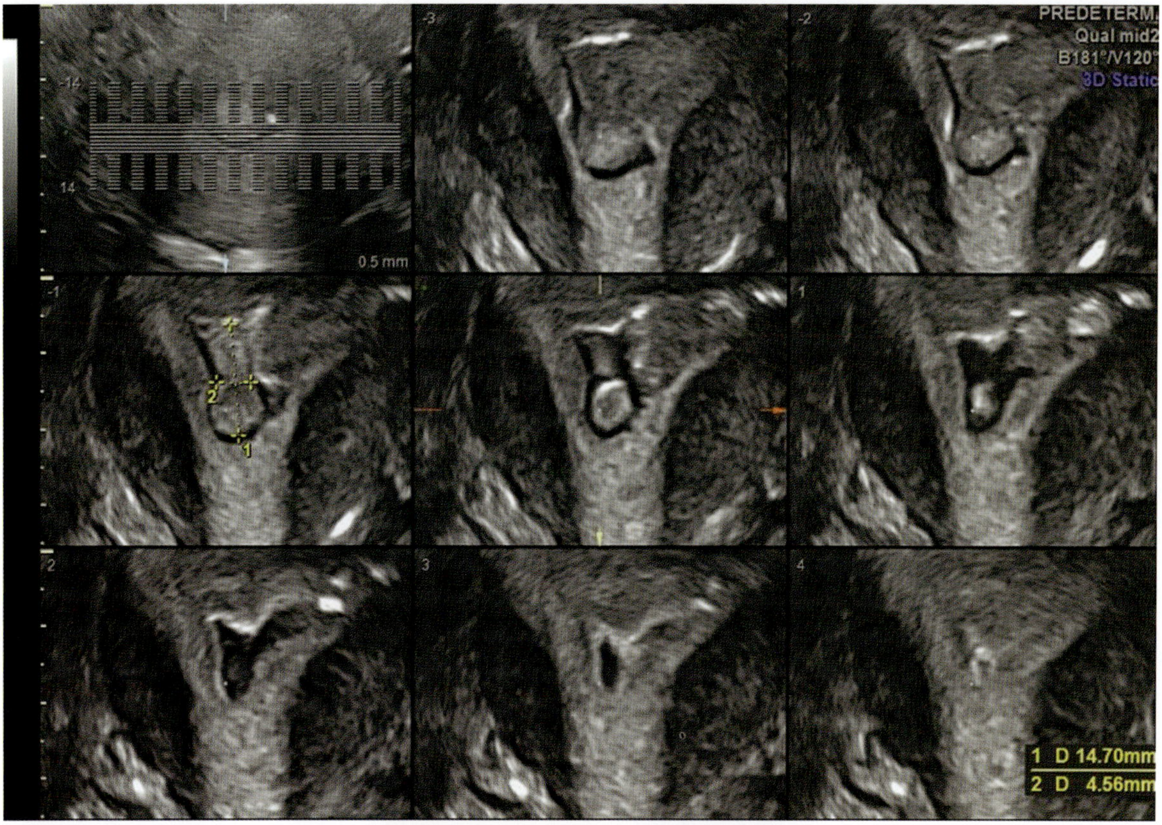

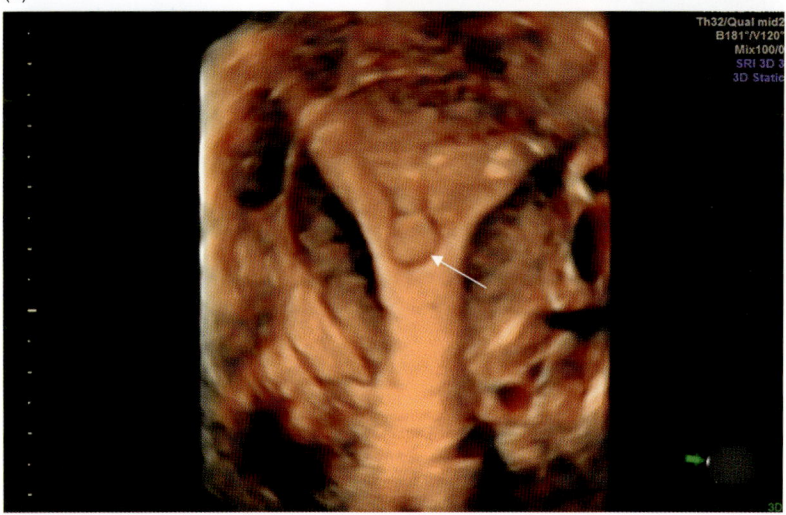

(b)

Figure 4.10 Hysterosonography for visualization of submucous myoma. 3D ultrasound is used to improve the delineation of the fibroid in two modalities: (a) with tomographic ultrasound imaging and (b) reconstruction in the coronal plane.

form of hyaline, cystic, fat or myxomatous. This will present with a complex ultrasound appearance of a homogeneous hyperechogenic lesion without acoustic shadowing or occasionally with posterior reinforcement and irregular hyperechoic or anechoic areas inside the fibroid, representing fat or myxoid

(a)

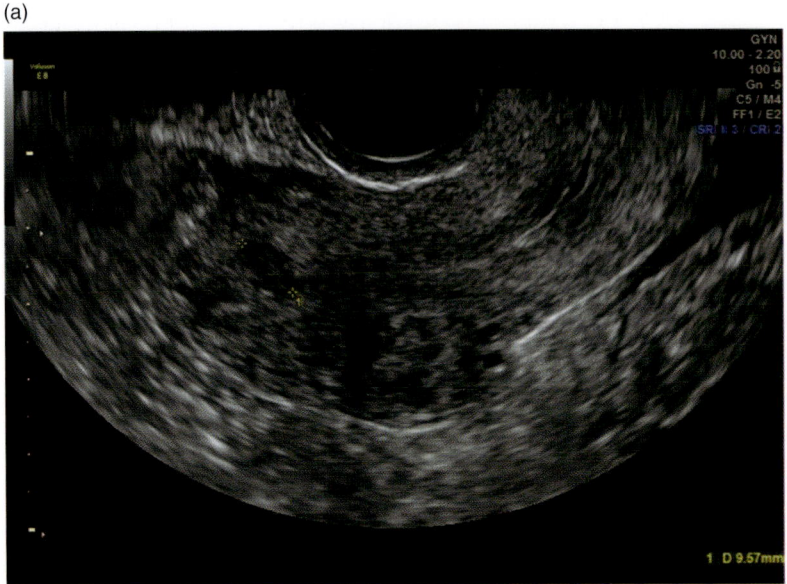

(b)

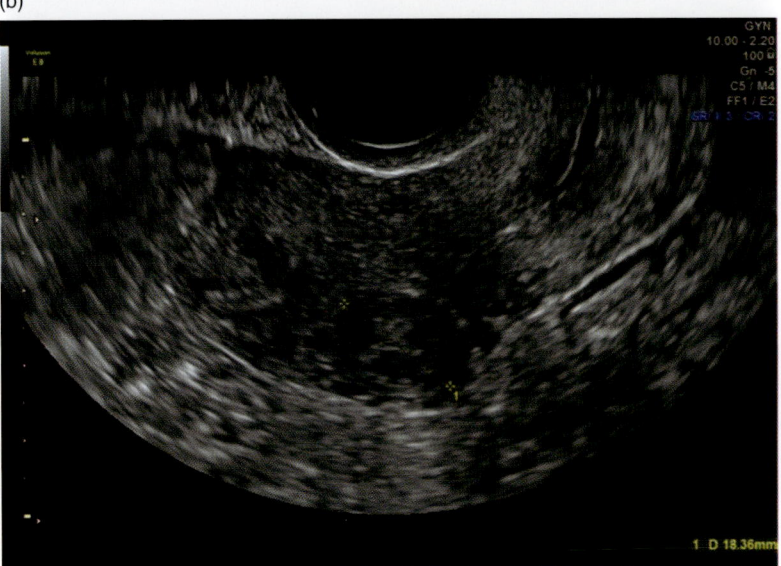

Figure 4.11 (a) Measurement of a small intramural myoma. In the cases of small, regular/globular fibroids, a single diameter measurement is sufficient. (b) Measurement of a subserous fibroid.

degeneration respectively. Hyaline degeneration is the most common and appears on ultrasound as anechoic foci within the myoma (Figure 4.16).

Fibroids should be distinguished from two conditions associated with the myometrium: adenomyosis, which will be described later in the chapter, and uterine sarcomas. The latter usually appear in menopausal women, the former can be present in any age group. Sonographic appearance should raise suspicion when a mass is visualized within the myometrium or distorts the uterine layers, has mixed echo density, a central necrosis and blood vessels with irregular distribution with low resistance as measured by pulse wave Doppler sonography (Figure 4.17). A rapidly growing fibroid should also raise suspicion of malignant transformation, and it is always useful to compare findings with prior imaging, if possible.

The histological structure of fibroids, with their concentric muscle fibre arrangement, drives the specific vascular pattern, which on Doppler imaging is mainly present on the periphery of the fibroid, with

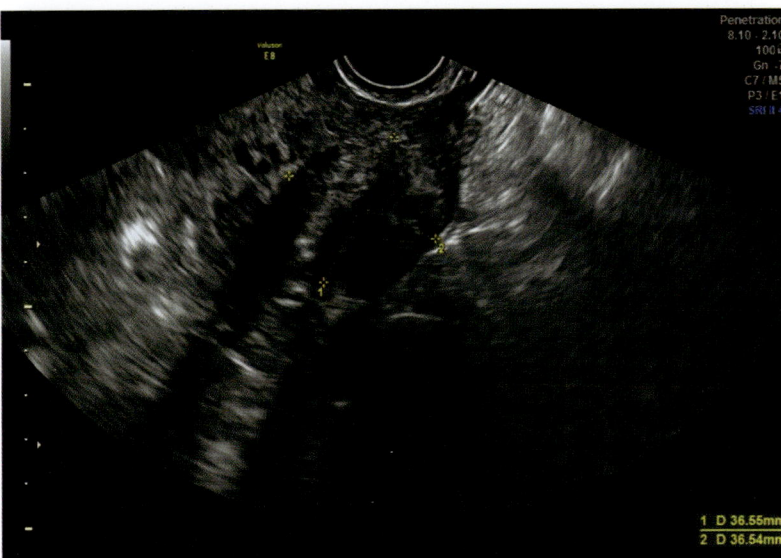

Figure 4.12 Measurement of larger fibroids should be carried out in at least two dimensions.

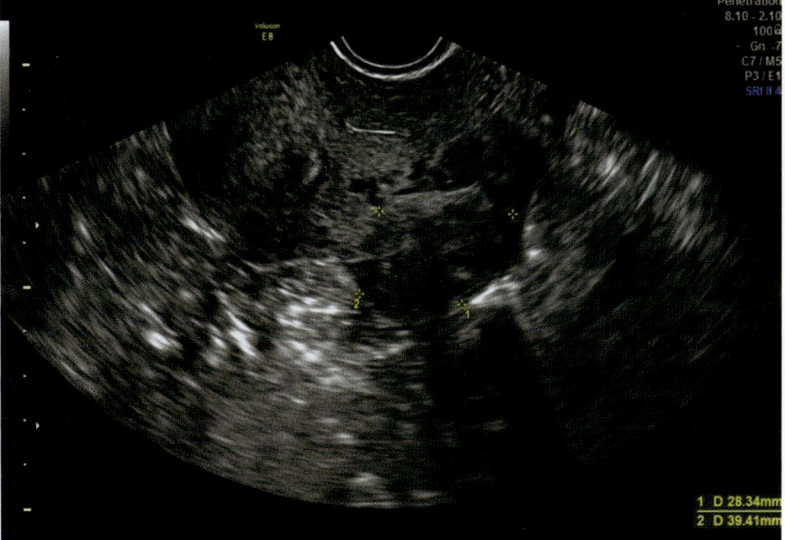

minimal observable vascularity within. This pattern allows us to differentiate fibroids from adenomyomas. Adenomyomas are composed of localized adenomyosis characterized by islands of ectopic endometrium interspersed by intense vascularization that crosses the structure in a disordered way; however, it often maintains its perpendicular course to the endometrium. Significant central vascularity in a fibroid may indicate sarcomatous change.

The application of 3D ultrasound imaging during transvaginal scanning allows for visualization of the coronal plane of the uterus. This plane has been especially useful as it allows definitive clarification of the exact position of the myoma in relation to the endometrial cavity, and the degree of cavity distortion can be determined. Fibroids may often cause uterine rotation along their axes, especially when they reach a considerable size, causing difficulties with endometrial assessment, but in some cases 3D analysis may be helpful as image manipulation may allow for some degree of cavity assessment (Figures 4.18 and 4.19). Colour or power Doppler ultrasound aids in difficult cases and helps to localize the myoma

(a)

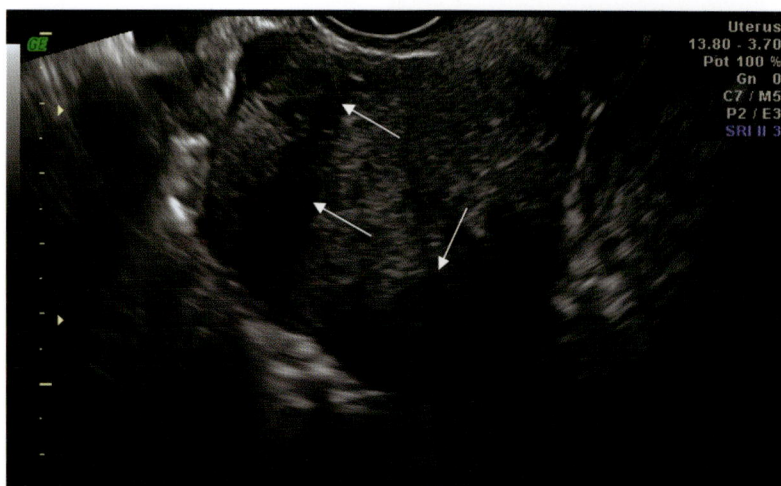

Figure 4.13 (a) Polymyomatous uterus. (b) Location and accurate measurement of each of the fibroids is indicated and helps with monitoring or response to treatment assessment.

(b)

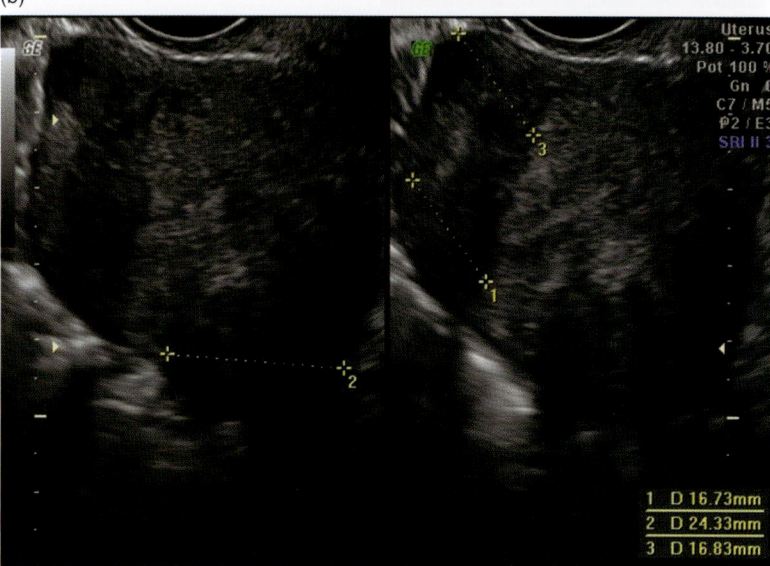

and its vascular supply, which may be useful for assessing the response to non-surgical treatments [15] (Figures 4.20 and 4.21), as well as monitoring the completeness of surgical resection and possible recurrence.

VOCAL (virtual organ computer-aided analysis) allows for accurate measurement of the volume of each myoma, which may be used for monitoring the size of the fibroids (Figure 4.22); however, this is not used in routine practice. Tomographic ultrasound imaging (TUI) integrated within the 3D software provides a single screen with multiple tomographic sections of the uterus of the multiplanar representation chosen for the exact delineation of the myoma (Figures 4.23 and 4.24). Applying various thickness settings to the sections and numbers of sections allows for accurate assessment of the fibroid in relation to anatomical landmarks, in a way not too dissimilar to how computed tomography (CT) allows for slicing through anatomical structures in a sequential manner.

It is important to monitor myomas in pregnancy, with accurate description of measurements and locations [16]. Large fibroids may contribute to the following obstetric complications: red degeneration due to the rapid growth of the fibroid with intense pain, foetal malpresentation at term, the possibility of obstruction of the birth canal, and postpartum

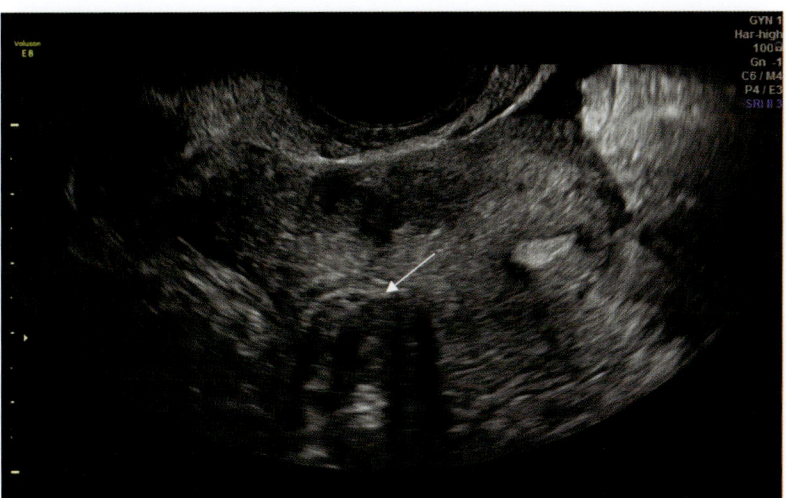

Figure 4.14 Myoma slightly calcified (arrow) on the posterior aspect of the uterus. An acoustic shadow is already noted.

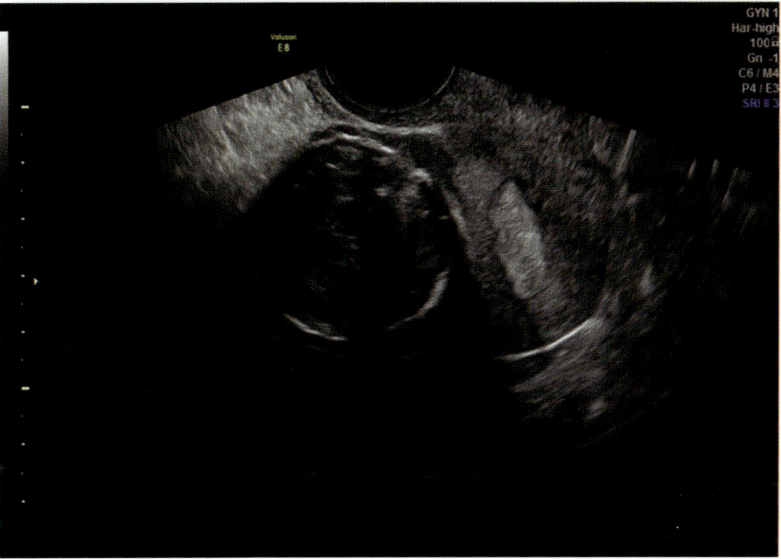

Figure 4.15 Large myoma on the right side of the uterus with a fully calcified surface and significant acoustic shadowing.

haemorrhage. All these conditions may be related to the distortion of the endometrial cavity produced by the myoma or by the alteration in the vascularization of the placenta when it is implanted over the fibroid. As mentioned earlier, during pregnancy the size of the fibroids may increase, especially in the first trimester, but may also be maintained or even decrease during the second half, and particularly in the immediate puerperium [17] (Figures 4.25–4.27).

Adenomyosis

Adenomyosis is a uterine condition where heterotopic endometrial glands are located within the myometrium, with hyperplasia of the adjacent smooth muscles [18]. Diagnosis of this condition is based on clinical data corroborated with imaging findings, although the definitive confirmatory test remains histological analysis of the uterus. MRI has traditionally been considered as the gold standard non-invasive diagnostic test; however, ultrasound – with its improved resolution and 3D capability – has now become the diagnostic modality of choice, as it is well tolerated, less expensive and widely available. While adenomyosis remains a diagnostic challenge, the finding of endo-myometrial junctional zone (JZ) thickening has been considered pathognomonic. Other described and recognized ultrasound findings

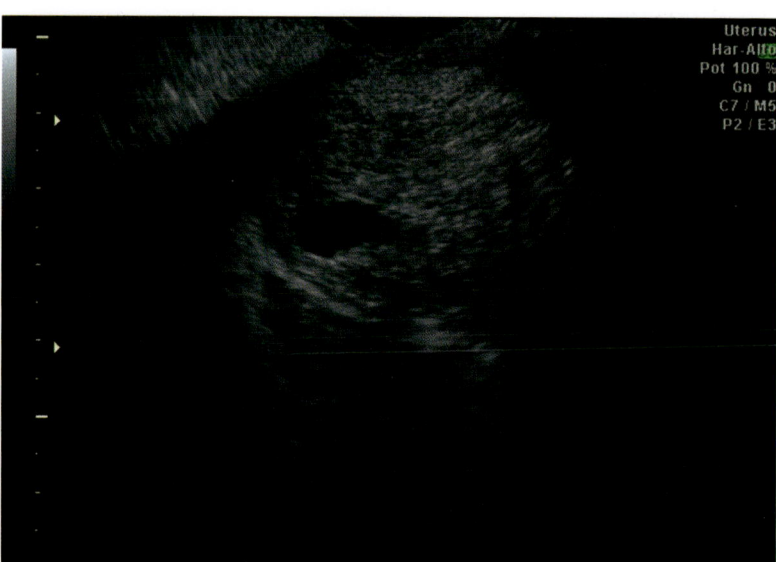

Figure 4.16 Hyaline degeneration within myoma (hypoechoic oval shape).

suggestive of adenomyosis include an irregular JZ diffusely or asymmetrically thickened with no relation to fibroids, distorted myometrium with heterogeneous hyperechogenicity, myometrial inclusion cysts in the form of anechoic lagoons, subendometrial linear striations with radial pattern, parallel shadowing or an adenomyoma (ill-defined, nodular and heterogeneous myometrial mass) [19,20] (Figure 4.28).

Some of the above ultrasound features, especially the hyperechogenic islands in the myometrial tissue, are more pronounced in the second half of the menstrual cycle owing to the secretory changes the tissue undergoes. The use of power Doppler allows for visualization of the straight blood vessels crossing the adenomyotic lesion, which follow a course completely perpendicular to the endometrium (Figure 4.29), thus differentiating it from the circumferential pattern of vascularity observed in fibroids. In the case of focal adenomyosis, or adenomyoma, the mass is contained within the myometrium, asymmetrically distorting the uterus, it is poorly delineated and has mixed echogenicity, with hyperechoic foci in the luteal phase representing ectopic endometrium. Blood vessels as seen on Doppler imaging traverse the mass freely (Figures 4.30 and 4.31).

The diagnosis of adenomyosis can be improved by using 3D ultrasound, as it allows for offline analysis with reconstruction of various anatomical planes, especially the coronal plane of the uterus. This particular view allows for subjective and objective assessment of the endo-myometrial JZ. A thickened JZ ($\geq$8 mm) with lack of defined boundaries and bridging of the JZ by echogenic endometrial foci are typical characteristics of adenomyosis on a 3D ultrasound multiplanar view or reconstruction [21–23] (Figure 4.32).

The authors propose a novel sonographic marker for diagnosis of adenomyosis using technology introduced by General Electric (Zipf, Austria) on their newest ultrasound machines – the HDLive mode (High Definition Live). The volume for analysis is obtained in a similar fashion as for any 3D volume and the image is manipulated to create a coronal view of the endometrial cavity (a detailed description of how to obtain 3D images is presented in Chapter 5).

Once the coronal plane is constructed, the 'Edit Light' functionality is activated, which allows directed trans-illumination of the object from different angles. In severe cases of adenomyosis, the authors observed the 'tree sign', with the cervical canal and the lower endometrial cavity simulating the trunk and the irregularities of the JZ with perpendicular blood vessels, and hypoechoic lagoons completing the image of the tree (see Figures 4.33 and 4.34). The study evaluating the reproducibility and reliability of this sign, as well as its association with reproductive outcomes, is ongoing.

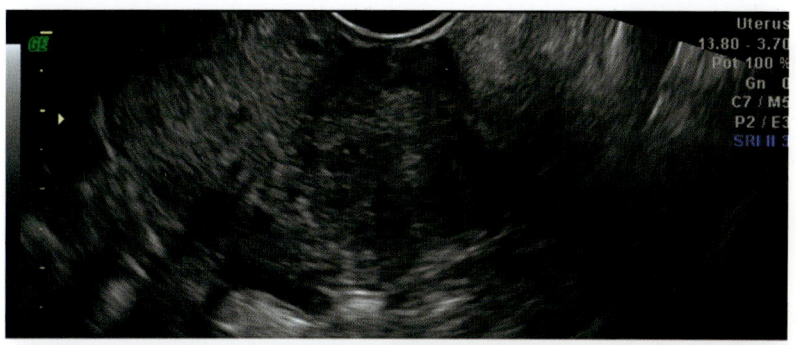

Figure 4.17 Case of a uterus with sarcoma: the entire uterine thickness is encompassed by a poorly defined lesion with central necrosis and abundant, irregular blood vessels.

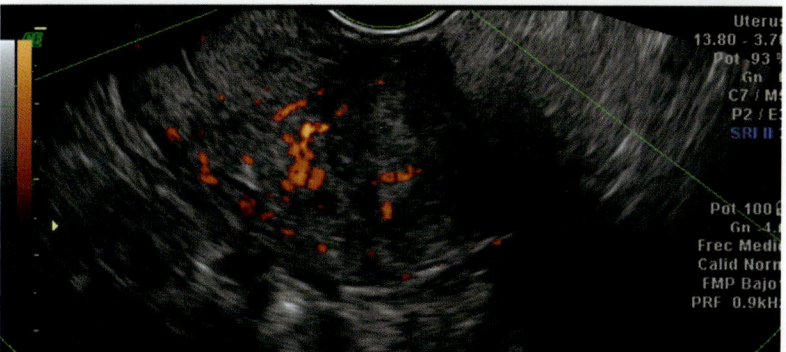

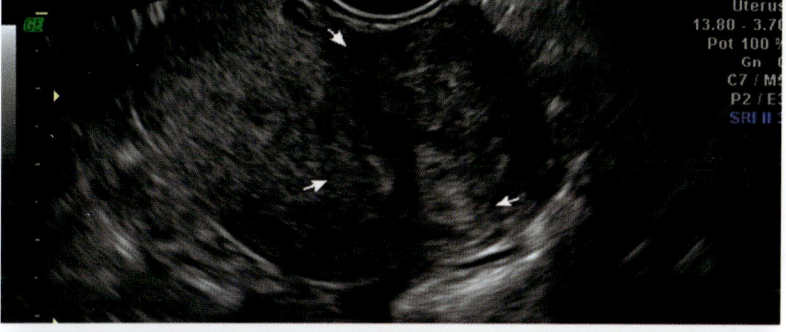

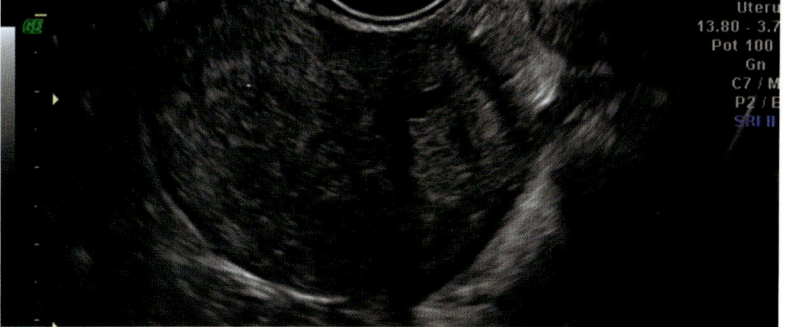

Tips and Tricks

- Transvaginal ultrasound is the diagnostic modality of choice for fibroids and adenomyosis.

- Transabdominal ultrasound may complement transvaginal ultrasound in cases of large fibroids or multifibroid uterus.
- Location of fibroids, especially in relation to the endometrium, may be best assessed with 3D ultrasound scan or TUI.

(a)

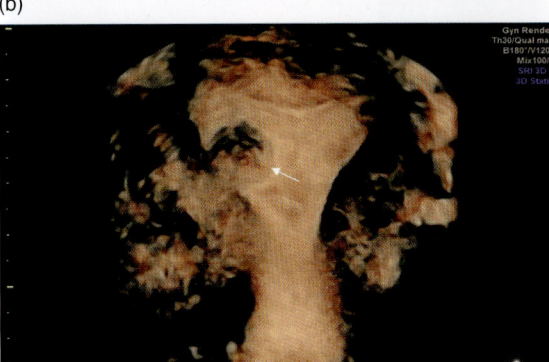

(b)

Figure 4.18 (a) Study of a submucous myoma (arrow) using 3D ultrasound with multiplanar representation. (b) Coronal plane of the uterus in the HDLive modality, with clear delineation of the myoma (arrow) in the cavity.

- Fibroids may change appearance over time due to various histological (physiological and pathological) changes and may develop anechoic spaces, acoustic shadowing or posterior reinforcement.

- Rapid increase in size should raise suspicion of sarcomatous transformation, especially if coupled with increased vascularity.

- Fibroid vascularity is mainly on the periphery, creating a 'ring of fire' appearance on Doppler imaging.

- Differentiation between type 0 fibroid and endometrial polyp may be achieved with Doppler imaging – feeding vessels will be present in both cases, but circular or semicircular patterns will be seen in the case of fibroids and a branching pattern (or just a feeding vessel) will be seen in polyps.

- Adenomyosis is best assessed in the luteal phase of the menstrual cycle.

- Asymmetrically enlarged uterus with inclusion cysts and parallel shadowing is a typical 2D sonographic appearance of adenomyosis.

- 3D imaging is very useful when assessing the endo-myometrial junction zone to help diagnose adenomyosis.

- Vascularity in adenomyosis is uninterrupted and traverses the lesion running perpendicular to the endometrium.

- Adenomyomas differ from fibroids in lack of a clear capsule and uninterrupted vascular pattern.

(a)

(b)

(c)

(d)

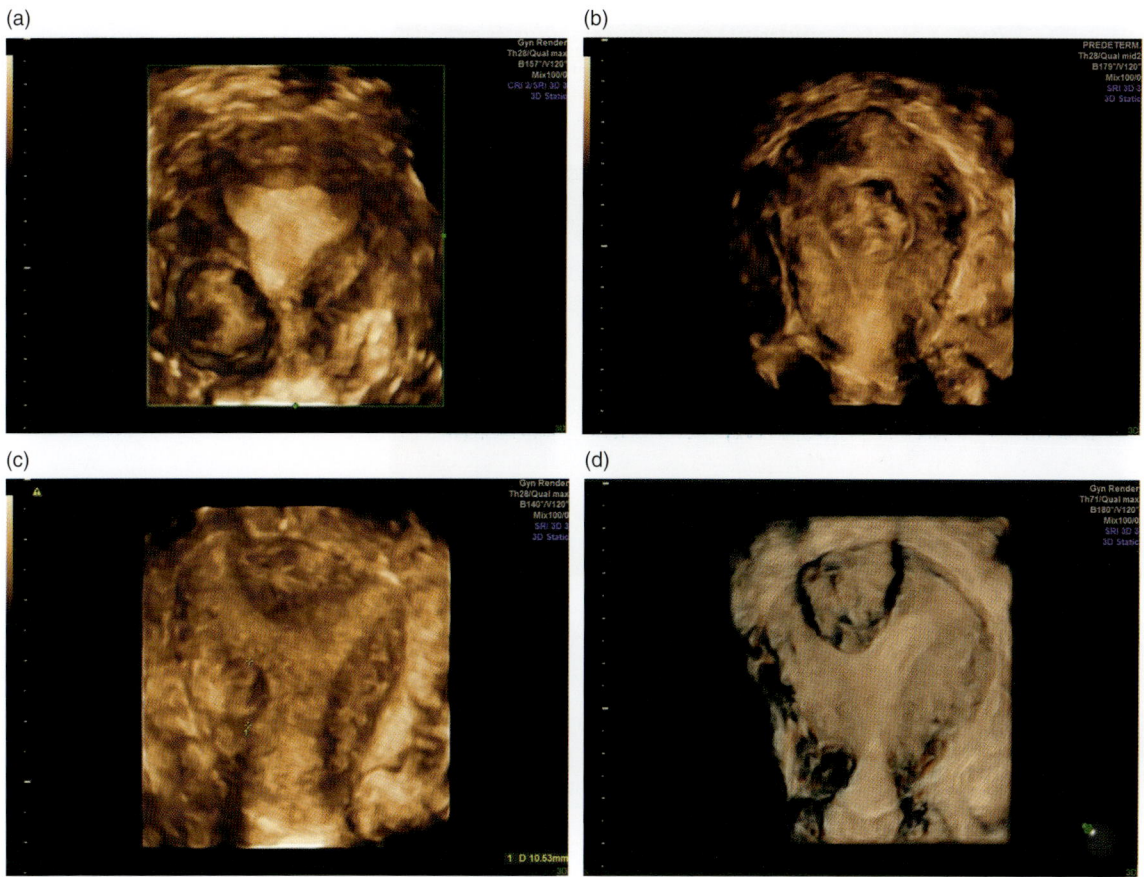

Figure 4.19 Several fibroids in 3D. (a) Intramural myoma, near the cervix. (b) Submucous myoma occupying much of the endometrial cavity. (c) Intramural myoma partially deforming the cavity. (d) Intramural myoma in the uterine fundus.

(a)

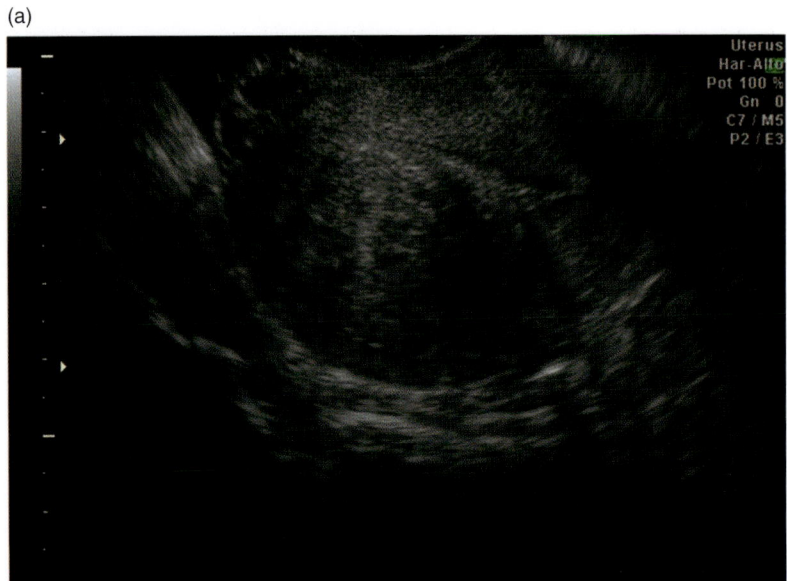

(b)

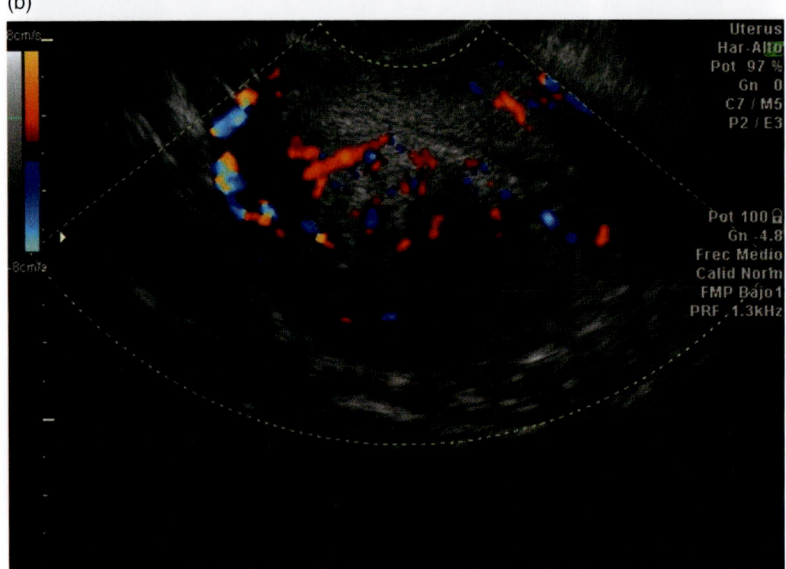

Figure 4.20 (a) Intramural myoma with poor delineation. (b) application of colour Doppler allows for a more accurate assessment of location and differentiation from adenomyosis, as the blood vessels show a peripheral distribution.

(a)

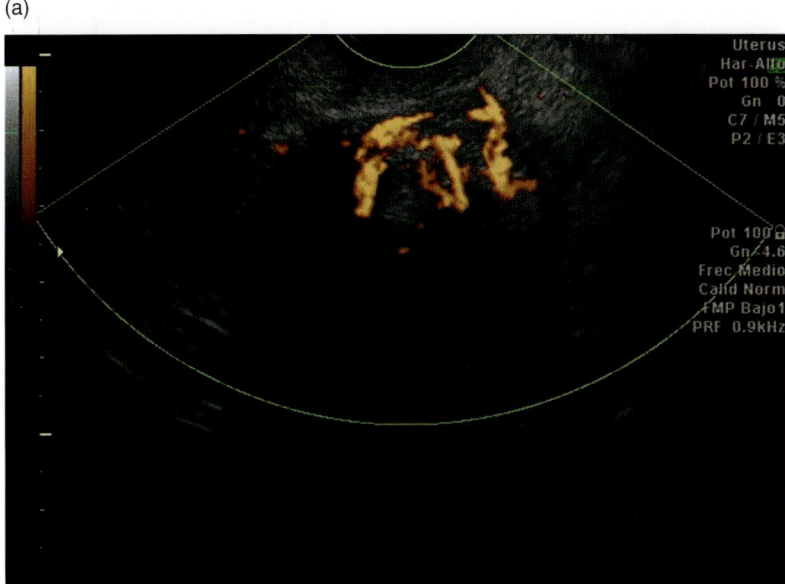

(b)

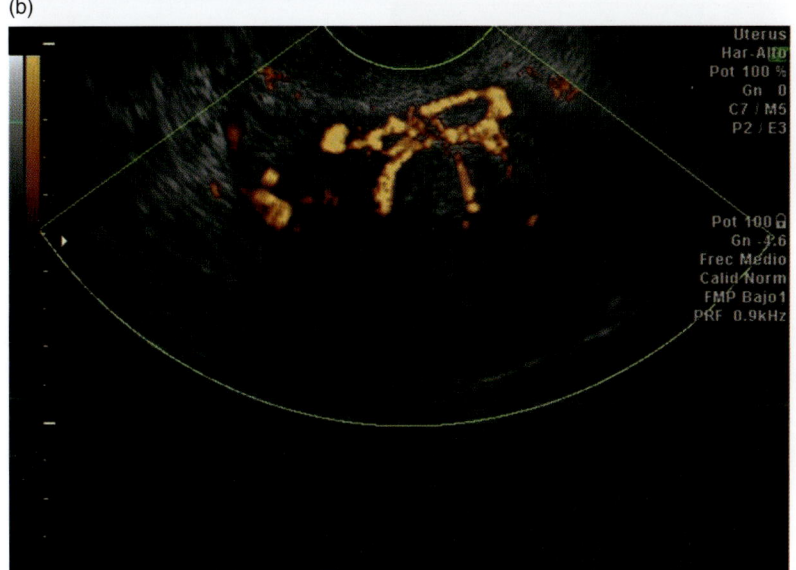

Figure 4.21 Power Doppler imaging of the same myoma as in Figure 4.20 in different planes.

(a)

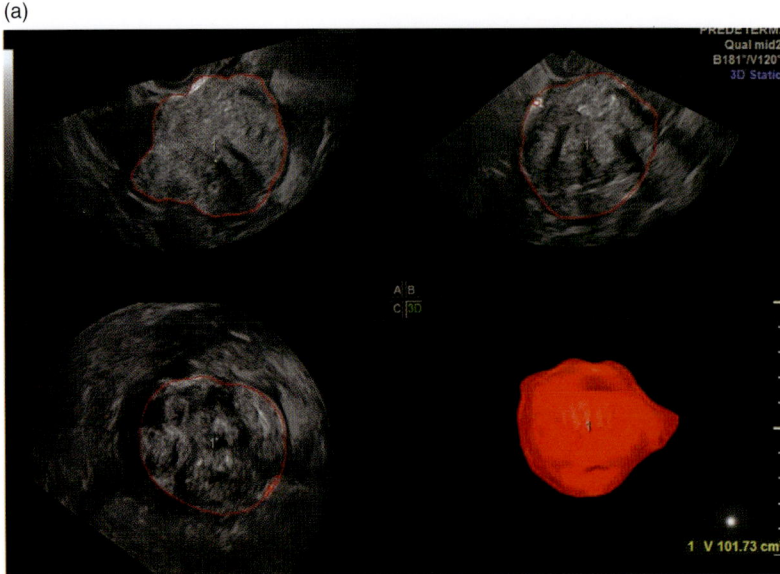

(b)

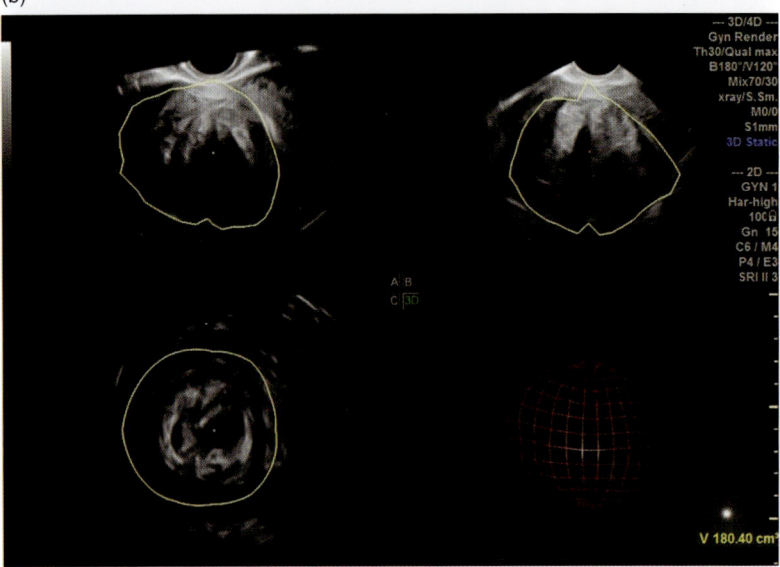

Figure 4.22 The VOCAL modality allows obtaining the volume of the myoma under study, as shown in the multiplanar representation of fibroids.

(a)

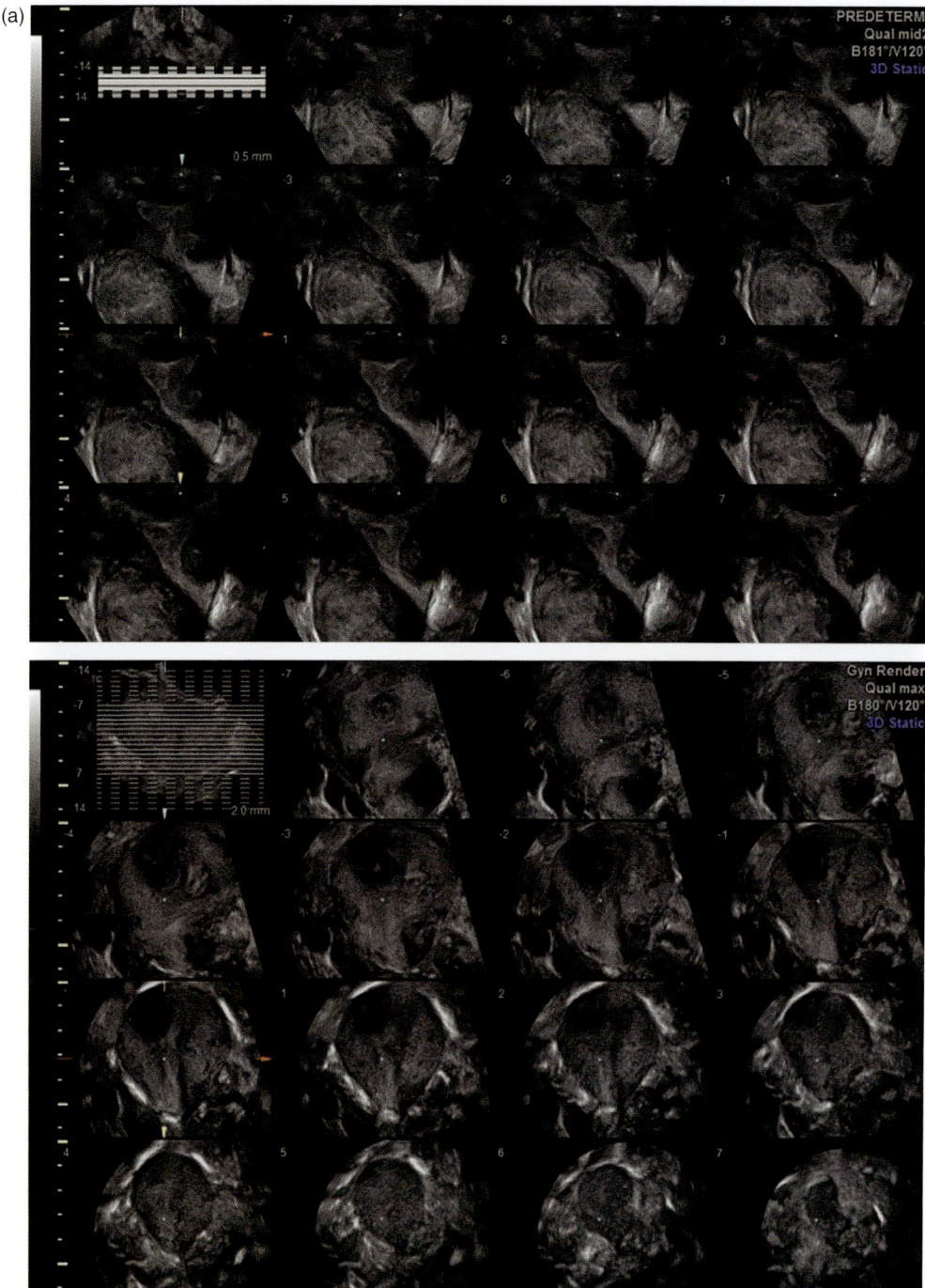

Figure 4.23 The TUI modality provides multiple tomographic sections of the uterus, allowing for exact delineation of the myoma within the myometrial wall and in relation to the endometrial cavity. Four examples are shown.

(b)

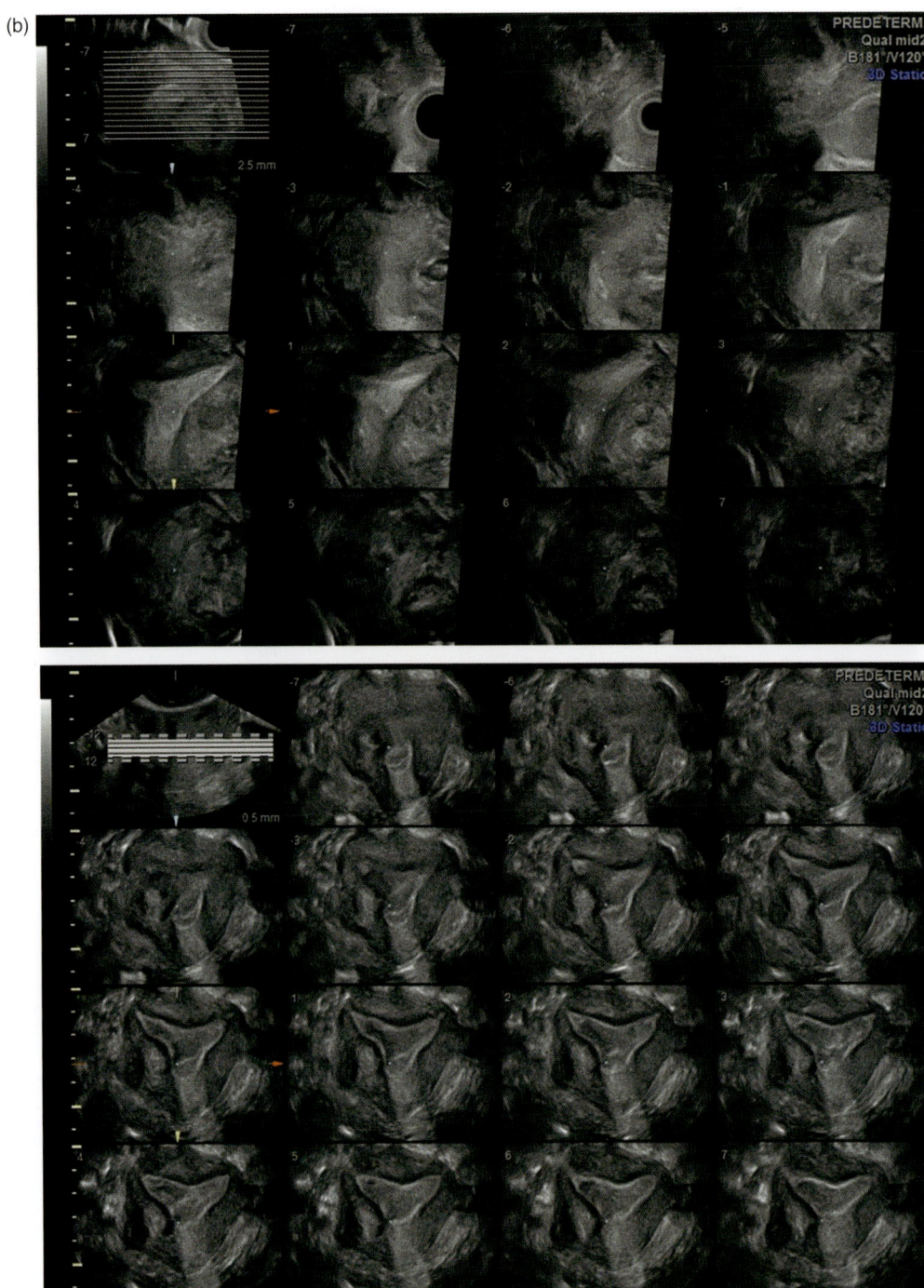

Figure 4.23 (cont.)

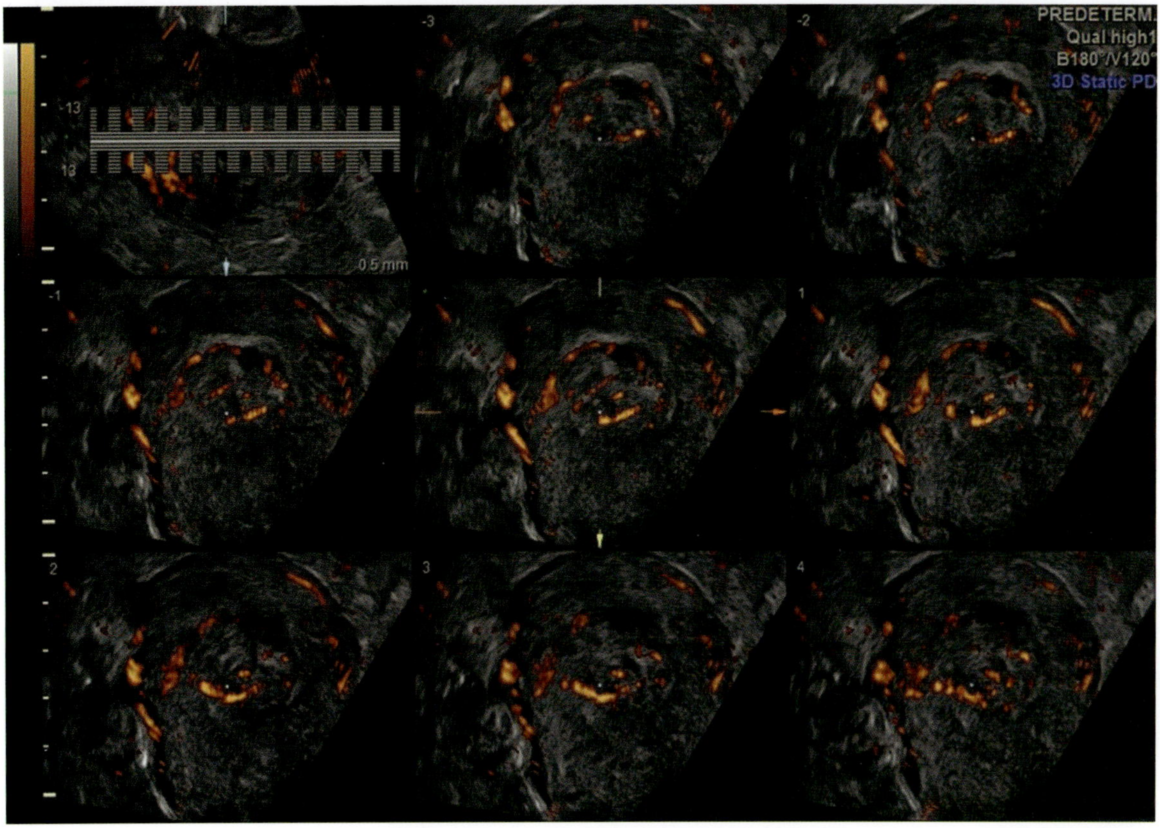

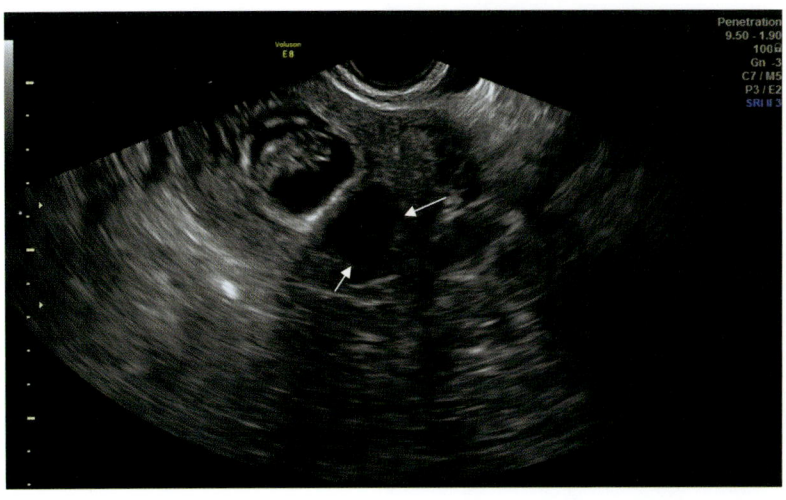

Figure 4.24 Several 3D modalities can be combined; for example, the 3D power Doppler and the TUI demonstrating a submucosal fibroid with peripheral vascularity.

Figure 4.25 A uterus containing a pregnancy of nine weeks' gestation with a single intramural myoma (arrows).

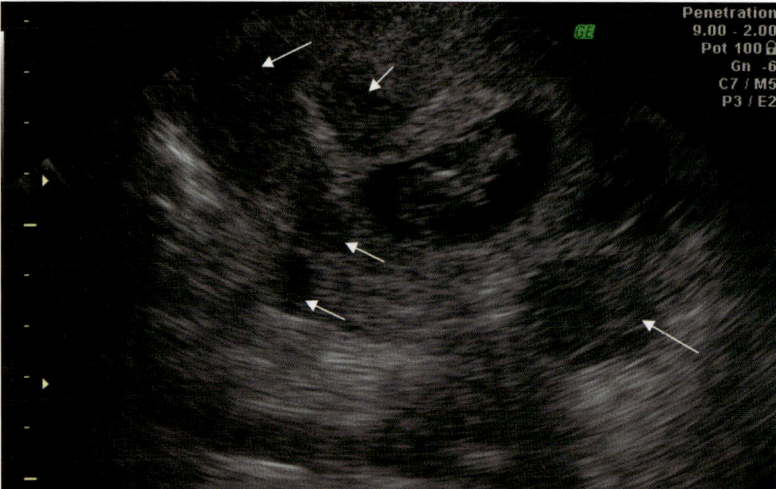

Figure 4.26 Gestation of nine weeks implanted in a polymyomatous uterus.

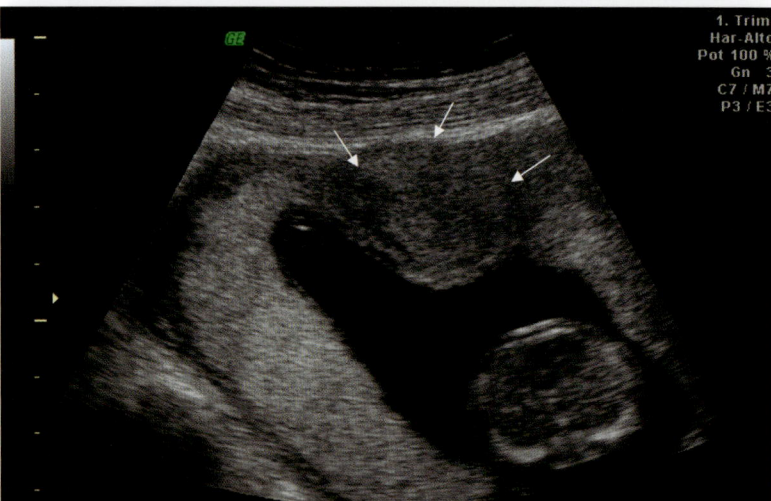

Figure 4.27 Gestation of 14 weeks, with myoma (arrows) deforming the amniotic cavity.

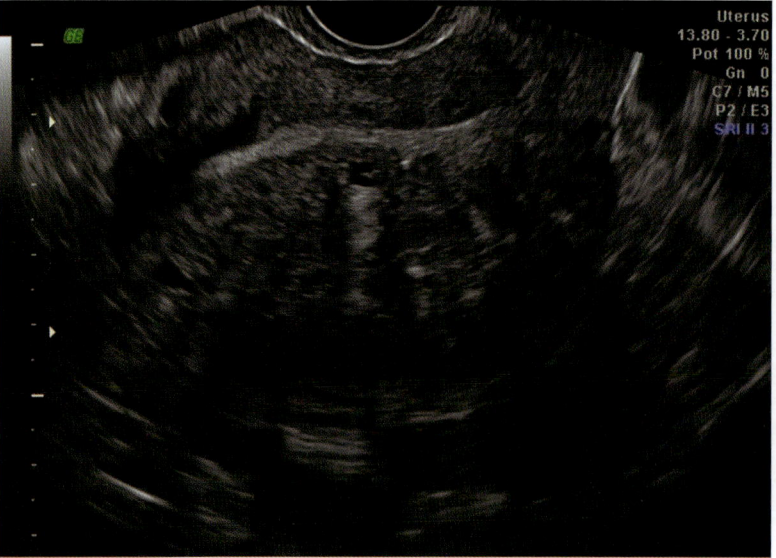

Figure 4.28 Classic signs of adenomyosis on 2D ultrasound scan: loss of endometrium–myometrium interface, thickening of the myometrium, differences in thickness of myometrial walls, heterogeneous hyperechogenicity, subendometrial cysts in the form of anechoic lagoons, and subendometrial striations.

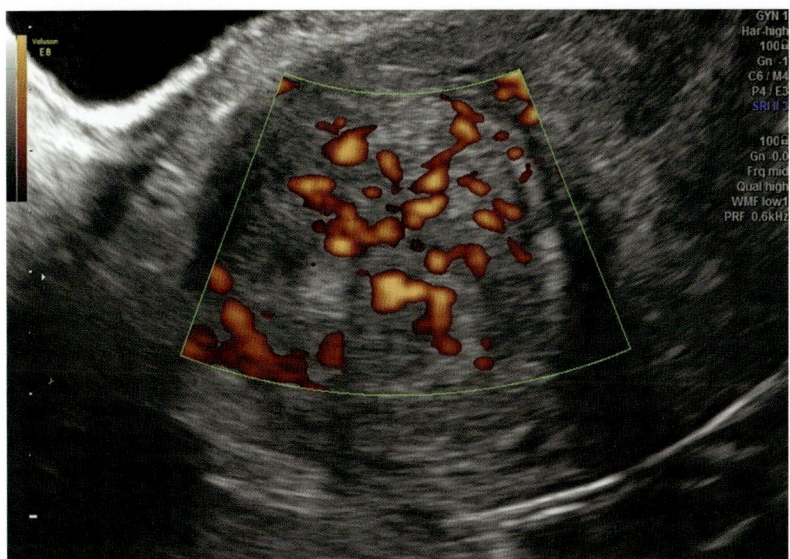

Figure 4.29 Power Doppler analysis demonstrates an uninterrupted vascular pattern in this case of adenomyosis, though the paths are irregular and not perpendicular to the endometrium as typically seen.

(a)

(b)

(c)

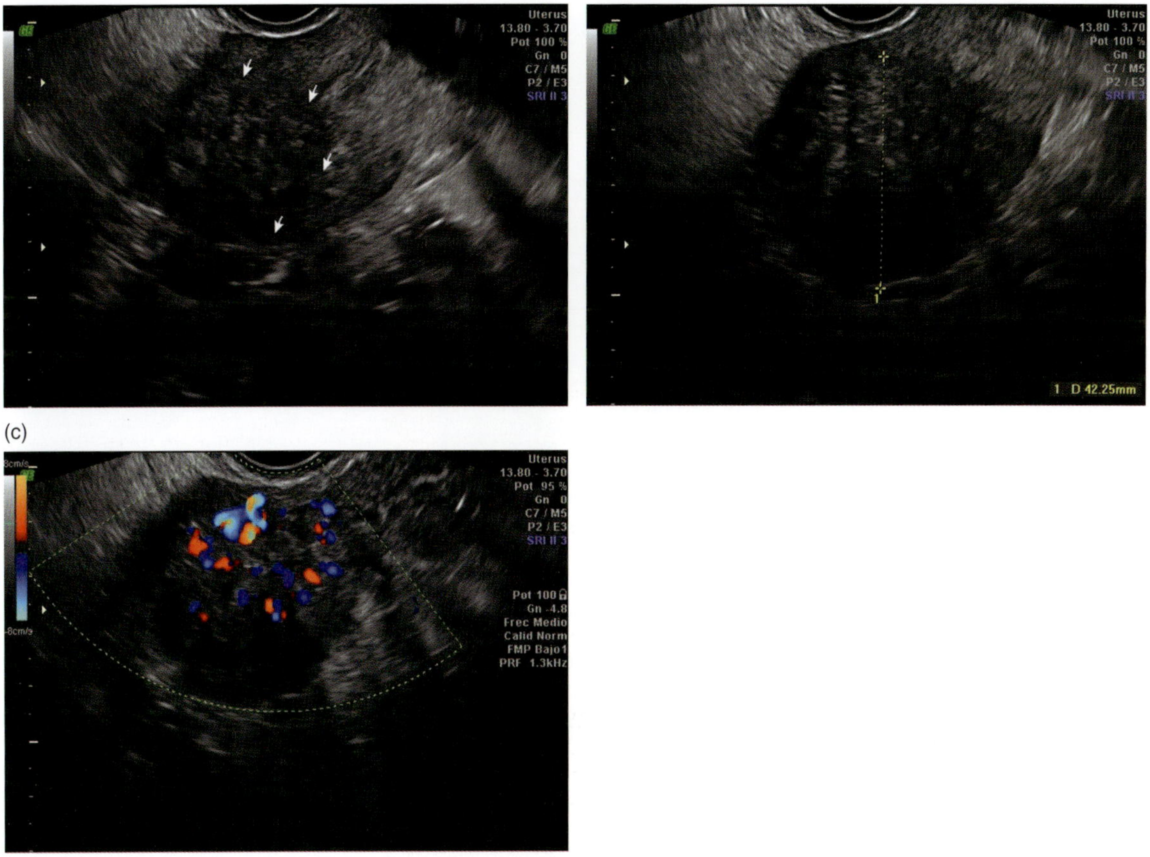

Figure 4.30 (a) Adenomyoma; arrows demonstrate a poorly defined border. (b) It is usually located within the uterine fundus. (c) Doppler modality helps to differentiate from fibroids.

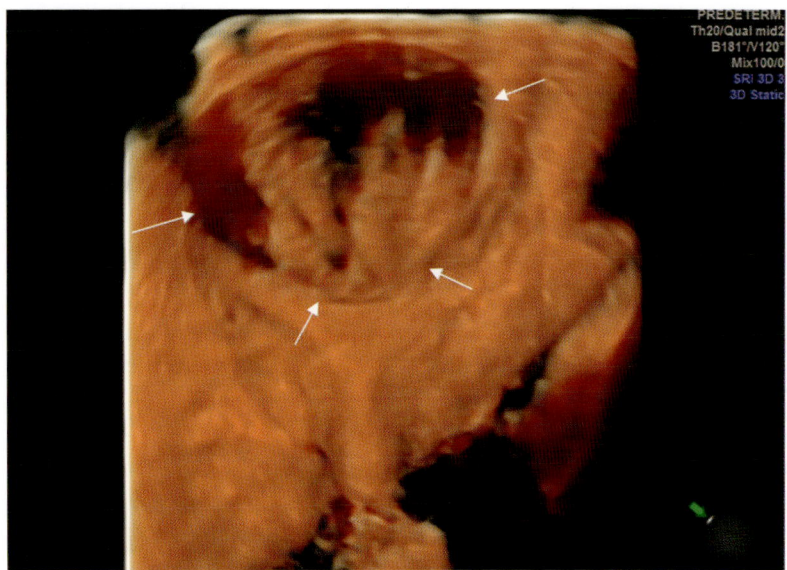

Figure 4.31 Adenomyoma (arrows) of the uterine fundus demonstrated with HDLive.

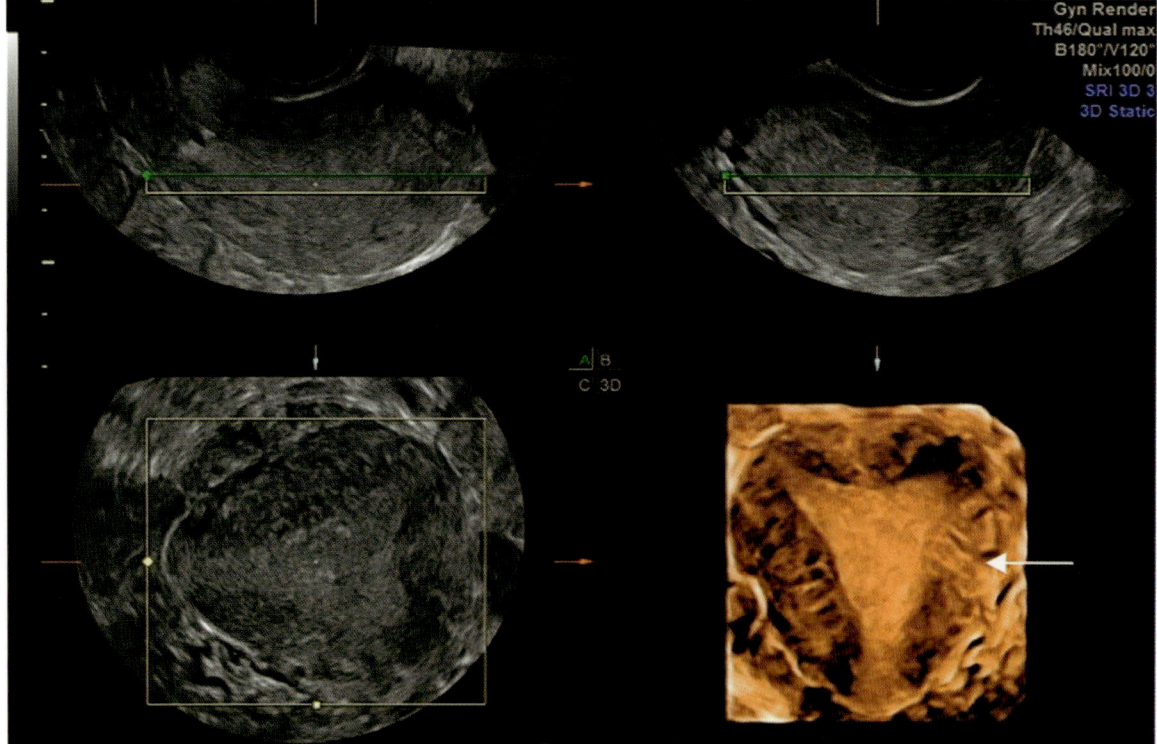

Figure 4.32 3D multiplanar view of a uterus with an area of adenomyosis located in the left lateral wall: effacement and lack of definition of the limits of the JZ, with infiltration towards the myometrium (arrow).

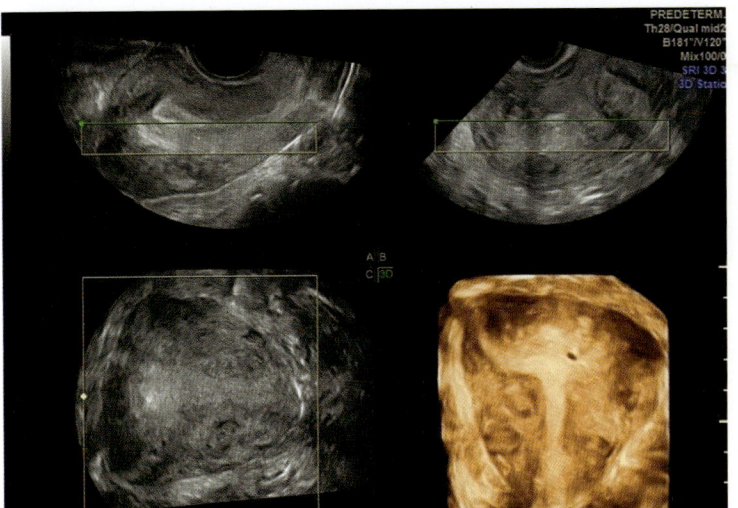

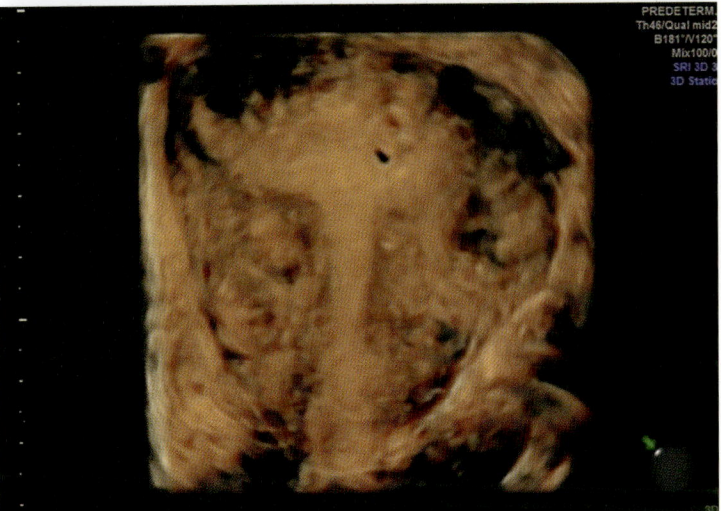

Figure 4.33 3D ultrasound multiplanar mode and reconstruction of images with the HDLive mode. Three cases of diffuse adenomyosis and 'tree sign' are shown. The right lower corner of the image demonstrates the direction of light. The trunk of the tree is formed by the cervical canal and the lower part of the endometrial cavity. Completing the image of this tree is the rest of the endometrial cavity and adenomyotic implants with feeding blood vessels.

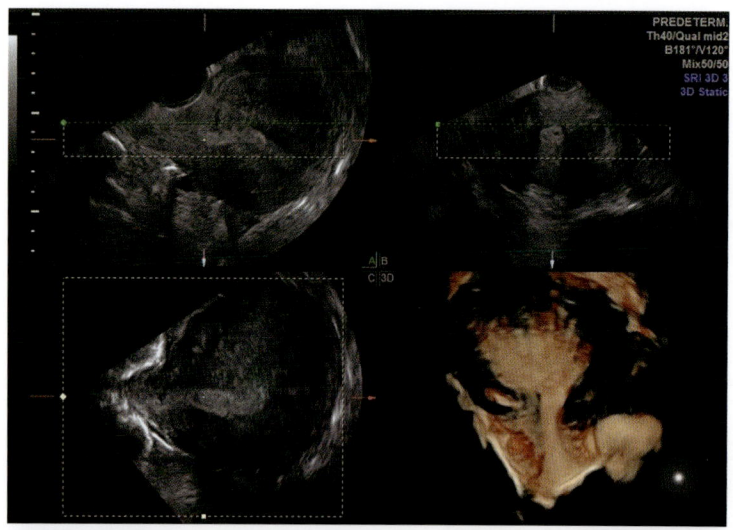

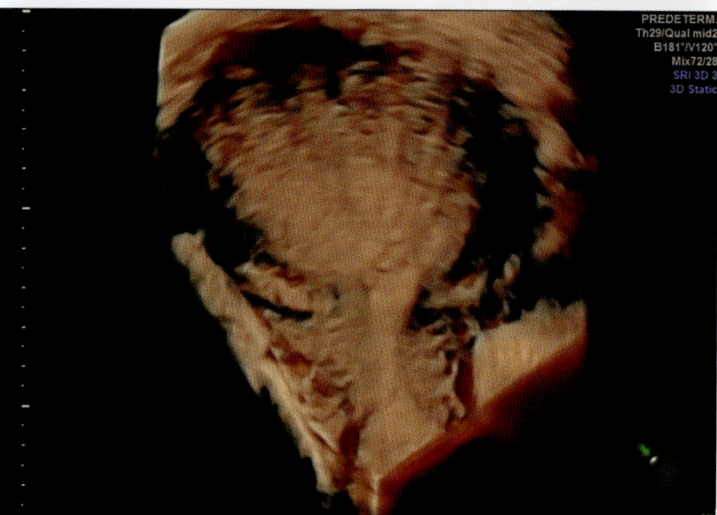

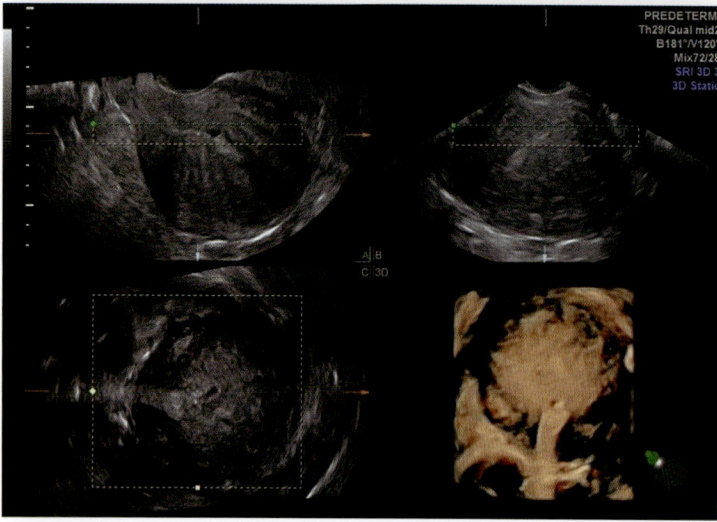

Figure 4.33 (cont.)

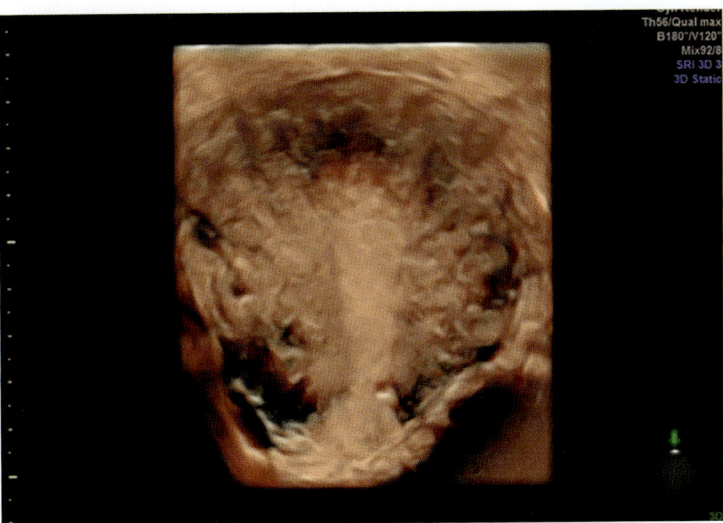

Figure 4.33 (cont.)

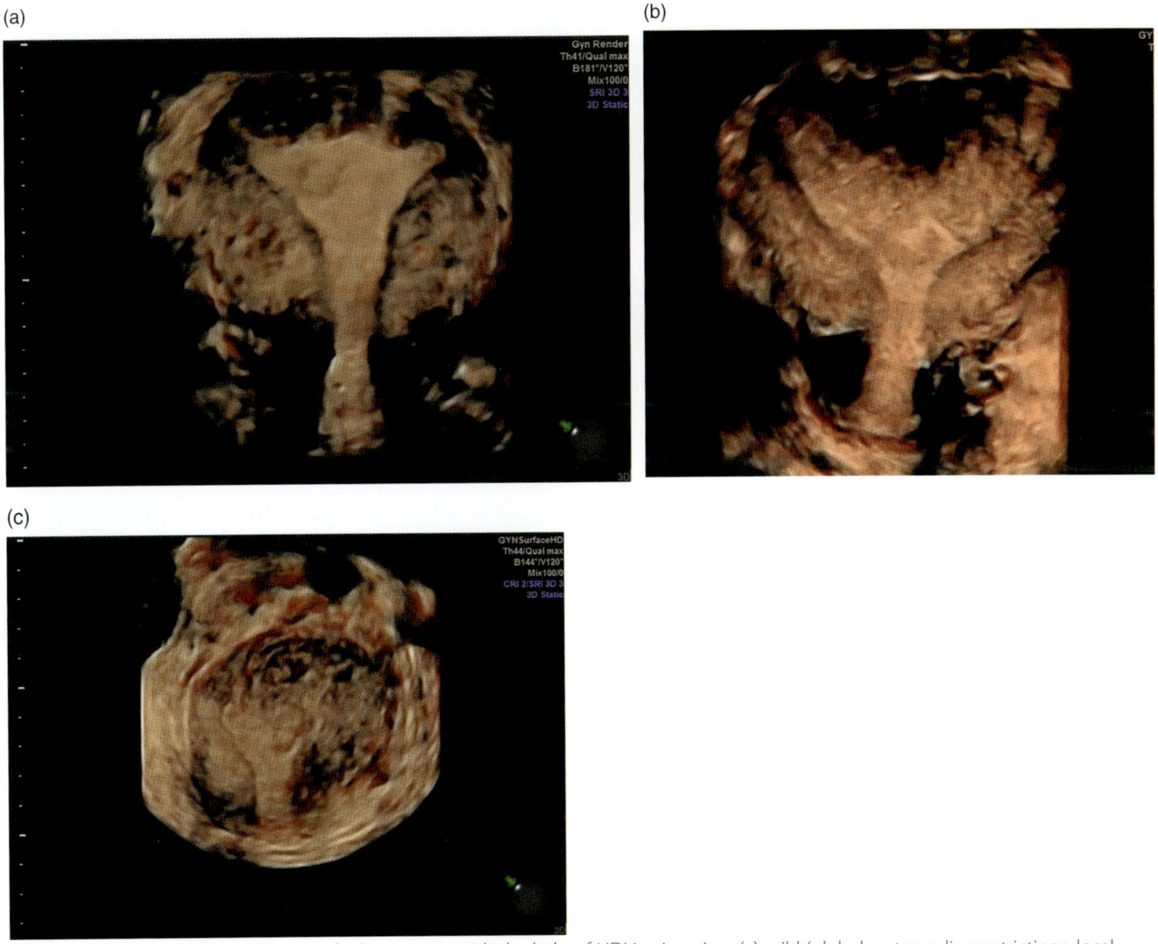

(a)

(b)

(c)

Figure 4.34 Proposed classification of adenomyosis with the help of HDLive imaging: (a) mild (globular uterus, linear striations, local disruptions and heterogeneous myometrium); (b) moderate (myometrial cysts and adenomyotic implants, or adenomyoma); (c) severe, with the described 'tree sign'.

References

1. Schwartz PE, Kelly MG. Malignant transformation of myomas: myth or reality? *Obstet Gynecol Clin North Am* 2006;**33**(1):183–98.

2. Bulletti C, Coccia ME, Battistoni S, Borini A. Endometriosis and infertility. *J Assist Reprod Genet* 2010;**27**(8):441–7.

3. Benaglia L, Cardellicchio L, Leonardi M, et al. Asymptomatic adenomyosis and embryo implantation in IVF cycles. *Reprod Biomed Online* 2014;**29**(5):606–11.

4. Vercellini P, Consonni D, Dridi D, et al. Uterine adenomyosis and in vitro fertilization outcome: a systematic review and meta-analysis. *Hum Reprod* 2014;**29**(5):964–77.

5. Tremellen K, Thalluri V. Impact of adenomyosis on pregnancy rates in IVF treatment. *Reprod Biomed Online* 2013;**26**(3):299–300.

6. Salim R, Riris S, Saab W, et al. Adenomyosis reduces pregnancy rates in infertile women undergoing IVF. *Reprod Biomed Online* 2012;**25**(3):273–7.

7. Maheshwari A, Gurunath S, Fatima F, Bhattacharya S. Adenomyosis and subfertility: a systematic review of prevalence, diagnosis, treatment and fertility outcomes. *Hum Reprod Update* 2012;**18**(4):374–92.

8. Pritts, E, Parker, W, Olive, D. Fibroids and infertility: an updated systematic review of the evidence. *Fertil Steril* 2009;**91**:1215–23.

9. Ivo Brosens I, Kunz G., Benagiano G. Is adenomyosis the neglected phenotype of an endomyometrial dysfunction syndrome? *Gynecol Surg* 2012;**9**(2):131–7.

10. Dueholm M, Lundorf E, Hansen ES, Ledertoug S, Olesen F. Evaluation of the uterine cavity with magnetic resonance imaging, transvaginal sonography, hysterosonographic examination, and diagnostic hysteroscopy. *Fertil Steril* 2001;**76**:350–7.

11. Munro MG, Critchley HO, Fraser IS, FIGO Menstrual Disorders Working Group. The FIGO classification of causes of abnormal uterine bleeding in the reproductive years. *Fertil Steril* 2011;**95** (7):2204–8.

12. Wamsteker K, Emanuel MH, de Kruif JH. Transcervical hysteroscopic resection of submucous fibroids for abnormal uterine bleeding: results regarding the degree of intramural extension. *Obstet Gynecol* 1993;**82**:736–40

13. Lasmar RB, Xinmei Z, Indman PD, Celeste RK, Di Spiezio Sardo A. Feasibility of a new system of classification of submucous myomas: a multicenter study. *Fertil Steril* 2011;**95**(6):2073–7.

14. Mavrelos D, Naftalin J, Hoo W, et al. Preoperative assessment of submucous fibroids by three-dimensional saline contrast sonohysterography. *Ultrasound Obstet Gynecol* 2011;**38**:350–4.

15. Mohan P, Hamblin M, Vogelzang RU. Artery embolization and its effect on fertility. *J Vasc Interv Radiol* 2013;**24**:925–30.

16. Qidwai IG, Caughey AB, Jacoby AF. Obstetric outcomes in women with sonographically identified uterine leiomyomata. *Obstet Gynecol* 2006;**107**:376–82.

17. Laughlin SK, Herring AH, Savitz DA, et al. Pregnancy-related fibroid reduction. *Fertil Steril* 2010;**94**:2421–3.

18. Reinhold C, Tafazoli F, Mehio A, et al. Uterine adenomyosis: endovaginal US and MR imaging features with histopathologic correlation. *Radiographics* 1999;**19**:S147–60.

19. Fedele L, Bianchi S, Dorta M, et al. Transvaginal ultrasonography in the diagnosis of diffuse adenomyosis. *Fertil Steril* 1992;**58**:94–7.

20. Jayaprakasan K, Panchal S. *Ultrasound in Subfertility: Routine Applications and Diagnostic Challenges.* Jaypee Brothers Medical Publishers, 2014.

21. Ludwin A, Ludwin I, Kudla M, et al. Diagnostic accuracy of three-dimensional sonohysterography compared with office hysteroscopic and its interrater/intrarater agreement in uterine cavity assessment after hysterocopicmetroplasty. *Fertil Steril* 2014;**101**(5) 1392–9.

22. Exacoustos C, Brienza L, Di Giovanni A, et al. Adenomyosis: three dimensional sonographic findings of the junction zone and correlation with histology. *Ultrasound Obstet Gynecol* 2011;**37**(4): 471–9.

23. Luciano DE, Exacoustos C, Albrecht L, et al. Three-dimensional ultrasound in diagnosis of adenomyosis: histologic correlation with ultrasound targeted biopsies of the uterus. *J Minim Invasive Gynecol* 2013;**20**(6):803–10.

Sonographic Assessment of Congenital Uterine Anomalies

5

Sotirios H. Saravelos and Tin-Chiu Li

Introduction

Congenital uterine anomalies (CUAs) are gaining increasing attention in the field of gynaecological ultrasound for a number of reasons: first, they appear to be of relatively high prevalence in both selected and unselected groups of women [1,2]; second, they appear to have a significant impact on reproductive outcomes and, on occasion, in adolescent symptomatology [3,4]; third, there has been a recent surge in relevant publications, which has culminated in a new international classification [5], and also a new international consensus for diagnosis [6]. Three-dimensional (3D) ultrasound is now recommended as the gold standard method for diagnosis, which implies that gynaecologists and/or sonographers may be expected to attain the correct diagnoses and classification of CUA for women presenting to them with, and even without, symptomatology.

The aim of the current chapter is to cover a number of areas relating to CUA. First, current and previous classifications of CUA will be described; second, the diagnostic accuracy of different diagnostic modalities will be presented; third, the prevalence of CUA will be outlined; fourth, the clinical implications of each CUA will be ascertained; and finally, a practical step-by-step guide to diagnosing CUA using 3D ultrasound will be suggested.

Which Classification Should Be Used?

One cannot set out to diagnose a CUA without knowledge of an appropriate classification system to apply to their findings. The evolution of the classifications for CUA has been interesting to observe. The very first attempts at classifying CUA appear to have originated from Cruveilher, Foerster and von Rokitansky in the mid-nineteenth century [7]. Following a series of further publications describing various patterns of CUA, Buttram and Gibbons presented a classification, which was based on both the anatomy of the anomaly and the degree of embryological failure that occurred at the Mullerian duct system [8]. This classification would later form the backbone of the most well-known classification used to date: the American Fertility Society (AFS; nowadays American Society for Reproductive Medicine (ASRM)) classification [9]. This classification contains a schematic graph of seven different types of anomalies, and has served the research and clinical community for almost 30 years. However, as imaging has become more accurate, new proposals of classifications emerged, which intended to be more comprehensive. This included the 'VCUAM classification', which individually described the anatomical anomalies of the vagina, cervix, uterus and associated malformations in order to systematically describe and report all genital anomalies [10]. It also included the 'Embryological clinical classification for female genitourinary problems' proposed by Acien and Acien originally in 1992 and subsequently updated in 2011 [7,11], which included as a basis the different embryological pathways and stages of development that have been observed.

Finally, most recently, the European Society for Human Reproduction and Embryology (ESHRE) and the European Society for Gynaecological Endoscopy (ESGE) jointly formed a working group in order to create the newest classification system. This ESHRE/ESGE classification was published jointly in 2013 and was achieved through a structured voting procedure (known as the Delphi procedure), involving a wider number of experts of the field [5]. This classification consists of descriptions for all female genital tract malformations (similar to the VCUAM classification) and also provides schematic guides to allow for diagnosis and differentiation between different anomalies (similar to the AFS classification). It also encourages objective measurements of the uterus, so as to accurately differentiate between subtypes of CUA. In particular, the septate uterus has been defined as the

Table 5.1 The percentage sensitivity, specificity, positive predictive value (PPV), negative predictive value (NPV) and overall accuracy along with the 95 per cent CI for each methodology commonly used to diagnose CUA.

Diagnostic method	Studies (n)	Sensitivity (%)	Specificity (%)	PPV (%)	NPV (%)	Accuracy (%)
Hysteroscopy Laparoscopy		Used as gold standard				
MRI		At least as accurate as 3D US				
3D US	11	98.3 (95.6–100)	99.4 (98.4–100)	99.2 (97.6–100)	93.9 (84.2–100)	97.6 (94.3–100)
SIS	13	95.8 (91.1–100)	97.4 (94.1–100)	97.8 (93.3–100)	94.6 (87.6–100)	96.5 (93.4–99.5)
2D US	9	67.3 (51.0–83.7)	98.1 (96.0–100)	94.6 (89.4–99.8)	86.0 (73.7–98.3)	86.6 (81.3–91.8)
HSG	16	84.6 (74.4–94.9)	89.4 (80.0–100)	83.6 (74.6–92.6)	89.1 (79.7–98.5)	86.9 (79.8–94.0)

Source: adapted from [6].

uterus with normal outline and an internal indentation at the fundal midline exceeding 50 per cent of the uterine wall thickness, while the bicorporeal (or bicornuate uterus) has been defined as a uterus with the presence of an external indentation at the fundal midline exceeding 50 per cent of the uterine wall thickness. The ESHRE/ESGE classification for the diagnosis of CUA is shown in Figure 5.1.

However, it is worth noting that although the most modern and updated classification is the ESHRE/ESGE classification, it has received criticism from a group of authors who observed an increase in the diagnosis of the septate uterus when using this classification compared with former classifications. These authors advised caution when using this new classification, as they fear it may cause confusion in terms of clinical management [12].

What Is the Most Accurate Investigation?

This is a question that has puzzled clinicians for several years. One of the reasons is that there are few anatomical organs that can be assessed with so many different investigative modalities. For the female genital tract this includes: 2D ultrasound, 3D ultrasound, saline infusion sonography (SIS), magnetic resonance imaging (MRI), hysterosalpingography (HSG), hysteroscopy and laparoscopy. Until recently, the methods used were primarily dependent on local availability and clinician preference, rather than rates of diagnostic accuracy [1]. However, recently an international consensus (coined the Thessaloniki Consensus) was published, which included a systematic review of 38 studies examining the

diagnostic accuracy of all the aforementioned methodologies against the historical gold standard of combined hysteroscopy and laparoscopy [6]. The most accurate methods in descending order (presented here as mean accuracy (95 per cent confidence interval)) were found to be: 3D ultrasound 97.6 per cent (94.3–100), SIS 96.5 per cent (93.4–99.5), HSG 86.9 per cent (79.8–94.0) and 2D ultrasound 86.6 per cent (81.3–91.8). Although no studies were found examining MRI as a screening tool (which is understandable due to the cost, frequent lack of availability and time required for assessment), in direct comparisons with 3D ultrasound it was considered to be at least as accurate [13]. The sensitivity, specificity, positive predictive value (PPV), negative predictive value (NPV) and overall accuracy for each methodology are presented in Table 5.1.

In view of these findings, the Thessaloniki Consensus concluded that 3D ultrasound should be considered as the gold standard for diagnosis of female genital anomalies, supplemented by MRI and/or hysteroscopy and laparoscopy for complex or inconclusive cases [6]. This should not come as a surprise, as in addition to the high diagnostic accuracy rates, 3D ultrasound offers other significant advantages such as being non-invasive, time efficient, cost-effective, readily available, objective and highly reproducible [14].

What Is the True Prevalence?

Until recently, the true prevalence of CUA had not been precisely determined. The reported prevalence in different populations was in fact so inconsistent that it was difficult to even ascertain whether it was

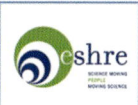

ESHRE/ESGE classification
Female genital tract anomalies

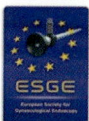

	Uterine anomaly		Cervical/vaginal anomaly	
	Main class	*Sub-class*	*Co-existent class*	
U0	Normal uterus		**C0**	Normal cervix
U1	Dysmorphic uterus	**a.** T-shaped	**C1**	Septate cervix
		b. Infantilis	**C2**	Double 'normal' cervix
		c. Others		
U2	Septate uterus	**a.** Partial	**C3**	Unilateral cervical aplasia
		b. Complete		
			C4	Cervical aplasia
U3	Bicorporeal uterus	**a.** Partial		
		b. Complete		
		c. Bicorporeal septate	**V0**	Normal vagina
U4	Hemi-uterus	**a.** With rudimentary cavity (communicating or not horn)	**V1**	Longitudinal non-obstructing vaginal septum
		b. Without rudimentary cavity (horn without cavity/no horn)	**V2**	Longitudinal obstructing vaginal septum
U5	Aplastic	**a.** With rudimentary cavity (bi- or unilateral horn)	**V3**	Transverse vaginal septum and/or imperforate hymen
		b. Without rudimentary cavity (bi- or unilateral uterine remnants/aplasia)	**V4**	Vaginal aplasia
U6	Unclassified malformations			
U			*C*	*V*

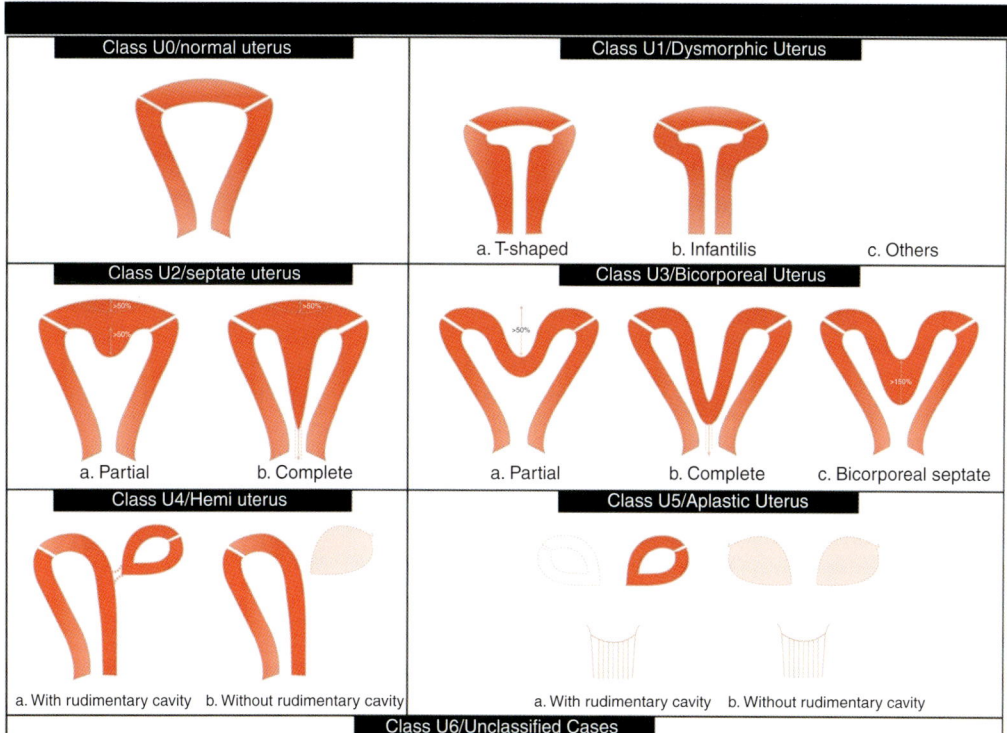

Figure 5.1 The ESHRE/ESGE classification of female genital tract anomalies (from [5]).

Table 5.2 Estimates of prevalence (mean percentage with 95 per cent CI) of subtypes of CUA according to population group

Population	Total (%)	Arcuate[a] (%)	Septate (%)	Bicorporeal (%)	Didelphys[b] (%)	Unicornuate (%)	Others (%)
General	5.5 (3.5–8.5)	3.9 (2.1–7.1)	2.3 (1.8–2.9)	0.4 (0.2–0.6)	0.3 (0.1–0.6)	0.1 (0.1–0.3)	0.1 (0–2.2)
Infertile	8.0 (5.3–12.0)	1.8 (0.8–4.1)	3.0 (1.3–6.7)	1.1 (0.6–2.0)	0.3 (0.2–0.5)	0.5 (0.3–0.8)	0.9 (0.4–1.8)
Recurrent miscarriage	13.3 (8.9–20)	2.9 (0.9–9.6)	5.3 (1.7–16.8)	2.1 (1.4–3)	0.6 (0.3–1.4)	0.5 (0.3–1.1)	0.9 (0.1–12.6)
Recurrent miscarriage and infertility	24.5 (18.3–32.8)*	6.6 (2.8–15.7)	15.4 (12.5–19)	4.7 (2.9–7.6)	2.1 (1.4–3.2)	3.1 (2–4.7)	0.3 (0–2.3)

[a] The arcuate uterus does not exist as an entity in the ESHRE/ESGE classification; therefore these anomalies would be expected to fall within either the normal group or the septate group.

[b] The didelphys uterus is considered as a bicorporeal uterus with a double cervix in the ESHRE/ESGE classification.

Source: adapted from [3].

a common or rare problem [1]. This was predominantly due to investigators using different methodologies with different diagnostic accuracy rates, as described above. However, recent meta-analyses have now managed to control for this bias, and at present, the prevalence (mean (95 per cent CI)) appears to be in the order of 5.5 per cent (3.5–8.5) in the unselected population, 8.0 per cent (5.3–12) in the infertile population, 13.3 per cent (8.9–20.0) in the recurrent miscarriage population and 24.5 per cent (18.3–32.8) in the combined recurrent miscarriage and infertility population [2]. The prevalence of CUA according to subtypes is presented in Table 5.2.

Are there Any Clinical Implications?

Perhaps the most important question that arises once a diagnosis of a CUA has been made is: does it affect the patient, and how? The answer can vary according to the type of anomaly, the woman's age and her fertility wishes. In adolescent gynaecology the commonest presentations encountered relating to CUA are primary amenorrhoea, cyclical pelvic pain or both. In the first case, the cause may be an aplastic or absent uterus, such as the Mayer–Rokitansky–Kuster–Hauser (MRKH) syndrome. In the second case, the cause may be an obstructive anomaly, such as an obstructive vaginal septum or the presence of unicornuate and active non-communicating rudimentary horn. In the third case, the cause may be vaginal or cervicovaginal agenesis with a functional uterus [15]. It must be noted that in women with significant CUA, there is a high rate of concurrent

renal tract abnormalities, which can reach up to 80 per cent [1]. Therefore, it is important to carry out urinary and renal system imaging if uterine anomalies are diagnosed. As adolescent gynaecology falls outside the remit of the present chapter, the clinical implications of CUA in women of reproductive age in particular will be expanded upon in more detail.

Recent meta-analyses have been conducted for women of reproductive age to ascertain the impact of CUA. They have, by and large, concluded that these anomalies are associated with reduced pregnancy rates, increased miscarriage rates, increased preterm delivery rates, increased rate of malposition at delivery, decreased birthweight and increased perinatal mortality rates [3,4]. Interestingly, case control studies have suggested that the resection of uterine septi is associated with a reduced risk of miscarriage when compared to women with untreated septi; however, it is important to note that this has yet to be tested within the context of a randomized controlled trial (RCT) [4,16]. The reproductive impact of each type of CUA is presented in Table 5.3.

How to Diagnose with Ultrasound

Conventional 2D transvaginal ultrasound is a less expensive way of assessing uterine morphology and screening for uterine anomalies. Timing the ultrasound evaluation during the second half of the cycle is more appropriate for evaluating the uterus for congenital anomalies as secretory endometrium, being

Table 5.3 The relative risk (with 95 per cent CI) of various reproductive outcomes according to subtypes of CUA

Anomaly	Conception rate	First trimester miscarriage	Second trimester miscarriage	Preterm labour	Foetal malpresentation at term
All anomalies	0.87 (0.68–1.11)	2.56 (0.89–7.38)	1.94 (0.92–4.09)	2.97 (2.08–4.23)***	3.87 (2.42–6.18)***
Arcuate	1.03 (0.94–1.12)	1.35 (0.81–2.26)	2.39 (1.33–4.27)**	1.53 (0.70–3.34)	2.53 (1.54–4.18)***
Septate	0.86 (0.77–0.96)*	2.89 (2.02–4.14)***	2.22 (0.74–6.65)	2.14 (1.48–3.11)***	6.24 (4.05–9.62)***
Bicornuate	0.86 (0.61–1.21)	3.40 (1.18–9.76)*	2.23 (1.05–5.15)*	2.55 (1.57–4.17)***	5.38 (3.15–9.19)***
Didelphys	0.9 (0.79–1.04)	1.10 (0.21–5.66)	1.39 (0.44–4.41)	3.58 (2.00–6.40)***	3.70 (2.04–6.70)***
Unicornuate	0.74 (0.39–1.41)	2.15 (1.03–4.47)*	2.22 (0.53–9.19)	3.47 (1.94–6.22)***	2.74 (1.30–5.77)**

* $p < 0.05$; ** $p < 0.01$; *** $p < 0.001$.
Source: adapted from [2].

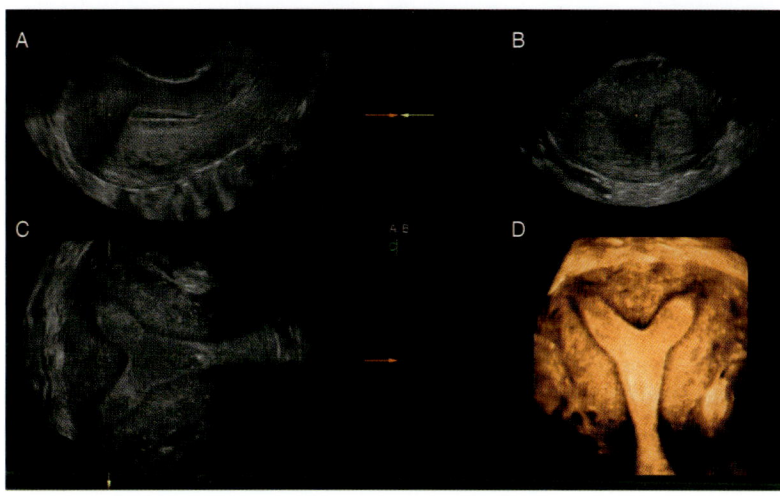

Figure 5.2 3D ultrasound scan of a subseptate uterus showing simultaneous display of longitudinal plane (a), transverse plane showing two endometrial echoes (b), and coronal plane (c), unique for 3D ultrasound. (d) Rendered view of coronal plane demonstrating a subseptate uterus.

more hyperechoic, is therefore easy to visualize, allowing for better visualization of the contours of the endometrial cavity. Seeing a double endometrial complex on a transverse plane is indicative of a uterine anomaly (Figure 5.2b), which could be a bicornuate (bicorporeal), septate, subseptate or arcuate (normal variant) uterus (Figure 5.3). Systematic scanning through the longitudinal plane of the uterus may reveal a uterine complex, which then disappears while moving to the opposite side, followed by appearance of a second uterine complex suggesting that the uterus may be bicornuate. The transverse plane provides more information and widely placed double endometrial echoes especially at the upper portion of the uterus (towards the fundus) and an indentation at the fundus on an oblique plane (if obtainable) are typical of a bicornuate or bicorporeal uterus. However, 3D ultrasound (described below in detail), through its unique feature of providing the coronal plane of the uterus (Figure 5.2c), facilitates simultaneous visualization of both external (serosal surface) and internal (endometrial) contours of the uterine fundus and can correctly classify the uterine anomaly into bicornuate, septate, subseptate or arcuate uterus [1,2].

Uterus didelphys (double uterus), although rare, also shows two endometrial complexes in the transverse plane of conventional 2D ultrasound, while 3D ultrasound and the clinical demonstration of two cervices confirm the diagnosis (Figure 5.4). Two uterine horns may be symmetrical or asymmetrical and two separate vaginas may be seen on speculum

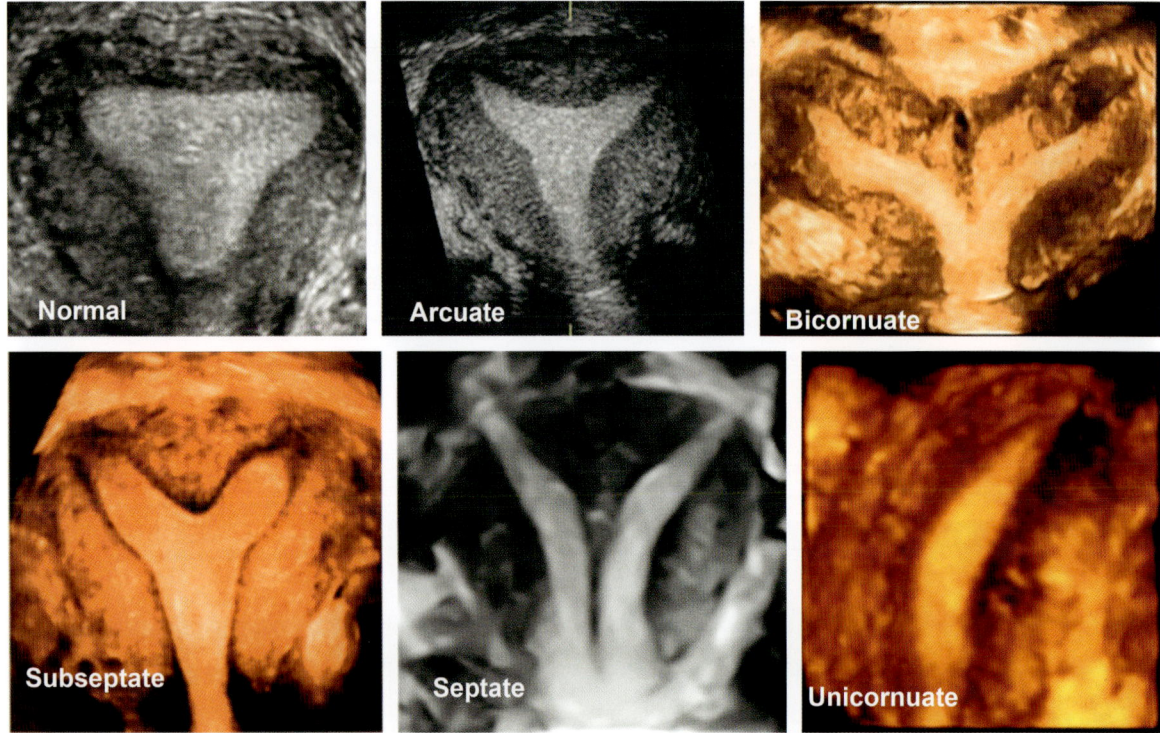

Figure 5.3 Coronal view of uteri showing uteri of different shapes.

examination. In cases of unicornuate/hemi-uterus, a normal-looking long axis of the uterus is seen on one side in the pelvis with no or a rudimentary uterine shadow on the other side. A rudimentary or severely hypoplastic uterine horn is seen as an isoechoic pear-shaped structure with or without a central thin echogenic endometrial line (Figure 5.5). On the transverse plane, at the level of the fundus, a beak-like projection from the endometrial shadow (cornua) is seen only on one side. 3D ultrasound, again, is confirmatory, demonstrating a banana-shaped uterine cavity and single interstitial portion of fallopian tube in the coronal plane (Figure 5.3). Saline infusion sonography has been suggested as a method for diagnosing rudimentary horns, as saline can be clearly seen in the unicornuate uterus, with no passage into the rudimentary horn.

As mentioned previously, 3D ultrasound is now the recommended method of diagnosing CUA, and has been recognized as the modern-day gold standard [6]. As a result, in this section a practical step-by-step guide will be presented on how to achieve a clear 3D ultrasound coronal image of the uterus, in order to correlate it with the ESHRE/ESGE classification and correctly classify CUA (Figure 5.6).

Step 1

An appropriate ultrasound machine with 3D capabilities and a functioning 3D transvaginal probe is required. For best image results, the gynaecological setting should be selected, with maximum quality of acquisition and maximum angle of sweep (typically 120 degrees).

Step 2

The uterus should be identified in the sagittal/longitudinal plane (unless it is a double/didelphis uterus, in which case it should be identified in the transverse plane). The depth of the window should be such that the uterine body occupies at least three-quarters of the screen. The focus should be aimed at the level of the endometrial cavity. The 3D function should be activated and both the operator and the patient should remain completely still while the acquisition takes place. The acquisition should incorporate the entire uterine body (or bodies).

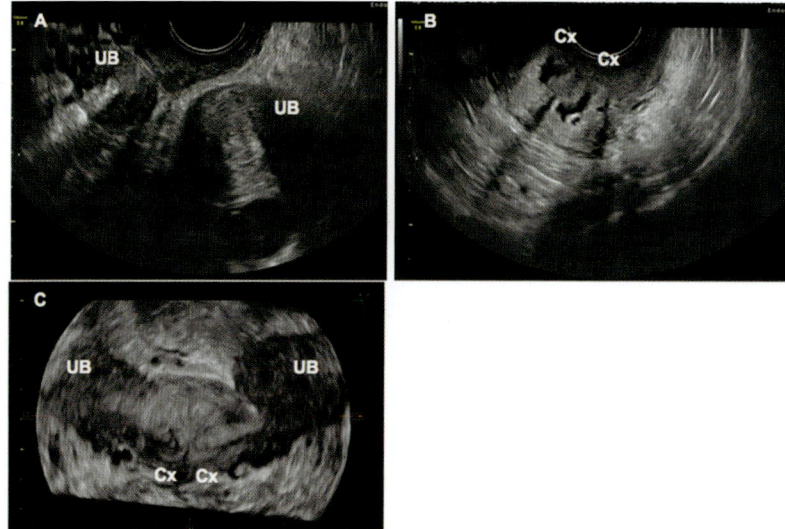

Figure 5.4 Transverse plane of two endometrial complexes with uterine body (UB) (a), two cervices (Cx) with anechoic mucous (b) in uterus didelphys (complete bicorporeal uterus). (c) 3D coronal plane of uterus didelphys demonstrating widely divergent uterine bodies (UB) and two cervices (Cx).

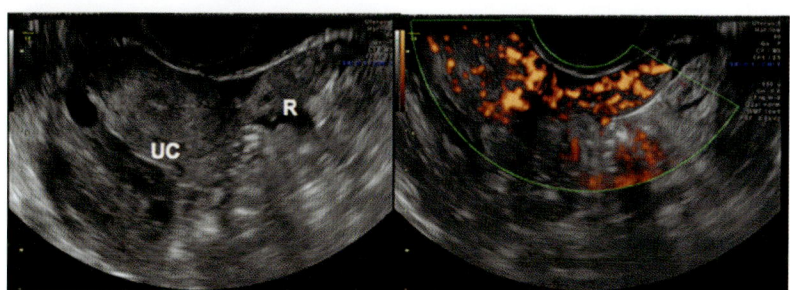

Figure 5.5 Unicornuate uterus (UC) with a rudimentary horn (R) in transverse view. Doppler picture on the right side showing vascular connection to the rudimentary horn.

Step 3

Following the 3D acquisition, the uterus will appear on screen in three separate planes (A, B, C) which can be viewed in various different modes according to the ultrasound machine used (most commonly the Sectional Planes mode and the Render mode). The operator should familiarize him/herself with manipulation of the uterus in the three planes using the X, Y and Z functions on the console.

Step 4

If Render mode is selected, a region of interest (ROI) box will appear on the screen. The ROI box should be manipulated so that it covers the endometrial cavity in its entirety. The green line of the ROI box indicates the direction of rendering and this should ideally be placed on top.

Step 5

Final adjustments can be made, such as curving the ROI box (ideally in the curvature of the endometrial cavity) and applying different render options (HDLive produces a realistic image). Once the operator is satisfied with the 3D image, this can be enlarged and compared to the CUA classification. The entire volume and individual image can be saved for later analysis. Operators are strongly encouraged to perform measurements to describe any CUA detected (e.g. length of uterine septum, interostial distance, thickness of the fundal myometrial wall and others). Further information regarding technical aspects can be seen in the Thessaloniki Consensus for diagnosing CUA [6].

Conclusion

There is an increasing interest in the literature with regard to CUA, which has culminated in the

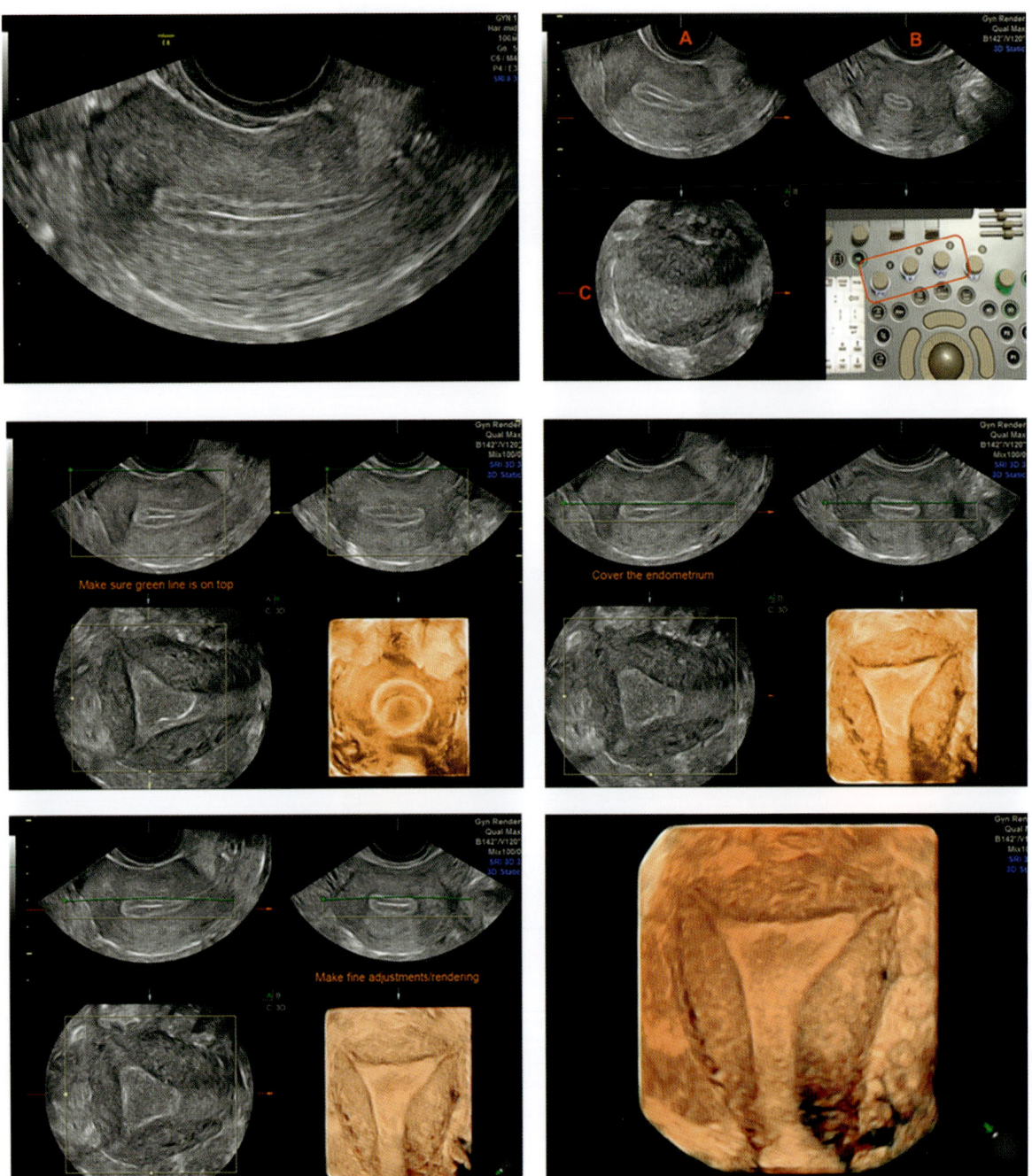

Figure 5.6 A step-by-step guide to diagnose CUA with 3D ultrasound. For 3D acquisition, the uterus should be visualized in its entirety in the sagittal plane (top left). Following acquisition, the uterus will appear in three different planes (A, B, C); the operator should be familiar with manipulating the uterus along the *x, y* and *z* axes using the functions on the console (top right). If Render mode is selected, the green segment of the region of interest (ROI) box should be placed at the top of the screen (middle left). The ROI box should then be adjusted so as to cover the endometrial cavity (middle right). Fine adjustments and rendering can be applied to improve the image quality (bottom left). Finally, the image can be enlarged and compared against the classification for CUA (bottom right).

description of several new classifications in recent years, the most recent being that of ESHRE/ESGE. Nowadays, in the modern work-up for diagnosis of CUA, 3D ultrasound has been recognized as the gold standard method of choice. Correct diagnosis and classification of the type of CUA is of utmost importance, as not only are they common in both selected and unselected groups of women, but they have significant adverse reproductive outcomes, which patients should be counselled about. In this chapter, a simple step-by-step approach for diagnosing CUA using 3D ultrasound has been presented to aid diagnosis.

Tips and Tricks

- Timing of assessment of uterine anomalies, should be scheduled for the luteal phase of the menstrual cycle, as this allows for better delineation of the contours of the endometrial cavity.
- Thorough scanning in 2D may provide some clues as to the presence of a congenital uterine anomaly.
- The presence of two endometrial complexes in the transverse plane indicates a possibility of a bicornuate, septate, subseptate or arcuate uterus.
- Beak-like appearance of the endometrium at the level of the fundus may indicate a unicornuate uterus. Careful scanning should be carried out to identify a rudimentary horn.
- Good-quality images are necessary to assure accurate diagnosis of uterine anomalies, and every effort should be made to achieve these.
- 3D ultrasound is the gold standard of diagnosis of congenital uterine anomalies, supplemented with MRI and/or hysteroscopy/laparoscopy in complex or inconclusive cases.
- When acquiring 3D volume, assure wide angle of acquisition and high resolution. Ask the patient to be as still as possible; if feasible, ask them to hold their breath – this minimizes respiratory motion artefacts.
- Adjust the magnification/zoom so that the corpus of the uterus occupies at least three-quarters of the screen.
- For very broad uteri, acquisition of the volume in the transverse plane allows for inclusion of the fundus and the entire uterine complex(es) necessary for accurate diagnosis.
- When analysing the 3D volume, consider curving the region of interest to ensure a true identification of the uterine anomaly.

References

1. Saravelos SH, Cocksedge KA, Li TC. Prevalence and diagnosis of congenital uterine anomalies in women with reproductive failure: a critical appraisal. *Hum Reprod Update* 2008;**14**:415–29.

2. Chan YY, Jayaprakasan K, Zamora J, et al. The prevalence of congenital uterine anomalies in unselected and high-risk populations: a systematic review. *Hum Reprod Update* 2011;**17**:761–71.

3. Chan YY, Jayaprakasan K, Tan A, et al. Reproductive outcomes in women with congenital uterine anomalies: a systematic review. *Ultrasound Obstet Gynecol* 2011;**38**:371–82.

4. Venetis CA, Papadopoulos SP, Campo R, et al. Clinical implications of congenital uterine anomalies: a meta-analysis of comparative studies. *Reprod Biomed Online* 2014;**29**:665–83.

5. Grimbizis GF, Gordts S, Di Spiezio Sardo A, et al. The ESHRE/ESGE consensus on the classification of female genital tract congenital anomalies. *Hum Reprod* 2013;**28**:2032–44.

6. Grimbizis GF, Di Spiezio Sardo A, Saravelos SH, et al. The Thessaloniki ESHRE/ESGE consensus on diagnosis of female genital anomalies. *Hum Reprod* 2016;**31**:2–7.

7. Acien P, Acien MI. The history of female genital tract malformation classifications and proposal of an updated system. *Hum Reprod Update* 2011;**17**:693–705.

8. Buttram VC, Jr., Gibbons WE. Mullerian anomalies: a proposed classification (an analysis of 144 cases). *Fertil Steril* 1979;**32**:40–6.

9. AFS. The American Fertility Society classifications of adnexal adhesions, distal tubal occlusion, tubal occlusion secondary to tubal ligation, tubal pregnancies, Mullerian anomalies and intrauterine adhesions. *Fertil Steril* 1988;**49**:944–55.

10. Oppelt P, Renner SP, Brucker S, et al. The VCUAM (vagina cervix uterus adnex-associated malformation) classification: a new classification for genital malformations. *Fertil Steril* 2005;**84**:1493–7.

11. Acien P. Embryological observations on the female genital tract. *Hum Reprod* 1992;**7**:437–45.

12. Ludwin A, Ludwin I. Comparison of the ESHRE-ESGE and ASRM classifications of Mullerian duct anomalies in everyday practice. *Hum Reprod* 2014; **30**:569–80.

13. Graupera B, Pascual MA, Hereter L, et al. Accuracy of three-dimensional ultrasound compared with magnetic resonance imaging in diagnosis of Mullerian duct anomalies using ESHRE-ESGE consensus on the classification of congenital anomalies of the female

genital tract. *Ultrasound Obstet Gynecol* 2015;**46**:616–22.

14. Saravelos SH, Li TC. Intra- and inter-observer variability of uterine measurements with three-dimensional ultrasound and implications for clinical practice. *Reprod Biomed Online* 2015;**31**:557–64.

15. Acien P, Acien M. The presentation and management of complex female genital malformations. *Hum Reprod Update* 2016;**22**:48–69.

16. Rikken JF, Kowalik CR, Emanuel MH, et al. Septum resection for women of reproductive age with a septate uterus. *Cochrane Database Syst Rev* 2017;**1**:CD008576.

Sonographic Assessment of Endometrial Pathology

Thierry Van den Bosch

Introduction

Endometrial pathology includes hyperplasia, polyps, cancer and infection. Intracavitary fibroids are *sensu stricto* not endometrial lesions, but should be included in the differential diagnosis.

Although intracavitary pathology may be found incidentally while scanning for an unrelated reason, most patients will be diagnosed during the evaluation of abnormal uterine bleeding. Ultrasound examination is the test of choice to triage patients for further management. If a thin and regular endometrium is seen after menopause, endometrial atrophy is the most likely diagnosis, while the risk for malignancy is very low [1,2] (Figure 6.1).

In those cases there is no need for further investigations. If a focal intracavitary lesion (e.g. an endometrial polyp or an intracavitary fibroid) is evidenced, the patient can be scheduled for an operative hysteroscopy. If the ultrasound image is suspicious for endometrial cancer or atypical hyperplasia, immediate endometrial sampling is indicated. If physiological endometrial changes or simple endometrial hyperplasia are anticipated, the clinician may choose endometrial sampling, hormonal therapy or expectant management.

This chapter gives an overview on how to assess the endometrium and the uterine cavity using ultrasonography.

Unenhanced Ultrasound Examination

The ultrasound scan starts with the visualization of the endometrium. The entire endometrium should be scanned from right to left and from fundus to isthmus. If the endometrium is clearly visible, it is measured in the sagittal plane, where it appears at its thickest (see Chapter 2). This is not necessarily the most fundal part of the endometrium.

If the endometrium cannot clearly be delineated, it must be recorded as 'not measurable'. A not measurable endometrium must be considered as potentially abnormal and warrants further testing (e.g. hydrosonography). In a series of 1220 women presenting with abnormal bleeding, almost 20 per cent of cancer cases had a non-measurable endometrium [3].

Merely reporting endometrial thickness is not enough. The ultrasonographic features should also be described [4]. The echogenicity of the endometrium may be uniform or non-uniform. During the menstrual cycle the endometrium in the follicular phase is typically uniform and hypoechogenic (three-layer type), and hyperechogenic in the secretory phase. The endometrium is reported as non-uniform if the background is heterogeneous (Figure 6.2) and/or in the presence of internal cysts (Figure 6.3).

The endometrial midline is reported as linear, non-linear, irregular or not visible. The endometrial–myometrial junction or junctional zone (JZ) is the hypoechogenic rim surrounding the endometrium. The JZ is the inner myometrium and is not part of the endometrium [5]. The JZ may be regular, irregular, interrupted or not defined. It is not always easy to see the JZ. The JZ visualization can be optimized using volume contrast imaging (VCI) set at 2 mm using 3D ultrasound [6].

Colour Doppler and power Doppler imaging to visualize the vascularization of the endometrium and of endometrial lesions may help in the diagnosis. While in most of the normal menstrual cycle no vessels can be seen in the endometrium, multiple peripheral vessels become visible at the end of the secretory phase. Intracavitary lesions have typical vascular patterns: a polyp has a single dominant vessel with or without branching [7], a fibroid circumferential flow and endometrial cancer multiple vessels from multifocal origins.

Polyp, Fibroid, Cancer or Clot?

An intracavitary lesion seen using hydrosonography may be an endometrial polyp, an intracavitary fibroid, a focal malignant lesion, a blood clot or caused by

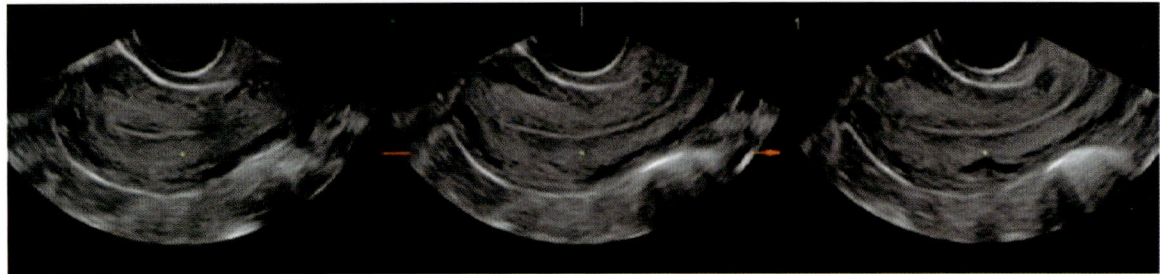

Figure 6.1 Tomographic ultrasound imaging (TUI) of a thin and regular endometrium.

(a)   (b)

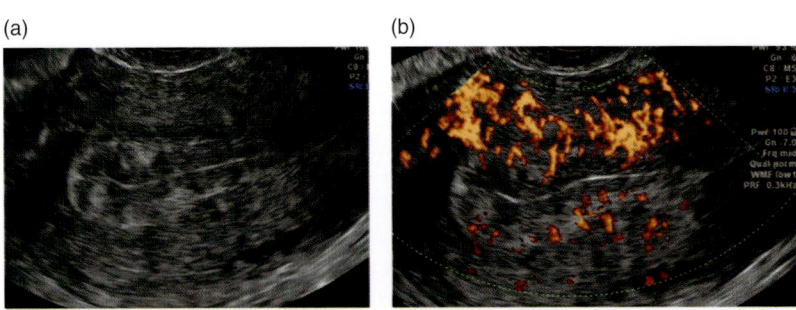

Figure 6.2 Non-uniform endometrium due to a heterogeneous background in a patient with focal complex hyperplasia without atypia: greyscale image (a) and power Doppler imaging (b) showing multiple vessels from multifocal origin.

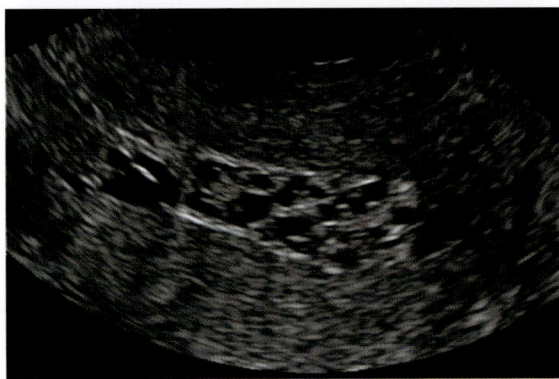

Figure 6.3 Non-uniform endometrium due to the presence of multiple endometrial cysts in a patient on tamoxifen.

polypoid endometrial growth. The outline of the lesion, its echogenicity and colour Doppler features may lead to the exact diagnosis. The outline of a polyp or an intracavitary fibroid is regular, as opposed to a clot or a focal malignant lesion. A polyp tends to be more hyperechogenic, occasionally with small internal cysts. A fibroid is habitually less echogenic and the overlying, more echogenic endometrium may be visible. The echogenicity of endometrial cancer varies according to the tumour type, a well-differentiated endometrioid cancer often being hyperechogenic. The endo-myometrial junction is typically interrupted in a FIGO type 1 or 2 fibroid as is often the case in endometrial cancer, while both an endometrial polyp and a clot are entirely intracavitary without affecting the JZ. The findings at colour Doppler are often helpful. A polyp (Figure 6.4) has typically a feeding vessel (pedicle), a fibroid (Figure 6.5) has circumferential flow, endometrial cancer (Figure 6.6) has multiple vessels from multifocal origin, while in a clot no flow can be detected. During fluid instillation a clot may move freely and its shape may even change during the examination. It is easier to visualize this using saline instillation. If a blood clot is suspected, it might be considered to aspirate the clot, e.g. using a pipelle sampler, and to check the cavity and the disappearance of the clot after aspiration.

In the presence of multiple 'polyps', the distinction from a polypoid endometrium should be made. Especially at the end of the secretory phase of the cycle, the endometrium can appear polypoid. In women of reproductive age, it may be advisable to repeat the scan in the week following the next menses. If by then the endometrium looks uniform, and typically showing a three-layer pattern, the diagnosis of physiological changes can be made. If not, multiple

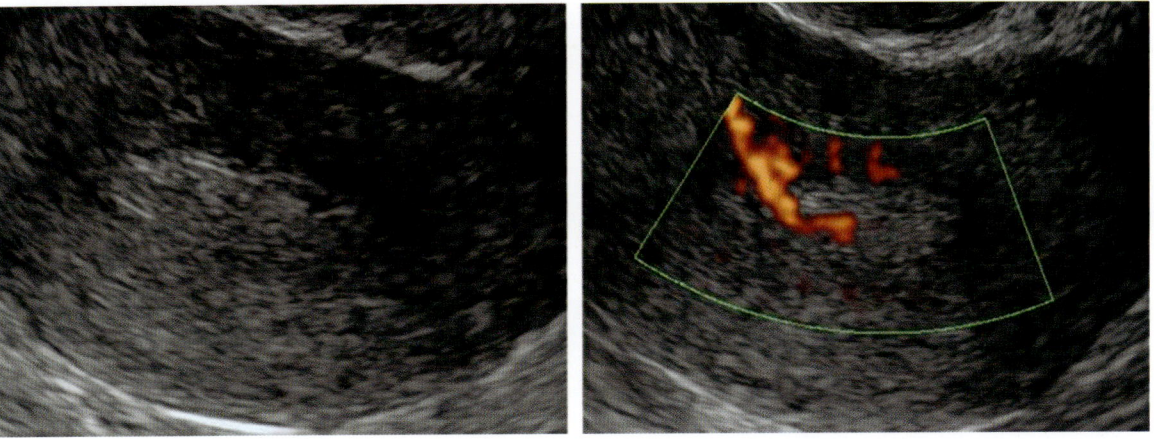

Figure 6.4 Endometrial polyp: greyscale ultrasonography (presence of a bright edge) and power Doppler imaging (presence of a single dominant – feeding – vessel).

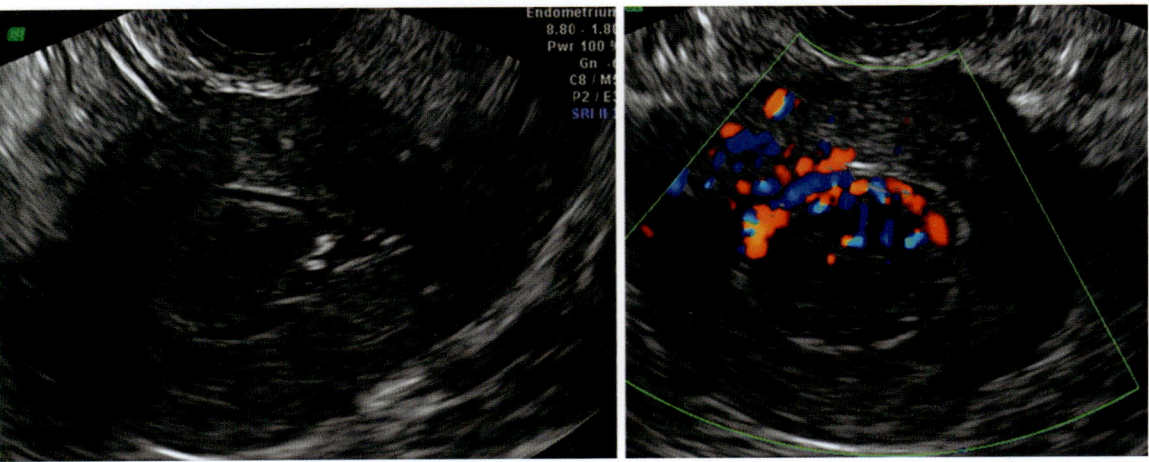

Figure 6.5 Gel instillation sonography: intracavitary fibroid at greyscale ultrasonography (right) and at colour Doppler imaging (presence of circular flow).

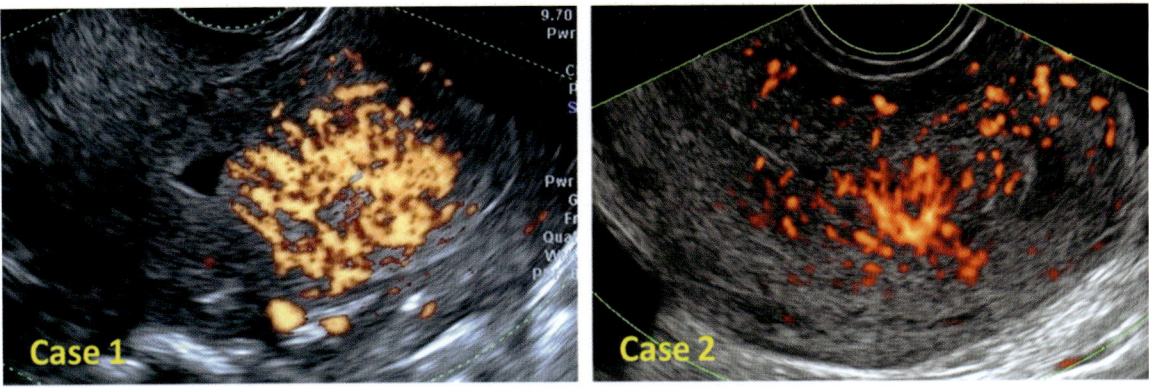

Figure 6.6 Endometrial cancer with multiple vessels form multifocal origin (case 1) and focal origin (case 2).

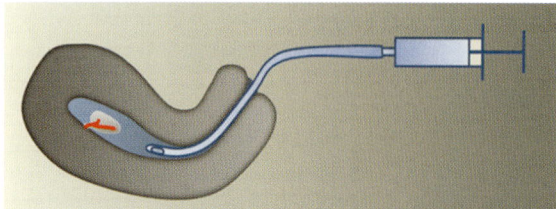

Figure 6.7 Schematic representation of fluid instillation sonography (hydrosonography).

(a)   (b)

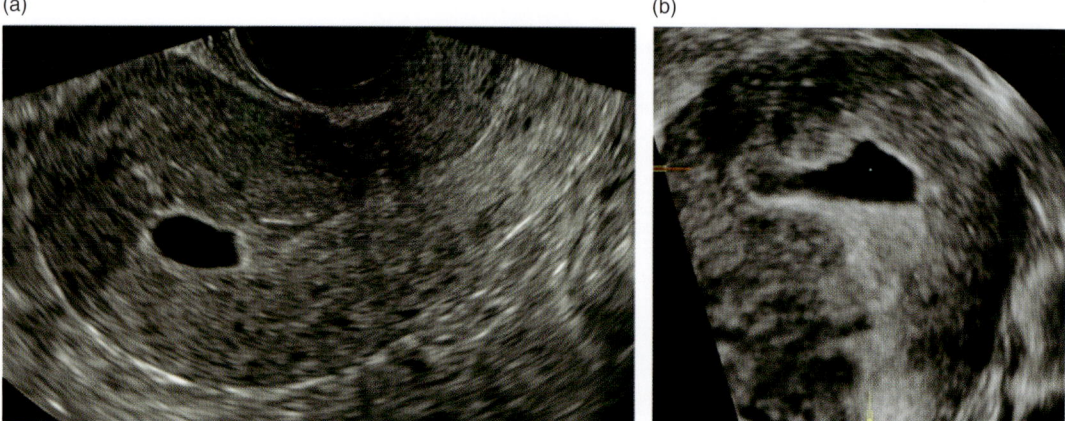

Figure 6.8 Intracavitary blood with a distinct dividing line between the serum and the sedimented erythrocytes: sagittal (a) and frontal (b) image.

polyps or endometrial disease, ranging from hyperplasia to cancer, are possible diagnoses. The finding of a feeding vessel in the stalk makes a polyp more plausible, whereas in case of multiple multifocal vessels, diffuse endometrial disease is more likely.

Fluid Instillation Sonography or Hydrosonography

The best way to diagnose intracavitary lesion is fluid instillation sonography or hydrosonography. Hydrosonography has proven to be as accurate as hysteroscopy in the diagnosis of endometrial polyps and intracavitary fibroids (Figure 6.7) [8].

Both saline (saline infusion sonography or SIS) and gel (gel instillation sonography or GIS) are used as negative (anechoic) contrast agents. While both have a similar diagnostic accuracy, gel has some advantages over saline [9,10]. Due to the gel's viscosity there is less backflow through the cervical canal, offering more stable cavity filling using a minimal amount of gel. This is particularly of importance when using simple catheters without a balloon. Moreover, the gel's higher viscosity impedes transtubal flow of gel

together with – potentially malignant – endometrial cells. The clinical significance of transtubal flow during SIS or hysteroscopy in terms of the patient's prognosis in the case of endometrial cancer is uncertain.

Reasons Not to Perform Hydrosonography

Before proceeding with fluid instillation, a formal unenhanced ultrasound examination is performed. In some cases, it may appear that fluid instillation is not necessary or not indicated.

In the case of pre-existing intracavitary anechoic fluid, the fluid may give sufficient contrast to assess the uterine cavity. Some clear serous intracavitary fluid is often seen in elderly women. In the case of blood, the echogenicity may be of a low level or inhomogeneous. From time to time the dividing line between the serum and the sedimented erythrocytes is clearly visible (Figure 6.8).

In the first half of the menstrual cycle, the endometrium is uniform and hypoechogenic, with an echogenic midline echo caused by the interphase between anterior and posterior endometrium. In the presence of an endometrial polyp or a fibroid, the lesion will be clearly seen against the hypo-echogenic endometrial background, making hydrosonography redundant.

If the endometrium is very thin, regular and clearly visible over the whole cavity, intracavitary pathology is most unlikely. Timmermans et al. reported that malignancy is most improbable if the total endometrial thickness is less than 3 mm [1]. In those cases, further tests such as fluid instillation sonography or hysteroscopy may be omitted. In cases of recurrent or persisting bleeding re-evaluation is warranted.

Fluid instillation is obviously contraindicated in pregnancy. This is one more reason why a formal unenhanced ultrasound examination is mandatory before proceeding with hydrosonography.

If endometrial malignancy is suspected, it is advisable to perform an office endometrial sampling first and await the histology results. The issue of seeding of malignant cells from the uterine cavity, through the fallopian tubes into the abdominal cavity, is still a matter of controversy. Although the flushing of malignant endometrial cells into the abdominal cavity during hysteroscopy or saline infusion sonography has been demonstrated, the clinical relevance in terms of cure or survival has not yet been established. However, out of caution, all guidelines recommend using the lowest pressure/flow possible during hysteroscopy or SIS. Therefore, out of caution, fluid instillation is best avoided if there is a strong suspicion of malignancy. If fluid instillation is to be performed, gel is preferred over saline because of the higher viscosity and hence lower risk for transtubal flow.

If cervicitis or pelvic infection is diagnosed, fluid instillation is not performed to avoid upwards spread of pathogens.

During the preliminary unenhanced ultrasound examination, extracavitary causes of bleeding from gynaecological or non-gynaecological origin are checked, including uterine fibroids, adenomyosis, ovarian pathology or bladder and rectum cancer.

Hydrosonography Step by Step

An appropriately sized open-sided (Collin type) speculum is used (Figure 6.9). The speculum's open side allows for swift speculum removal while the catheter is still inserted in the uterus. If a closed (Cuzco type) speculum is used great care should be taken that the catheter does not slip out of the uterus while the speculum is removed over the catheter and the fluid syringe.

The cervix is inspected and cleaned using small swabs and some disinfectant. Some causes of abnormal bleeding may become apparent during inspection, including cervicitis, an ectropion, cervix carcinoma, an endocervical polyp, a pedunculated fibroid or endometrial polyp protruding through the cervix.

Different types of catheters can be used for hydrosonography. Some catheters, such as balloon catheters and cone catheters, impede backflow. We use simple neonatal suction catheters. They are thin (2 mm outer diameter), relatively soft, though rigid enough to be easily threaded through the cervical canal, and long enough not to hamper the handling of the vaginal probe. Moreover, they are cheap.

Using a Rampley sponge-holding forceps or a similar device, the catheter is held about 1 cm from the catheter tip. The tip is pushed through the ectocervical ostium and the catheter is moved slowly upwards till it is felt touching the fundus of the uterus. The patient is asked to tell the examiner as soon as she feels some pain in the lower abdomen, meaning the catheter touched the uterus fundus.

If the external cervical ostium is too narrow to insert the catheter tip, the use of a small dilator will often be helpful. Once the catheter tip is inserted over 2 mm, the injection of a small bolus of gel may help find the way through the endocervical canal. In some cases, the catheter does not slide through the endocervical canal. There is no use in pushing hard, but rather try to push the catheter gently in different directions. In some cases it may be decided to use a tenaculum to grip the cervix and straighten the utero-cervical angle. Performing transabdominal scanning during the catheter insertion may prove of value to indicate the direction to follow.

If the endocervical canal is so stenotic that it is hardly visible at speculum inspection, not allowing even the smallest dilator, hydrodilation may be attempted. For hydrodilation, use a 5 or 10 cc syringe with saline and a 50 mm long 21 G intramuscular needle. Place the tip of the needle in the ostium while injecting saline. Take care not to puncture in the cervix.

Before removing the speculum, inject a very small amount of gel (0.5–1 cc), to check that the catheter is high in the cavity and not curled in the endocervical canal. In the latter case the gel will immediately flow back through the cervix.

The speculum is removed; the vaginal probe is inserted while the catheter is still in the uterine cavity.

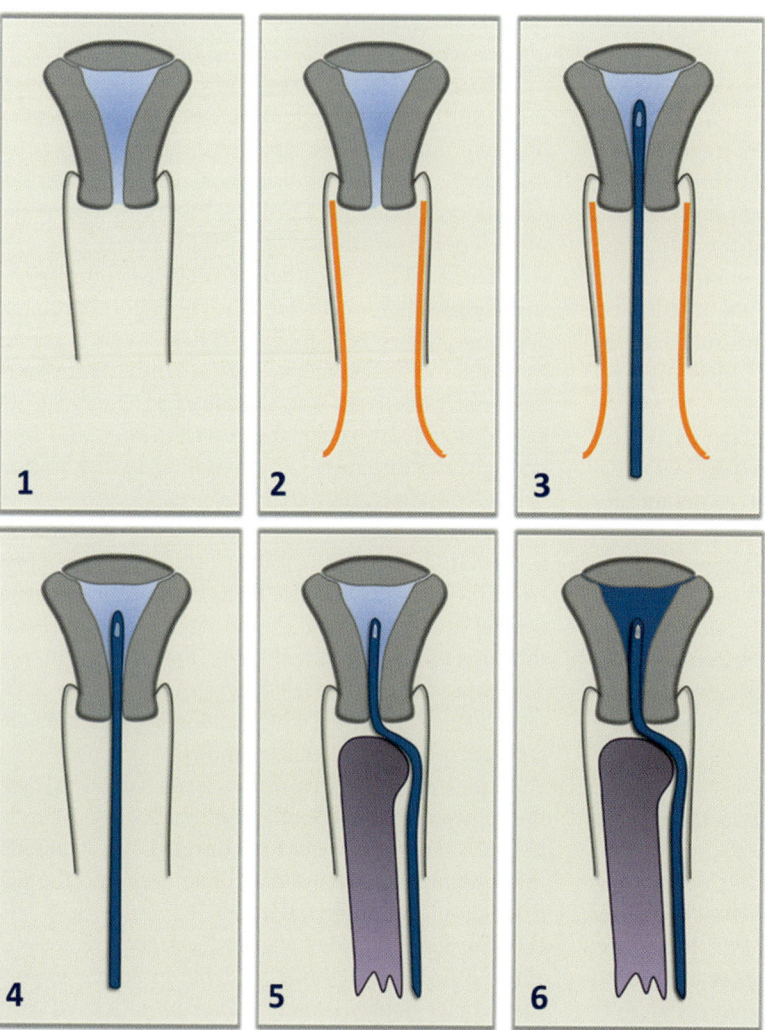

Figure 6.9 Hydrosonography step by step: schematic representation.

If there is an assistant available, the assistant holds the syringe and injects some gel while looking at the ultrasound machine screen, taking care to avoid over-inflation of the uterine cavity. In the absence of an assistant, the syringe is placed on the patient's abdomen and, while scanning, the examiner injects small aliquots of gel.

Starting the scanning, the catheter is followed from the cervix to the catheter tip. On one hand, this confirms the correct position of the catheter; on the other, especially in a highly distorted cavity, it may help orientation. It is also important to know where the catheter is and not to mistake it for endometrial abnormality. If the catheter disturbs the imaging, it can be slowly pulled out of view.

While holding the probe in a sagittal plane, small aliquots of fluid are injected. If the cavity is distorted it might be necessary to slightly move the probe to obtain a proper view of the cavity. It is of utmost importance to inject the fluid slowly to avoid sudden painful overstretching of the cavity. Talk to your patient while instilling fluid and ask her to tell you if she feels any discomfort or pain. Usually 2–3 cc is sufficient to separate both endometrial layers and to rule out intracavitary lesion. It is not necessary to aim for a highly dilated cavity.

It is of extreme importance to avoid air bubbles. Air bubbles are very echogenic and severely disturb the ultrasound image. Therefore, make sure to flush the syringe as well as the catheter before insertion. Hold

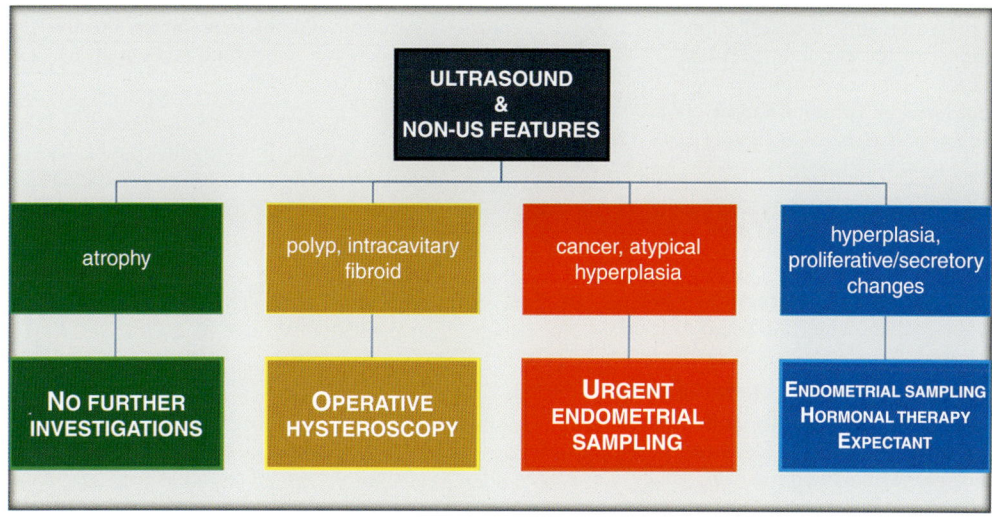

Figure 6.10 Management of abnormal uterine bleeding.

the syringe upright and flush the air. Connect the catheter and flush the air out of the total length of the catheter.

At the end of the procedure, remove the catheter slowly while scanning the lower part of the uterine cavity. During the passage through the endocervical canal, some gel may be injected to evidence the canal lining.

Some women, especially those with a history of severe dysmenorrhoea, may experience lower abdominal cramping after the completion of the procedure. Patients are advised to take a non-steroidal anti-inflammatory drug in the event of pain or discomfort.

Conclusions

In the management of women with abnormal uterine bleeding, ultrasonography allows for an efficient triage, between those suspicious for malignancy who need to be prioritized, those in whom operative hysteroscopy is indicated and those who do not need additional tests (Figure 6.10).

Ultrasonography does not substitute histology. If there is a contradiction between the ultrasound images, the clinical presentation and the histological results of an endometrial biopsy, the diagnosis should be reconsidered [11].

> **Tips and Tricks**
>
> • If the endometrium is thin, regular, uniform and well visible, malignancy is most unlikely.

• Unless at the end of the secretory phase, there are no vessels visible within the endometrium.
• Colour imaging facilitates the differential diagnoses between a polyp, an intracavitary fibroid, endometrial cancer and a blood clot.
• If you do not see the entire endometrium do not measure it, but perform a hydrosonography.
• For hydrosonography, use gel and inject slowly. Often, no more than 3 cc is sufficient.
• Air bubbles severely disturb the image quality at hydrosonography: flush the air out of the syringe and the catheter before inserting the catheter!
• Use an open-sided speculum for hydrosonography.

References

1. Timmermans A, Opmeer BC, Khan KS, et al. Endometrial thickness measurement for detecting endometrial cancer in women with postmenopausal bleeding: a systematic review and meta-analysis. *Obstet Gynecol* 2010;**116**(1):160–7.

2. Van den Bosch T, Van Schoubroeck D, Domali E, et al. A thin and regular endometrium on ultrasound is very unlikely in patients with endometrial malignancy. *Ultrasound Obstet Gynecol* 2007;**29**(6):674–9.

3. Van den Bosch T, Ameye L, Van Schoubroeck D, Bourne T, and Timmerman D. Intra-cavitary uterine pathology in women with abnormal uterine bleeding: a prospective study of 1220 women. *Facts Views Vis Obgyn* 2015;7(1):17–24.

4. Leone FP, Timmerman D, Bourne T, et al. Terms, definitions and measurements to describe the sonographic features of the endometrium and intrauterine lesions: a consensus opinion from the International Endometrial Tumor Analysis (IETA) group. *Ultrasound Obstet Gynecol* 2010;**35**(1):103–12.

5. Naftalin J, Jurkovic D. The endometrial–myometrial junction: a fresh look at a busy crossing. *Ultrasound Obstet Gynecol* 2009;**34**(1):1–11.

6. Votino A, Van den Bosch T, Installe AJ, et al. Optimizing the ultrasound visualization of the endometrial–myometrial junction (EMJ). *Facts Views Vis Obgyn* 2015;**7**(1):60–3.

7. Timmerman D, Verguts J, Konstantinovic ML, et al. The pedicle artery sign based on sonography with color Doppler imaging can replace second-stage tests in women with abnormal vaginal bleeding. *Ultrasound Obstet Gynecol* 2003;**22**(2):166–71.

8. de Kroon CD, de Bock GH, Dieben SW, et al. Saline contrast hysterosonography in abnormal uterine bleeding: a systematic review and meta-analysis. *BJOG* 2003;**110**(10):938–47.

9. Van den Bosch T, Betsas G, Van Schoubroeck D, et al. Gel infusion sonography in the evaluation of the uterine cavity. *Ultrasound Obstet Gynecol* 2009;**34**(6):711–14.

10. Werbrouck E, Veldman J, Luts J, et al. Detection of endometrial pathology using saline infusion sonography versus gel instillation sonography: a prospective cohort study. *Fertil Steril* 2011;**95**(1):285–8.

11. Van den Bosch T, Van Schoubroeck D, Van Calster B, Cornelis A, Timmerman D. Pre-sampling ultrasound evaluation and assessment of the tissue yield during sampling improves the diagnostic reliability of office endometrial biopsy. *J Obstet Gynaecol* 2012;**32**(2):173–6.

Sonographic Assessment of Polycystic Ovaries

Tarek Elshamy and Kanna Jayaprakasan

Introduction

Polycystic ovary syndrome (PCOS) is the most common endocrine disorder among women in the reproductive age group. The reported prevalence of PCOS ranges between 5 and 15 percent [1]. This variation is largely dependent on the population studied and the diagnostic criteria used to establish the diagnosis [2]. Obesity, infertility, menstrual disorders and signs of hyperandrogenism are common clinical presentations of this syndrome. Women with PCOS are also at increased risk of long-term health problems such as cardiovascular disease and type-2 diabetes. In addition, it is associated with increased risk of endometrial hyperplasia and endometrial cancer secondary to exposure to unopposed oestrogen.

Polycystic ovary syndrome is a diagnosis of exclusion. However, several sets of diagnostic criteria were proposed by different expert groups to make a diagnosis, namely the National Institute of Health (NIH) criteria, the Rotterdam criteria and the Androgen Excess and Polycystic Ovary Syndrome (AE-PCOS) Society criteria [3] (Table 7.1). The NIH PCOS consensus compiled in 1990 was largely based on expert opinion rather than evidence from clinical trials. According to the NIH consensus, both chronic anovulation and signs of hyperandrogenism (clinical or biochemical) must be present to establish the diagnosis of PCOS. Other disorders, including non-classic congenital adrenal hyperplasia (NC-CAH), Cushing's syndrome, androgen secreting tumours, hyperprolactinaemia, and thyroid dysfunction, need to be excluded [4].

Thirteen years later, the Rotterdam ESHRE/ASRM-sponsored PCOS Consensus Workshop Group revised the NIH consensus and added the polycystic ovary (PCO) ultrasound appearances to the diagnosis of PCOS. The 2003 Rotterdam consensus includes three criteria: (1) oligo- or anovulation; (2) clinical or biochemical signs of hyperandrogenism; and (3) polycystic-appearing ovaries on imaging.

In order to make the diagnosis of PCOS, two of the three criteria must be present. The diagnosis of PCOS is by exclusion and other disorders of hyperandrogenaemia and ovulatory dysfunction must be first excluded [5]. The Rotterdam criteria for polycystic ovaries on ultrasound are 12 or more follicles measuring 2–9 mm and/or ovarian volume more than 10 cm^3 in one or both ovaries.

More recently, an international evidence-based guideline for the assessment and management of PCOS has identified the most effective ultrasound criteria to diagnose PCOS considering the recent advances with improved resolution ultrasound [6]. We discuss these criteria later in this chapter.

Polycystic Ovary Syndrome Phenotypes

Four clinical phenotypes of PCOS have been recognized according to the combination of PCOS manifestations. These phenotypes are illustrated in Table 7.1. The phenotypes are classified into: (1) classic PCOS which includes groups A and B, and (2) newer PCOS which comprises groups C and D; both include the PCO morphology as a feature in contrast to the classic PCOS group [7,8].

The addition of the morphological appearance of polycystic ovary to the Rotterdam diagnostic criteria resulted in identifying two additional PCOS phenotypes: (1) women with ovulatory dysfunction and polycystic ovaries but without hyperandrogenism; and (2) ovulatory women with hyperandrogenism and polycystic ovaries [10]. In 2009, the AE-PCOS society expert review reassessed the key features of PCOS and compiled a new consensus. The AE-PCOS diagnostic criteria include: (1) hyperandrogenism, including hirsutism and/or hyperandrogenaemia; (2) ovarian dysfunction, including oligo-anovulation and/or polycystic-appearing ovaries; and (3) exclusion of other related disorders [3].

87

Table 7.1 Phenotypes of PCOS according to the Androgen Excess and PCOS Society (AE-PCOS)

Parameter	Phenotype A	Phenotype B	Phenotype C	Phenotype D
Hyperandrogenism	+	+	+	−
Ovulatory dysfunction	+	+	−	+
Polycystic ovarian morphology	+	−	+	+

Source: [9].

According to the AE-PCOS consensus, hyperandrogenism is a necessary criterion for the diagnosis of PCOS. Therefore, the PCOS phenotype of ovulatory dysfunction and polycystic ovaries but without hyperandrogenism (previously acceptable by the Rotterdam criteria) does not qualify for the diagnosis of PCOS [3].

Polycystic Ovary Morphology on Ultrasound

Pelvic ultrasound is considered an essential tool in the evaluation of women with suspected PCOS. Since the first ultrasound study of the female pelvis in the 1970s [11], several attempts have been made to identify ultrasound criteria to define PCO. However, there has been no complete consensus on these ultrasound criteria to date.

One of the early and widely used definitions was proposed in 1985 and defined PCO as the presence of 10 or more cysts measuring 2–8 mm in diameter, arranged peripherally around a dense core of stroma or scattered through an increased amount of stroma [12]. Other ultrasound studies reported enlarged ovaries with the follicle arranged peripherally or scattered throughout hyperechogenic stroma in 70 per cent of symptomatic women with PCOS [13]. These criteria were based on transabdominal ultrasound. Further studies have shown that the ovaries cannot be adequately assessed in 42 per cent of the cases by using transabdominal ultrasound [14]. Several limiting factors have been identified, such as obesity, low resolution, the full bladder distorting the pelvic anatomy and loops of bowel masking the ovaries [15].

The introduction of transvaginal ultrasound, with its improved resolution, has led to better visualization of the pelvic structures and development of more precise ultrasound criteria for the diagnosis of PCO [16]. The 2003 ESHRE/ASRM meeting in Rotterdam compiled a consensus definition for PCO. According to the Rotterdam criteria, polycystic ovaries are present when (1) one or both ovaries demonstrate 12 or more follicles measuring 2–9 mm in diameter; or (2) the ovarian volume exceeds 10 cm^3. Only one ovary meeting either of these criteria is sufficient to establish the presence of polycystic ovaries [17]. This definition recognized two important parameters: (1) ovarian volume and (2) number of follicles.

Ovarian Volume and Area

There are several reports in the literature comparing ovarian volume in women with PCOS to those of healthy women. A volume of 10 cm^3 was set as the threshold volume for PCO [18,19]. However, some reports suggest that ovarian volume alone is not enough for the diagnosis of PCO due to the high degree of volume overlap between normal ovaries and PCO [15]. There are many formulas for calculation of the ovarian volume [20]. Several studies proposed that ovarian volume should be calculated on the basis of the simplified formula for an ellipsoid (0.5 × length × width × thickness of the ovary) [18,21] (Figure 7.1). It is worth mentioning that increased total ovarian area has been proposed as an ultrasound criterion for the diagnosis of PCO. In a study of 48 control cases, the ovarian stroma was quantified by subtracting the cyst area from the total ovarian area on a longitudinal plane of the ovary and the upper normal limit (95th percentile) of the stromal area was set at 380 mm^2/ovary. This study also observed a correlation between the total ovarian area and the stromal area [22]. The advantages of such an approach include reliable acquisition from transabdominal or transvaginal ultrasound, and it does not require a computerized-assisted analysis as the modern ultrasound machine software can readily measure the area of any outlined structure. In a large observational study, the sum of the areas of both ovaries was less than 11 cm^2 in normal women and an ovarian area above this cutoff was found exclusively in women with PCOS [22]. Other authors set this cutoff at 5.5 cm^2 per ovary [23].

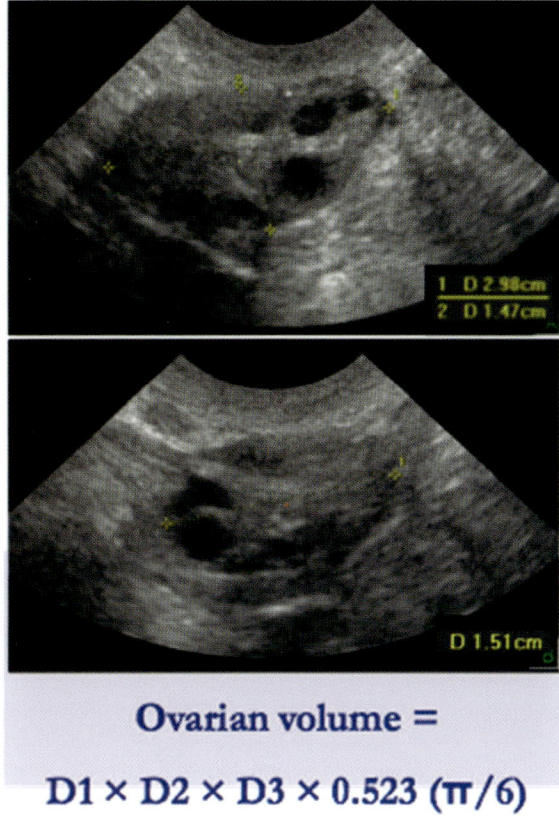

$$\text{Ovarian volume} =$$

$$D1 \times D2 \times D3 \times 0.523 \; (\pi/6)$$

Figure 7.1 Ovarian volume measurement by 2D ultrasound: three diameters (maximum longitudinal and antero-posterior diameter in longitudinal plane and maximum transverse diameter in transverse plane).

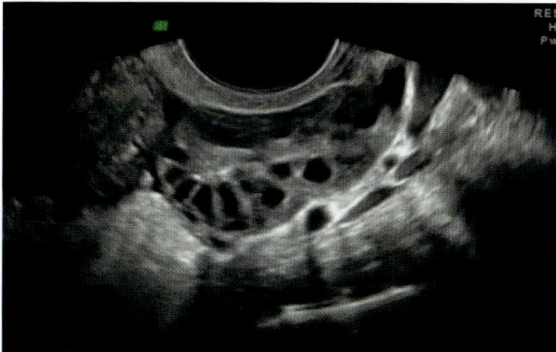

Figure 7.2 Classic PCO morphology: peripherally arranged follicles with bright echogenic stroma.

Follicle Distribution

Two types of PCO have been identified based on their follicle distribution on ultrasound: (1) peripheral cystic pattern (PCP), where the follicles are distributed in the subcapsular region (pearl necklace appearance) (Figure 7.2); and (2) general cystic pattern (GCP), where the follicles are scattered throughout the entire ovarian parenchyma [10] (Figure 7.3). This peripheral distribution is usually observed in younger patients, while in older women the follicle distribution is more generalized [27]. In addition, each appearance reflects a specific endocrine pattern [16].

Multifollicular Ovary

The term multifollicular ovary (MFO) describes normal-sized or slightly enlarged ovaries with multiple (12 or more) follicles (4–10 mm in diameter) and having a normal stromal size [12] (Figure 7.4). Multifollicular ovary is a common ultrasound finding and can be seen in normal pubertal girls, girls with central precocious puberty, hyperprolactinaemia and in women with hypothalamic amenorrhoea. Therefore, the whole clinical picture should be considered before rushing into a diagnosis of PCOS when MFO is recognized on ultrasound.

Stromal Echogenicity and Stromal Volume

Ovarian stromal hyperechogenicity (Figures 7.5 and 7.6) has been reported as one of the earliest ultrasound criteria for the diagnosis of PCO [12]. Another study has shown no difference in stromal echogenicity between PCO and normal ovaries using transvaginal ultrasound, and suggested that the subjective impression of hyperechogenic stroma may

Number of Follicles

The Rotterdam consensus identified the threshold to diagnose PCO on ultrasound as the presence of 12 or more follicles measuring 2–9 mm in diameter per ovary. This cutoff was based on a study published by Jonard et al. in 2003, which reported that 12 or more follicles offered the best compromise between 99 per cent specificity and 75 per cent sensitivity in detection of PCOS [19]. However, more recent studies have challenged this cutoff and showed high prevalence of ovaries with more than 12 follicles in healthy women [24,25]. The AE-PCOS sponsored a task force to review results from more recent studies and proposed increasing the threshold to 25 or more follicles [26]. A recent international guideline has recommended [6] a threshold of ≥20 follicles, measuring 2–9 mm, per ovary, to diagnose PCO.

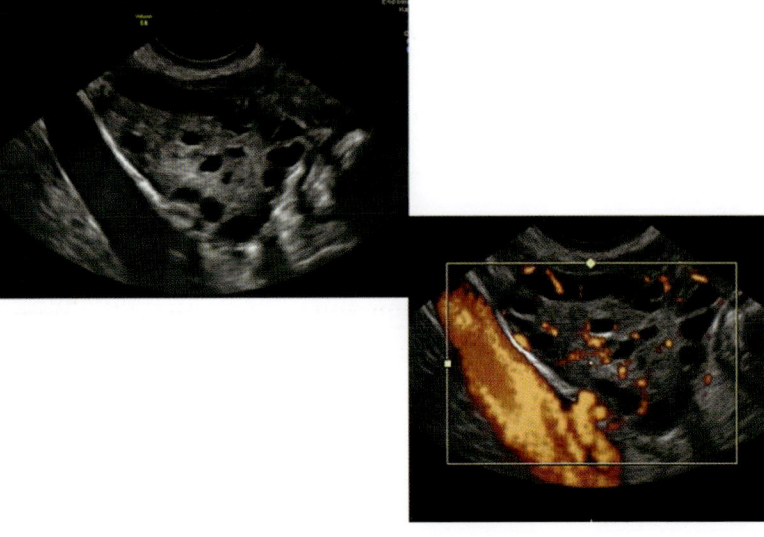

Figure 7.3 PCO morphology: follicles are scattered throughout ovary (greyscale image and with Doppler applied).

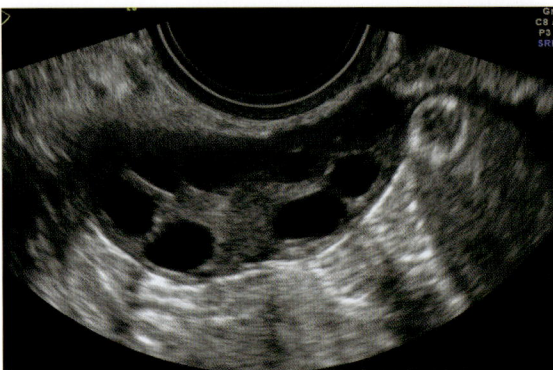

Figure 7.4 Multi-follicular ovary.

be due to an increased stromal volume [28]. The role of stromal hypertrophy and hyperechogenicity has been emphasized as a reliable ultrasound sign to differentiate PCO from other causes of MFO with a reported sensitivity of 94 per cent [18,29]. However, hyperechogenicity is highly subjective and is dependent on the settings of the ultrasound machine. Total ovarian volume has largely replaced stromal volume as a parameter to diagnose PCO by ultrasound as it is easily measured in clinical practice and correlates well with stromal volume [30].

Stromal Blood Flow

The use of Doppler ultrasound allows for the detection of the vascularity of the ovarian stroma. Polycystic ovaries are characterized by increased stromal vascularity

which contributes to the hyperechogenic appearance of the ovarian stroma. These findings were supported by observations from histological studies of PCO, which showed a twofold increase in the density of cortical stromal blood vessels compared to normal ovaries [31]. Several ultrasound parameters of the ovarian stromal blood flow have been proposed for the diagnosis of PCO, including 2D ultrasound pulse wave Doppler indices of ovarian stromal vessels (Figure 7.7) and 3D ultrasound power Doppler vascular indices: vascularization index (VI), flow index (FI) and vascularization flow index (VFI) (Figure 7.8). Some studies reported significant increase in these 3D power Doppler indices in PCO compared to normal ovaries [32,33]. However, there are other reports that did not find any significant difference in these indices between the PCO and normal ovaries [34,35]. A major limiting factor of the 3D power Doppler indices is that they are significantly dependent on the ultrasound machine settings [36].

Polycystic Ovaries in Women without PCOS

The presence of PCO on ultrasound scan does not automatically establish a diagnosis of PCOS. It is estimated that polycystic ovaries are present in 25 per cent of normal ovulating women [37] and in 27–39 per cent of adolescent girls [38]. It has also been postulated that girls with PCO may have a genetic predisposition to the syndrome [39]. Some authors associated the presence of PCO with

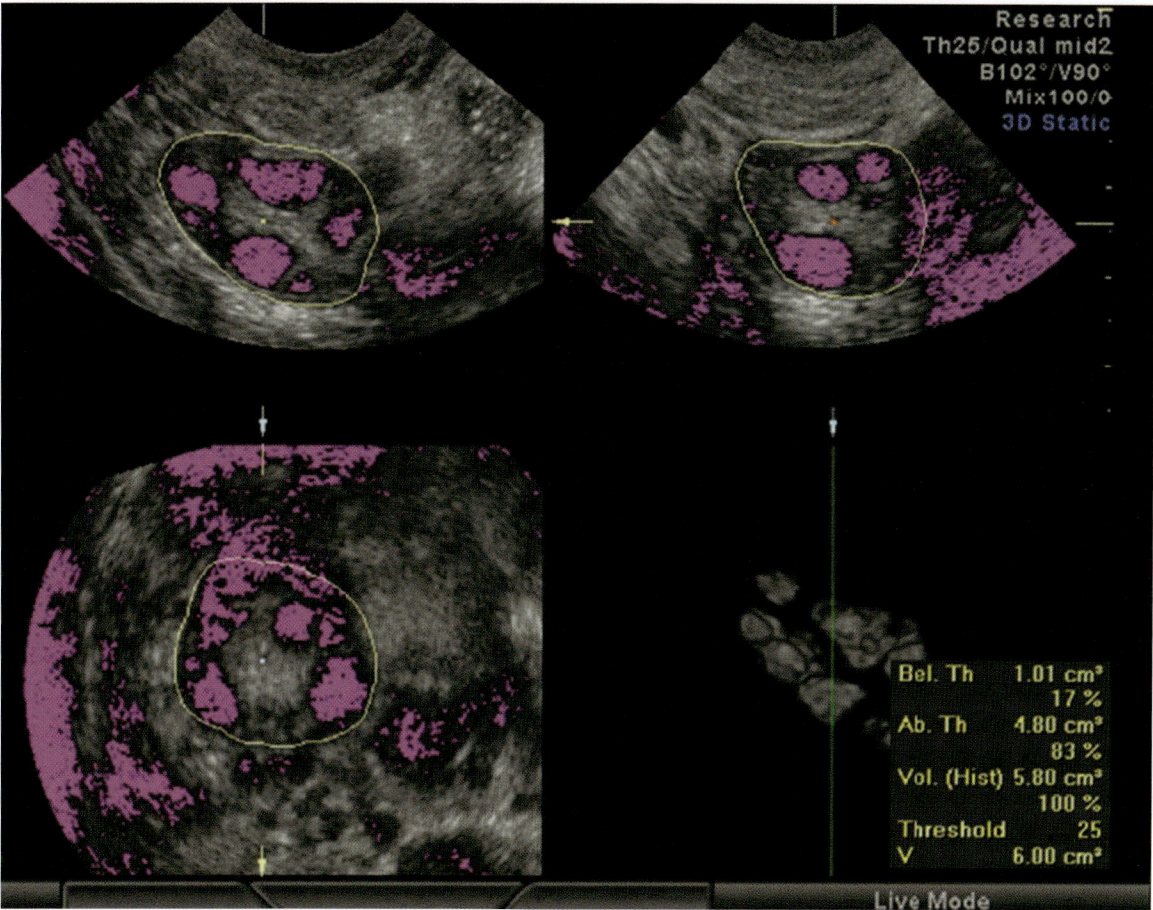

Figure 7.5 Ovarian stromal volume can be measured using 3D ultrasound (VOCAL software). Clinical application is limited, however.

menstrual irregularities [38]. Others suggested that the presence of PCO in ovulatory women is associated with increased risk of recurrent miscarriage [40] and subfertility [41]. Therefore, it remains unclear whether PCO appearance on ultrasound represents a normal variant or an unexpressed form of PCOS.

3D Ultrasound Application

The current ultrasound criteria for the diagnosis of PCO are based on 2D ultrasound. However, 2D ultrasound has some limitations. First, there is significant inter- and intra-observer variability when making the diagnosis of PCO on ultrasound [42]. Second, the inter-observer agreement for follicle count was reported to be poor [43].

The introduction of 3D ultrasound in reproductive medicine has provided new methods for the assessment of antral follicle count (AFC), ovarian volume, and stromal vascularity.

Antral Follicle Count

There are two methods for assessment of follicle count: (1) 3D multiplanar view and (2) SonoAVC (sonography-based automated volume count). In the 3D multiplanar view method, the three orthogonal planes (longitudinal or A, transverse or B and coronal or C) of a stored 3D ovarian volumetric dataset are displayed simultaneously (Figure 7.9). Then, the observer counts the number of the follicles using the three perpendicular planes shown in the multiplanar view. The inter-observer reliability was significantly improved by utilizing this method [44] (Figure 7.9).

In the SonoAVC method, the 3D ovarian volume dataset is obtained first. Then, it is processed by the SonoAVC software, which identifies every single

91

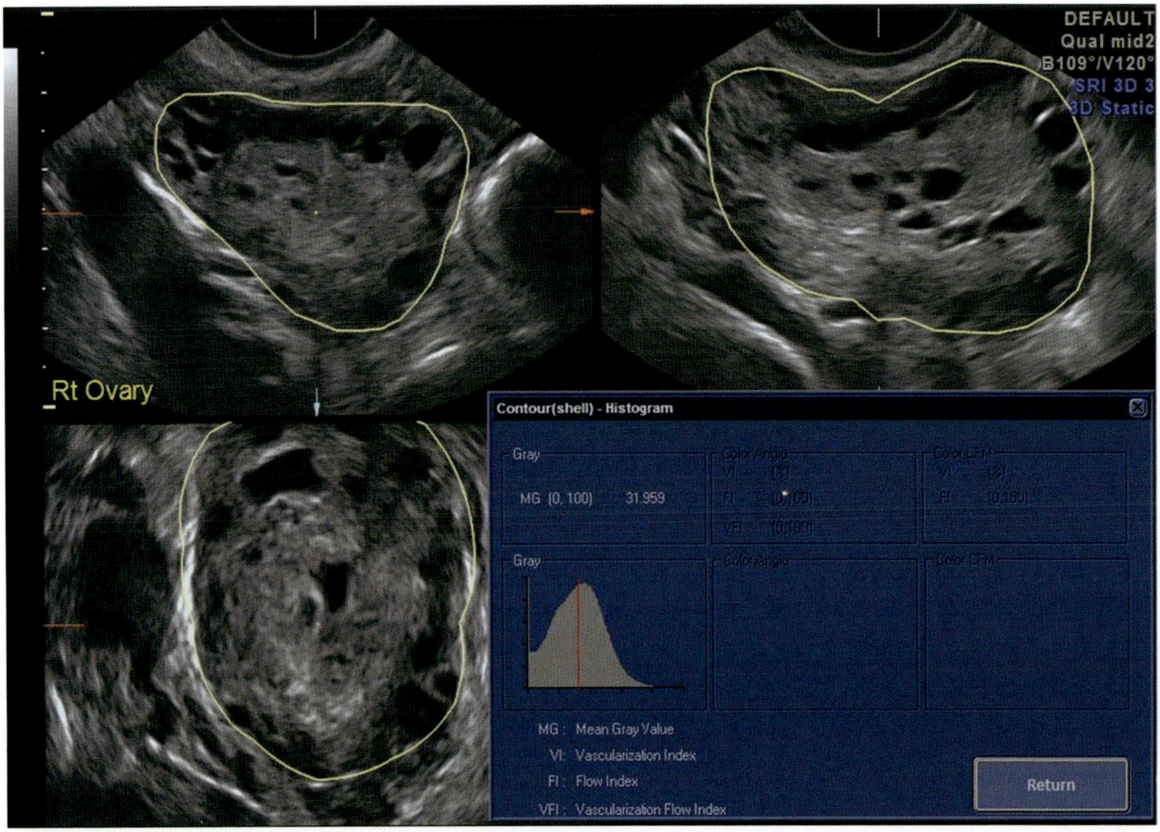

Figure 7.6 Ovarian stromal echogenicity can be measured using the histogram facility within the 3D ultrasound VOCAL software. It is expressed as mean grey value (MGV).

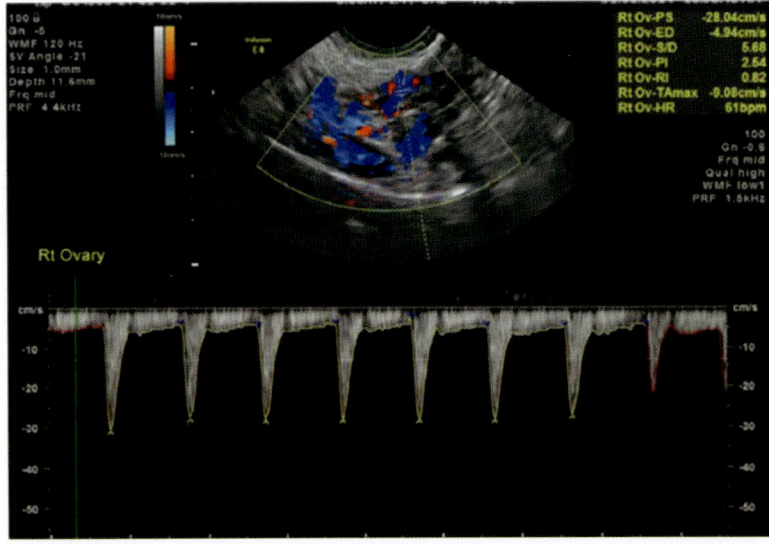

Figure 7.7 Ovarian stromal blood flow assessment with 2D pulse wave Doppler. The vascular indices measurements are in the top right-hand corner of the image

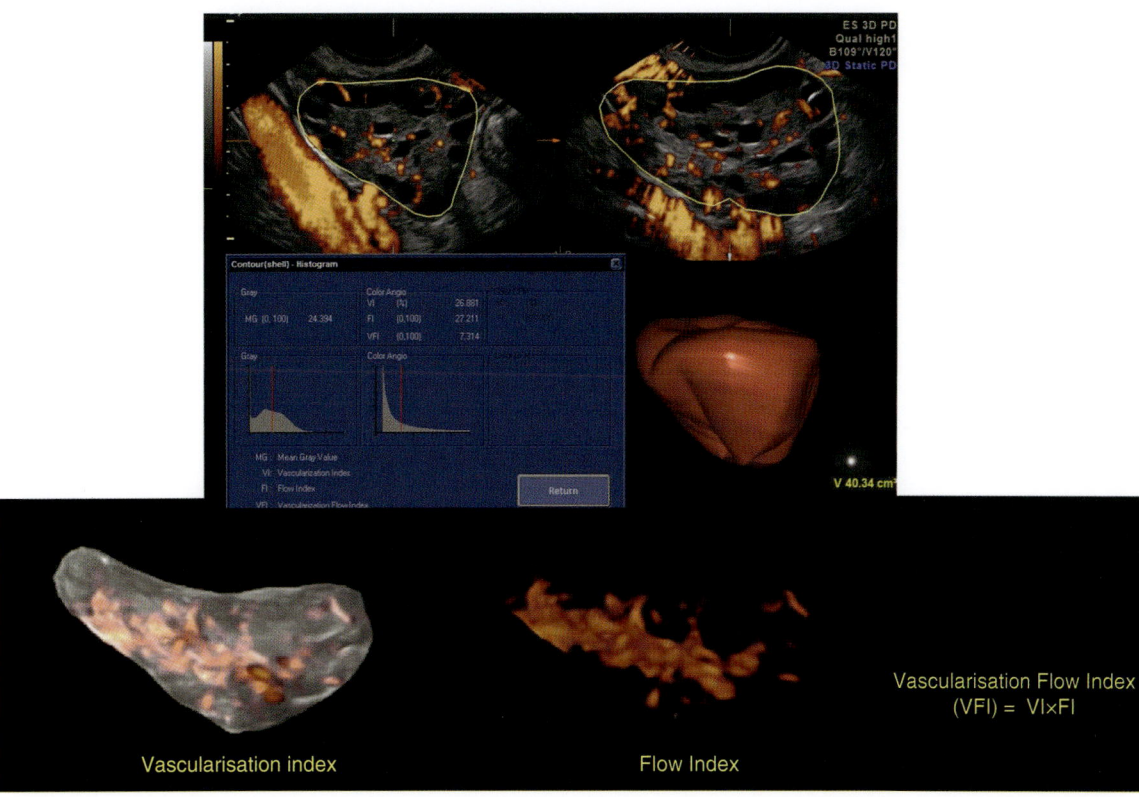

Figure 7.8 3D power Doppler measurement of the ovarian blood flow. It measures three vascular indices – vascularization index (total Doppler signal, i.e. total blood flow), flow index (Doppler signal intensity) and vascularization flow index.

follicle, codes it with a specific colour and automatically measures the follicle diameters and volumes (Figure 7.10). This method is not robust or accurate enough currently and requires further post-processing to select or delete some follicles or hypoechoic areas that are falsely missed or recognized by the software, respectively. This automated method is highly valid and provides more accurate values than those obtained from 2D measurements [45].

Ovarian Volume

Another useful application of 3D ultrasound is the ability to calculate the ovarian volume more accurately and reliably compared to 2D ultrasound. This has been attributed to the capability of 3D ultrasound to correct for any ovarian shape irregularities [44,46] (Figure 7.11). The virtual organ computer-aided analysis (VOCAL) imaging program has been used to obtain the ovarian volume calculation with high reliability and validity in the *in vitro* setting [36]. However, its application in routine practice is limited due to limited

availability of the software and need for more time for its application [47].

Assessment of Blood Flow

Power Doppler angiography has been utilized in a number of studies to quantify the ovarian stromal blood flow from 3D ovarian volumes (Figure 7.8). Three vascular indices have been used: the VI, the FI, and the VFI. These indices are measured using 'histogram' facilities within the VOCAL software. However, they do have some limitations, such as poor reproducibility, the need for offline evaluation and that these indices are largely influenced by ultrasound machine settings [35,48,49]. Therefore, advances in 3D ultrasound technology are required to overcome these limitations and make the modality more robust and reproducible.

PCO Morphology in Adolescents

Polycystic ovary syndrome usually manifests during the peri-pubertal years and the clinical and

93

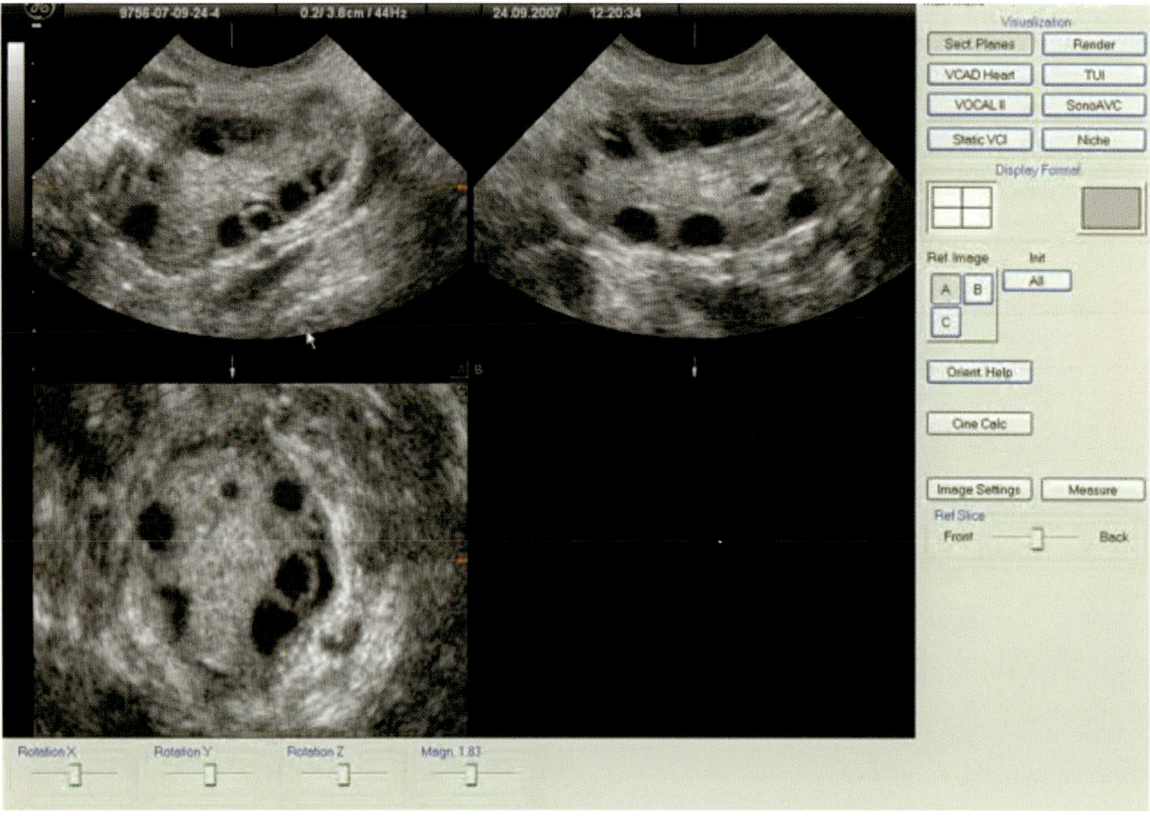

Figure 7.9 3D multiplanar view of an ovary.

biochemical features of PCOS seen in adolescent girls are similar to those in adults [50]. The diagnosis of PCOS in adolescents is problematic as the morphological changes in the ovary can mimic the appearance of PCO in adults. Therefore, when the Rotterdam criteria for PCO were applied to adolescents, the prevalence of PCO was reported to be between 35.4 and 54 per cent within this population of healthy, young women [51,52].

In addition, the differentiation between PCO and MFO can be difficult, as the ultrasound examination is usually done transabdominally in adolescents [53]. Some authors report an ovarian volume of more than 10 cm³ on transabdominal ultrasound as a diagnostic criterion, because follicle count is unreliable for the diagnosis of PCO with this method [26]. Some authors compared ovarian morphology in adolescent girls with and without PCOS using magnetic resonance imaging (MRI) and reported that the follicle count and the ovarian volume were greater in girls with PCOS compared to the control group [54].

Recent Recommendations for Ultrasound Diagnosis of PCOS

A recent international guideline has recommended utilizing the following evidence-based criteria for the diagnosis of PCOS [6]. When transvaginal ultrasound is utilized, on either ovary, a threshold of ≥20 follicles, measuring 2–9 mm, per ovary and/or an ovarian volume of ≥10 cm³, after excluding dominant follicles and corpora lutea, should be utilized to diagnose PCO. When transabdominal ultrasound is utilized, PCO can be diagnosed based on ovarian volume ≥10 cm³ for one or both ovaries.

Tips and Tricks

How to Calculate the Ovarian Volume Using 2D Ultrasound

- Perform transvaginal 2D ultrasound scan (D2–5 of the cycle).
- Identify one of the ovaries.

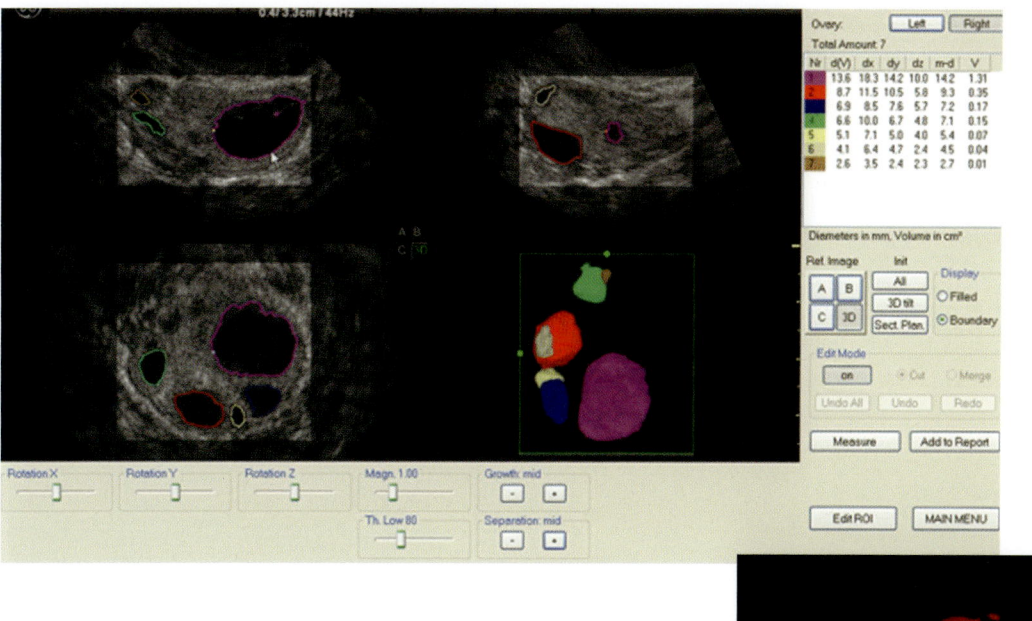

Figure 7.10 SonoAVC semi-automated method of follicle assessment: follicles are colour-coded and diameters and volume of each follicle are displayed in its output on the right-hand side.

- Examine the ovary in both longitudinal and transverse planes and rule out any pathology. Measure the maximum longitudinal diameter (length 'L') and maximum antero-posterior diameter (thickness 'H') in the longitudinal plane and the maximum transverse diameter (width 'W').
- At this stage, you can calculate the ovarian volume from the following formula (L × W × H × 0.5). The scanning machine automatically calculates this when these three measurements are done.

How to Calculate the Ovarian Volume Using VOCAL Integrated within 3D Ultrasound

- Obtain a good-quality 3D volume of the ovary and display it in the multiplanar mode.
- Select A or B plane. The authors prefer B plane.
- Activate VOCAL.
- Under 'define contour', select 'manual'.

- Under 'contour finder', select 'trace'.
- Select a rotational step of 30, 15 or 9 degrees. The narrower the angle, the more accurate the volume of the measured ovary, but more time-consuming is the analysis.
- With each rotation of the 3D volume, manually trace around the ovary.
- Repeat this step 6, 12 or 20 times, depending on the angle of rotation (30, 15 or 9 degrees, respectively).
- Once the tracings are carried out, select 'done' and the volume will be calculated automatically and displayed on the output pane.

How to Count the Antral Follicles in 2D Ultrasound

- Perform transvaginal 2D ultrasound scan (preferably D2–5 of the cycle, although it can be done in any part of the cycle).
- Identify the ovary.

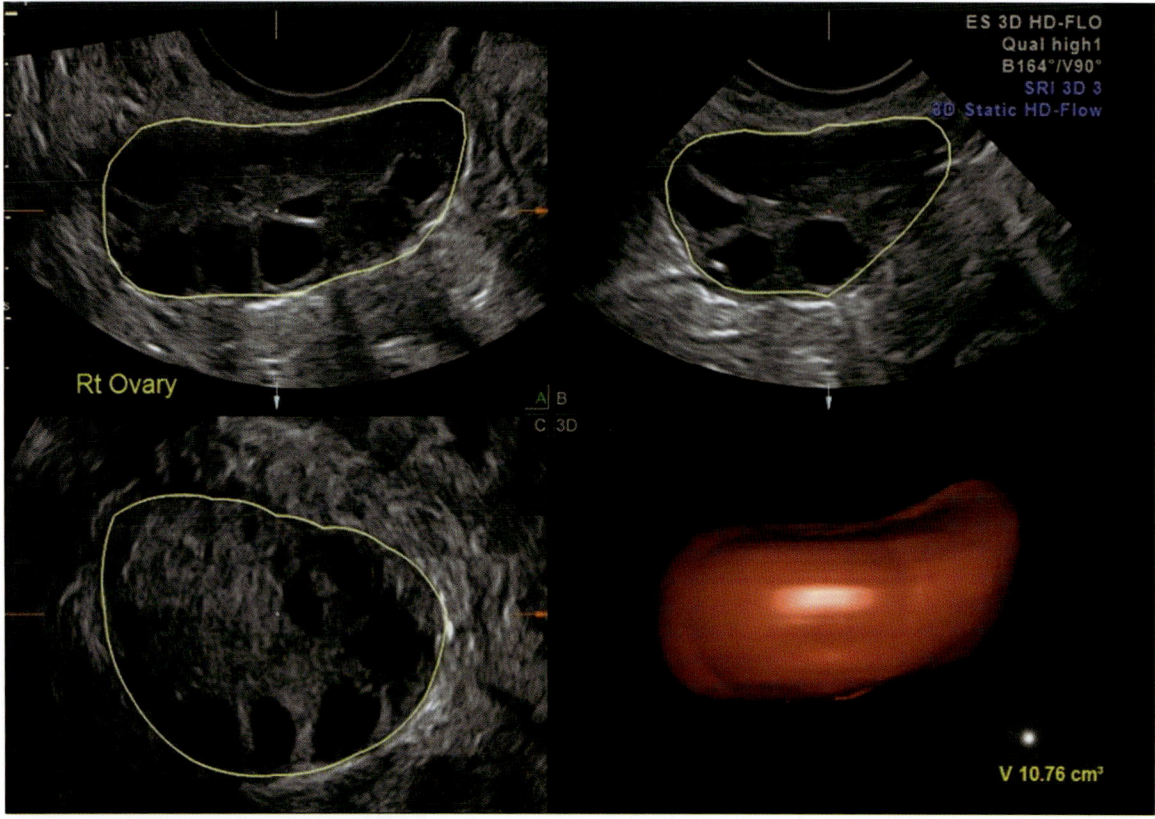

Figure 7.11 Ovarian volume: 3D ultrasound measurement using VOCAL software.

- In the longitudinal plane, start from the outer surface of the ovary and sweep through to the opposite surface.
- Count all antral follicles (rounded anechoic cystic structures of 2–10 mm).
- Repeat the steps on the left side. Calculate the total antral follicle count by adding the right and left antral follicle counts.

How to Count the Antral Follicles in Multiplanar Mode in 3D Ultrasound

- Obtain a 3D volume of the ovary and display it in the multiplanar mode.
- The three orthogonal planes (longitudinal 'A', transverse 'B' and coronal 'C' planes) of the 3D ovarian volume are displayed simultaneously.
- Select A or B plane and scroll through the ovary in one plane.
- Start from the outer surface of the ovary and sweep through to the opposite surface.

- Count the number of antral follicles (2–10 mm) from both ovaries and add both to obtain the total antral follicle count.
- To increase reliability, count the number of follicles in the other plane (i.e. 'B' if 'A' was assessed first); if discrepant, take the average of the two measurements.

How to Assess Ovarian Stromal Blood Flow Using 2D Pulse Wave Doppler Ultrasound

- Perform a transvaginal 2D ultrasound scan.
- Identify the ovary and obtain a longitudinal view.
- Activate the colour flow control (labelled 'C'); the colour box will appear.
- Position and adjust the colour box over the ovary to visualize the arteries within the ovarian stroma.
- Activate the pulse wave control (labelled 'PW'); a vertical sampling line will appear on the screen with a gate (represented by two horizontal lines).

- Adjust the sampling line and the gate (1 mm width) correctly on the blood vessel. Avoid vessels near the surface of the ovary, aim for angle of insonation <30 degrees.
- Press the 'update' control to obtain the spectral trace.
- Observe the spectral trace for a few seconds and obtain at least three waveforms.
- Activate the 'freeze' control.
- Use the automatic frequency follower to trace the outline of the waveforms and press 'set'. Peak systolic velocity (PSV), resistance index (RI) and pulsatility index (PI) are automatically measured.

How to Calculate 3D Power Doppler Indices

- Identify the ovary in a 2D ultrasound and activate the power Doppler to identify the blood vessels in the ovarian stroma.
- Obtain a 3D volume of the ovary and display it in the multiplanar mode.
- Select A or B plane. The authors prefer B plane.
- Activate VOCAL.
- Under 'define contour', select 'manual'.
- Under 'contour finder', select 'trace'.
- Select a rotational step of 30, 15 or 9 degrees.
- With each rotation of the 3D volume, manually trace around the ovary.
- Repeat this step as many times as required.
- Once the tracings are carried out, select 'done' and the volume will be calculated automatically.
- Select the 'Histogram' function.
- A box with graphs will appear in the upper quadrant of the image known as the volume histogram where the mean grey volume (MGV), colour angiogram and the 3D power Doppler vascular indices (vascularization index (VI), flow index (FI) and vascularization flow index (VFI)) are displayed.

References

1. Azziz R, Carmina E, Dewailly D, et al. Criteria for defining polycystic ovary syndrome as a predominantly hyperandrogenic syndrome: an Androgen Excess Society guideline. *J Clin Endocrinol Metab* 2006;**91**(11):4237–45.

2. March WA, Moore VM, Willson KJ, et al. The prevalence of polycystic ovary syndrome in a community sample assessed under contrasting diagnostic criteria. *Hum Reprod* 2009;**25**(2):544–51.

3. Azziz R, Carmina E, Dewailly D, et al. The Androgen Excess and PCOS Society criteria for the polycystic ovary syndrome: the complete task force report. *Fertil Steril* 2009;**91**(2):456–88.

4. Kawadzki J, Dunaif A, Givens J, Haseltine F, Merriam G. Diagnostic criteria for polycystic ovary syndrome: a rational approach, in *Polycystic Ovary Syndrome*, A Dunaif, JR Givens, F Haseltine, editors. Blackwell Scientific, 1992;377–84.

5. ESHRE TR, Group A-SPCW. Revised 2003 consensus on diagnostic criteria and long-term health risks related to polycystic ovary syndrome. *Fertil Steril* 2004;**81**(1):19–25.

6. Teede HJ, Misso ML, Costello MF, et al. Recommendations from the international evidence-based guideline for the assessment and management of polycystic ovary syndrome. *Fertil Steril* 2018;**110**:364–79.

7. Shaw LJ, Bairey Merz CN, Azziz R, et al. Withdrawn: postmenopausal women with a history of irregular menses and elevated androgen measurements at high risk for worsening cardiovascular event-free survival: results from the National Institutes of Health—National Heart, Lung, and Blood Institute Sponsored Women's Ischemia Syndrome Evaluation. *J Clin Endocrinol Metab* 2008;**93**(4):1276–84.

8. Diamanti-Kandarakis E, Dunaif A. Insulin resistance and the polycystic ovary syndrome revisited: an update on mechanisms and implications. *Endocrine Rev* 2012;**33**(6):981–1030.

9. Lizneva D, Suturina L, Walker W, et al. Criteria, prevalence, and phenotypes of polycystic ovary syndrome. *Fertil Steril* 2016;**106**(1):6–15.

10. Matsunaga I, Hata T, Kitao M. Ultrasonographic identification of polycystic ovary. *J Obstet Gynaecol Res* 1985;**11**(2):227–32.

11. Kratochwil A, Urban G, Friedrich F. Ultrasonic tomography of the ovaries. *Obstet Gynecol Survey* 1973;**28**(7):501–2.

12. Adams J, Polson D, Abdulwahid N, et al. Multifollicular ovaries: clinical and endocrine features and response to pulsatile gonadotropin releasing hormone. *The Lancet* 1985;**326**(8469–8470):1375–9.

13. Parisi L, Tramonti M, Derchi LE, et al. Polycystic ovarian disease: ultrasonic evaluation and correlations with clinical and hormonal data. *J Clin Ultrasound* 1984;**12**(1):21–6.

14. Hull M. Polycystic ovarian disease: clinical aspects and prevalence. *Res Clin Forums* 1989;**11**(1):989.

15. Battaglia C. The role of ultrasound and Doppler analysis in the diagnosis of polycystic ovary syndrome. *Ultrasound Obstet Gynecol* 2003;**22**(3):225–32.

16. Takahashi K, Ozaki T, Okada M, Uchida A, Kitao M. Relationship between ultrasonography and histopathological changes in polycystic ovarian syndrome. *Hum Reprod* 1994;**9**(12):2255–8.

17. Balen AH, Laven JS, Tan SL, Dewailly D. Ultrasound assessment of the polycystic ovary: international consensus definitions. *Hum Reprod Update* 2003;**9**(6):505–14.

18. Pache T, Wladimiroff J, Hop W, Fauser B. How to discriminate between normal and polycystic ovaries: transvaginal US study. *Radiology* 1992;**183**(2):421–3.

19. Jonard S, Robert Y, Dewailly D. Revisiting the ovarian volume as a diagnostic criterion for polycystic ovaries. *Hum Reprod* 2005;**20**(10):2893–8.

20. Nardo LG, Buckett WM, Khullar V. Determination of the best-fitting ultrasound formulaic method for ovarian volume measurement in women with polycystic ovary syndrome. *Fertil Steril* 2003;**79**(3):632–3.

21. Fulghesu AM, Ciampelli M, Belosi C, et al. A new ultrasound criterion for the diagnosis of polycystic ovary syndrome: the ovarian stroma/total area ratio. *Fertil Steril* 2001;**76**(2):326–31.

22. Dewailly D, Robert Y, Helin I, et al. Ovarian stromal hypertrophy in hyperandrogenic women. *Obstet Gynecol Survey* 1995;**50**(4):293–6.

23. Robert Y, Dubrulle F, Gaillandre L, et al. Ultrasound assessment of ovarian stroma hypertrophy in hyperandrogenism and ovulation disorders: visual analysis versus computerized quantification. *Fertil Steril* 1995;**64**(2):307–12.

24. Duijkers IJ, Klipping C. Polycystic ovaries, as defined by the 2003 Rotterdam consensus criteria, are found to be very common in young healthy women. *Gynecol Endocrinol* 2010;**26**(3):152–60.

25. Jokubkiene L, Sladkevicius P, Valentin L. Number of antral follicles, ovarian volume, and vascular indices in asymptomatic women 20 to 39 years old as assessed by 3-dimensional sonography. *J Ultrasound Med* 2012;**31**(10):1635–49.

26. Dewailly D, Lujan ME, Carmina E, et al. Definition and significance of polycystic ovarian morphology: a task force report from the Androgen Excess and Polycystic Ovary Syndrome Society. *Hum Reprod Update* 2014;**20**(3):334–52.

27. Battaglia C, Artini P, Salvatori M, et al. Ultrasonographic patterns of polycystic ovaries: color Doppler and hormonal correlations. *Ultrasound Obstet Gynecol* 1998;**11**(5):332–6.

28. Buckett W, Bouzayen R, Watkin K, Tulandi T, Tan S. Ovarian stromal echogenicity in women with normal and polycystic ovaries. *Hum Reprod* 1999;**14**(3):618–21.

29. Ardaens Y, Robert Y, Lemaitre L, Fossati P, Dewailly D. Polycystic ovarian disease: contribution of vaginal endosonography and reassessment of ultrasonic diagnosis. *Fertil Steril* 1991;**55**(6):1062–8.

30. Kyei-Mensah AA, LinTan S, Zaidi J, Jacobs HS. Relationship of ovarian stromal volume to serum androgen concentrations in patients with polycystic ovary syndrome. *Hum Reprod* 1998;**13**(6):1437–41.

31. Delgado-Rosas F, Gaytán M, Morales C, Gómez R, Gaytán F. Superficial ovarian cortex vascularization is inversely related to the follicle reserve in normal cycling ovaries and is increased in polycystic ovary syndrome. *Hum Reprod* 2009;**24**(5):1142–51.

32. Lam PM, Johnson IR, Raine-Fenning NJ. Three-dimensional ultrasound features of the polycystic ovary and the effect of different phenotypic expressions on these parameters. *Hum Reprod* 2007;**22**(12):3116–23.

33. Mala YM, Ghosh SB, Tripathi R. Three-dimensional power Doppler imaging in the diagnosis of polycystic ovary syndrome. *Int J Gynecol Obstet* 2009;**105**(1):36–8.

34. Järvelä I, Mason H, Sladkevicius P, et al. Characterization of normal and polycystic ovaries using three-dimensional power Doppler ultrasonography. *J Assist Reprod Genet* 2002;**19**(12):582–90.

35. Pascual MA, Graupera B, Hereter L, et al. Assessment of ovarian vascularization in the polycystic ovary by three-dimensional power Doppler ultrasonography. *Gynecol Endocrinol* 2008;**24**(11):631–6.

36. Raine-Fenning N, Nordin N, Ramnarine K, et al. Evaluation of the effect of machine settings on quantitative three-dimensional power Doppler angiography: an in-vitro flow phantom experiment. *Ultrasound Obstet Gynecol* 2008;**32**(4):551–9.

37. Polson D, Wadsworth J, Adams J, Franks S. Polycystic ovaries: a common finding in normal women. *The Lancet* 1988;**331**(8590):870–2.

38. Michelmore K, Balen A, Dunger D, Vessey M. Polycystic ovaries and associated clinical and biochemical features in young women. *Obstet Gynecol Survey* 2000;**55**(8):494–6.

39. Battaglia C, Regnani G, Mancini F, et al. Polycystic ovaries in childhood: a common finding in daughters of PCOS patients. A pilot study. *Hum Reprod* 2002;**17**(3):771–6.

40. Sagle M, Bishop K, Ridley N, et al. Recurrent early miscarriage and polycystic ovaries. *BMJ* 1988;**297**(6655):1027.

41. Kousta E, White D, Cela E, McCarthy M, Franks S. The prevalence of polycystic ovaries in women with infertility. *Hum Reprod* 1999;**14**(11):2720–3.

42. Amer S, Li T, Bygrave C, et al. An evaluation of the inter-observer and intra-observer variability of the ultrasound diagnosis of polycystic ovaries. *Hum Reprod* 2002;**17**(6):1616–22.

43. Lujan ME, Chizen DR, Peppin AK, Dhir A, Pierson RA. Assessment of ultrasonographic features of polycystic ovaries is associated with modest levels of inter-observer agreement. *J Ovarian Res* 2009;**2**(1):6.

44. Jayaprakasan K, Campbell B, Clewes J, Johnson I, Raine-Fenning N. Three-dimensional ultrasound improves the interobserver reliability of antral follicle counts and facilitates increased clinical work flow. *Ultrasound Obstet Gynecol* 2008;**31**(4):439–44.

45. Deb S, Campbell B, Clewes J, Raine-Fenning N. Quantitative analysis of antral follicle number and size: a comparison of two-dimensional and automated three-dimensional ultrasound techniques. *Ultrasound Obstet Gynecol* 2010;**35**(3):354–60.

46. Raine-Fenning N, Campbell B, Clewes J, Johnson I. The interobserver reliability of ovarian volume measurement is improved with three-dimensional ultrasound, but dependent upon technique. *Ultrasound Med Biol* 2003;**29**(12):1685–90.

47. Brett S, Bee N, Wallace W, Rajkhowa M, Kelsey T. Individual ovarian volumes obtained from 2-dimensional and 3-dimensional ultrasound lack precision. *Reprod Biomed Online* 2009;**18**(3):348–51.

48. Martins W. Three-dimensional power Doppler: validity and reliability. *Ultrasound Obstet Gynecol* 2010;**36**(5):530–3.

49. Raine-Fenning N, Nordin N, Ramnarine K, et al. Determining the relationship between three-dimensional power Doppler data and true blood flow characteristics: an in-vitro flow phantom experiment. *Ultrasound Obstet Gynecol* 2008;**32**(4):540–50.

50. Hickey M, Doherty D, Atkinson H, et al. Clinical, ultrasound and biochemical features of polycystic ovary syndrome in adolescents: implications for diagnosis. *Hum Reprod* 2011;**26**(6):1469–77.

51. Hickey M, Sloboda D, Atkinson H, et al. The relationship between maternal and umbilical cord androgen levels and polycystic ovary syndrome in adolescence: a prospective cohort study. *J Clin Endocrinol Metab* 2009;**94**(10):3714–20.

52. Mortensen M, Rosenfield RL, Littlejohn E. Functional significance of polycystic-size ovaries in healthy adolescents. *J Clin Endocrinol Metab* 2006;**91**(10):3786–90.

53. Carmina E, Oberfield SE, Lobo RA. The diagnosis of polycystic ovary syndrome in adolescents. *Am J Obstet Gynecol* 2010;**203**(3):201.e1–e5.

54. Brown M, Park AS, Shayya RF, et al. Ovarian imaging by magnetic resonance in adolescent girls with polycystic ovary syndrome and age-matched controls. *J Magn Reson Imaging* 2013;**38**(3):689–93.

Sonographic Assessment of Ovarian Cysts and Masses

Shama Puri

Pelvic ultrasound remains the single most effective method for detection and characterization of adnexal masses [1]. While transvaginal ultrasound provides optimal visualization, it has limited field of view; larger masses, which extend up into the abdomen, are best assessed by both transvaginal and transabdominal scan. Colour or power Doppler is useful in detecting flow in apparent solid areas and septations. The majority of adnexal masses are benign, particularly in premenopausal women. The vast majority of benign adnexal masses have characteristic ultrasound features to allow correct diagnosis in 90 per cent of women [2]. Ultrasound assessment of the morphological and vascular features of a mass has been shown to be highly effective for predicting whether a mass is benign or malignant. Accurate characterization of adnexal masses is essential for optimal patient management. Correctly identifying a benign mass enables the patient to be discharged or treated accordingly in general gynaecology departments, whereas patients with suspected malignancy should be referred appropriately to subspecialist gynaecology oncology units, which has been shown to optimize care and improve survival [3].

Ovarian Masses that Can Usually be Diagnosed on Ultrasound

Simple Cyst

These are usually hormone-dependent functional cysts.

Ultrasound features. Criteria for a simple cyst are: well circumscribed, anechoic with smooth, thin walls and posterior acoustic enhancement. No septations or solid elements are seen and there is no internal blood flow (Figure 8.1). They are usually less than 5 cm in size. Simple cysts less than 5 cm in premenopausal and less than 1 cm in postmenopausal women do not require a follow-up ultrasound scan [4]. A cyst that is otherwise simple but has a single thin septation or a small

calcification in the wall is almost always benign and should be followed in a similar fashion as a simple cyst [4].

Clinical significance. It is a common incidental finding in premenopausal women and most are follicular cysts, which regress spontaneously in one or two cycles. Rarely, simple ovarian cysts, particularly the larger ones or those in older women, are serous cystadenomas. In a study of postmenopausal women, no cancers were detected in 3259 simple cysts smaller than 10 cm, estimating the risk of malignancy in simple cysts as 0.1 per cent [5].

Ovarian Inclusion Cyst

These occur due to invagination of the ovarian cortical surface, resulting in cyst formation.

Ultrasound features. These are small, less than 10 mm simple cysts most commonly seen in postmenopausal women (Figure 8.2). In premenopausal women these cannot be differentiated from a follicle. They are typically located immediately beneath or within 1–2 mm of the ovarian surface. No internal blood flow is seen.

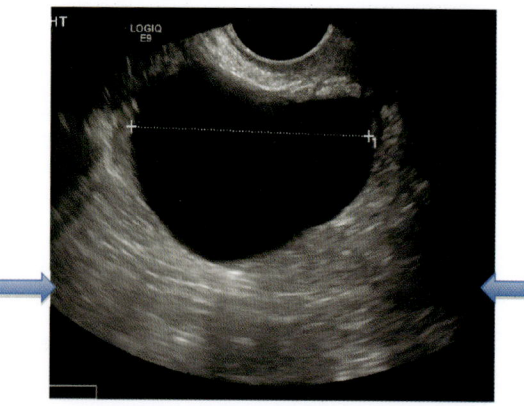

Figure 8.1 Follicular cyst in 30-year-old patient. It is completely anechoic, thin-walled and shows posterior acoustic enhancement (arrows).

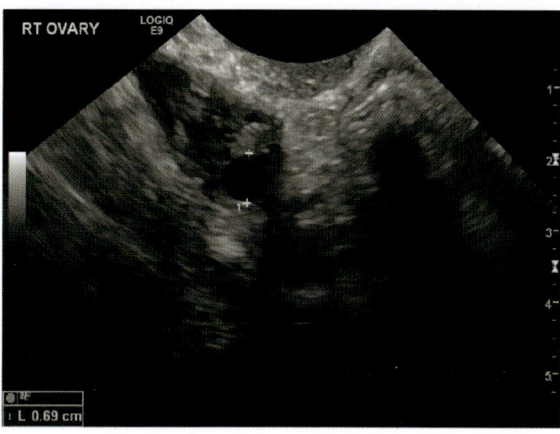

Figure 8.2 Ovarian inclusion cyst. Clinically inconsequential postmenopausal simple cyst less than 1 cm. It is anechoic and thin-walled with no solid elements or blood flow.

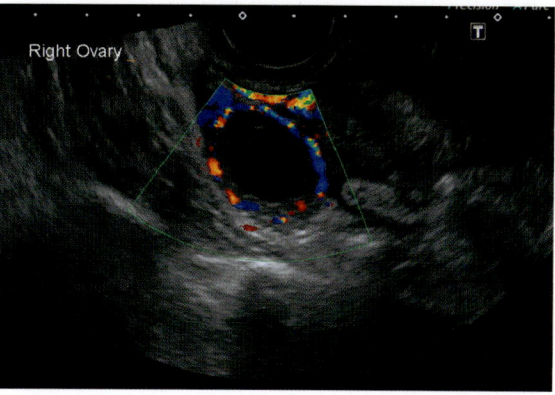

Figure 8.3 Corpus luteal cyst. Thick-walled cyst showing peripheral blood flow ('ring of fire'). It can have internal echoes and look more solid with internal haemorrhage.

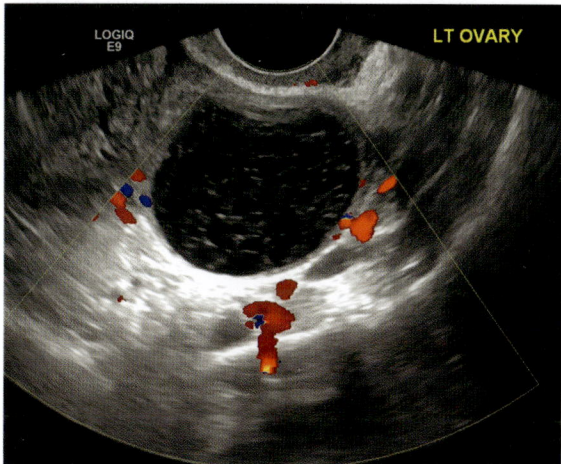

Figure 8.4 Haemorrhagic cyst in a 42-year-old patient. There is a reticular pattern of internal echoes due to fibrin strands giving a fishnet appearance. Fibrin strands are thin, weakly echogenic and do not extend completely across the cyst, unlike true septations.

Clinical significance. Common incidental finding with no clinical significance. They typically remain stable or involute and require no follow-up. The presence of ovarian inclusion cysts has no significance in identifying patients with increased risk of malignancy.

Corpus Luteum

Corpus luteum is a physiological structure that develops after ovulation and is a normal finding on ultrasound.

Ultrasound features. These are unilocular cysts typically less than 3 cm which can be simple/ anechoic or haemorrhagic. They have a thick, crenellated wall. Haemorrhage may produce internal echoes or mimic a solid mass [6]. There is no internal blood flow, but prominent vascular flow is noted in the cyst wall, described as a 'ring of fire' [7] (Figure 8.3).

Clinical significance. The majority regress spontaneously within two months. Mostly asymptomatic although can present with acute pelvic pain.

Haemorrhagic Cyst

This is a functional cyst with internal haemorrhage. Haemorrhage usually occurs during ovulation secondary to rupture of germinal epithelium. These are seen in premenopausal women or sometimes in early postmenopausal women due to occasional ovulation.

Ultrasound findings. A complex cystic mass with reticular pattern of internal echoes due to fibrin strands creating a net- or mesh-like appearance described as: lace-like, fishnet or cobweb (Figure 8.4). The clot can be seen as a solid-appearing area usually with concave margins, showing no internal blood flow (Figure 8.5). An echogenic, retracting clot may be confused as a solid mural nodule. Fluid–fluid levels may sometimes be seen, with echogenic blood products layered at the bottom [8] (Figure 8.6). A haemorrhagic cyst may overlap with endometrioma if imaged acutely before the fibrin strands or clot develop (Figure 8.7). If the cyst ruptures, echogenic free fluid in the pelvis may be seen.

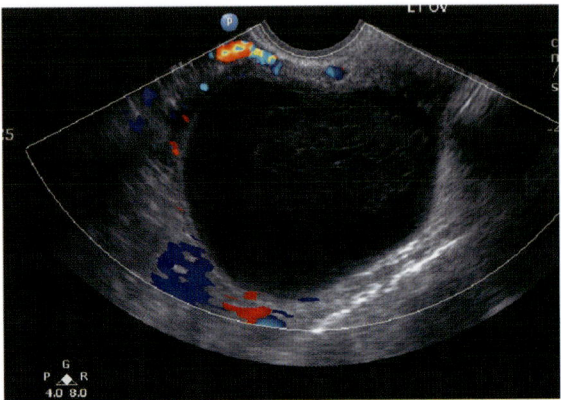

Figure 8.5 Haemorrhagic cyst with clot retraction. The clot could be mistaken for a solid component of a neoplasm. This structure had no internal blood flow and the cyst resolved at follow-up ultrasound at six weeks.

Tips and Tricks

Fibrin strands are thin, weakly echogenic and do not extend completely across the cyst, unlike true septations.

Clinical significance. Haemorrhagic cysts may be asymptomatic or present with acute pelvic pain. When large, these may serve as a lead point for ovarian torsion. No follow-up is necessary in asymptomatic women with cysts less than 5 cm. If more than 5 cm, a short-term follow-up in 6–12 weeks is recommended as they usually disappear or reduce significantly in size in 6–8 weeks. Ideally, the follow-up scan should be done in the follicular phase (day 3–10) of the menstrual cycle.

(a)

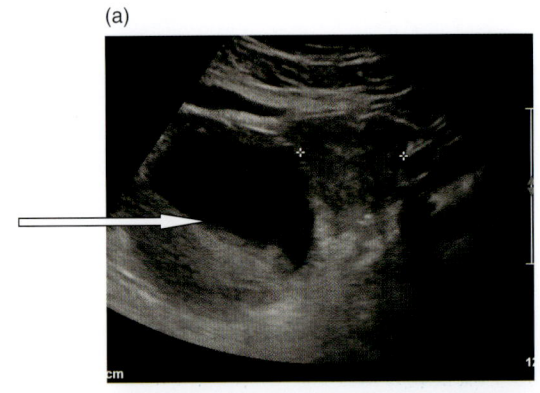

(b)

Figure 8.6 (a) Transabdominal scan of a haemorrhagic cyst showing fluid–fluid level (arrow) with blood products at the bottom. No blood flow was evident. Uterus marked by callipers. (b) Transvaginal scan of a haemorrhagic cyst with fluid–fluid level (arrow). Note that the level is almost horizontal on the abdominal scan and vertical on the transvaginal scan (the left of the screen is anterior, the right is posterior).

(a)

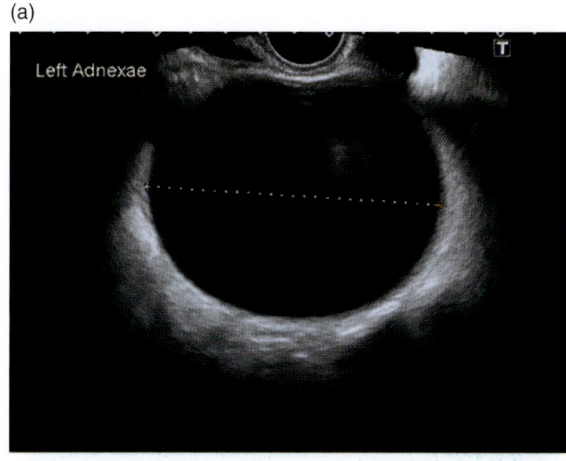

(b)

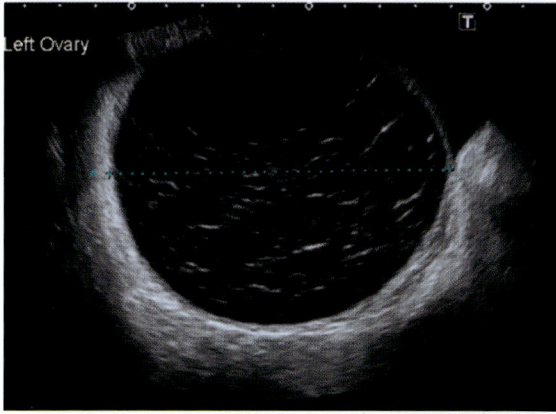

Figure 8.7 This young, five-weeks-pregnant lady had an ultrasound scan for spotting and lower abdominal pain. (a) Cyst with fine internal echoes due to acute haemorrhage. Scan repeated after one week (b) due to ongoing PV bleed shows fibrin strands typical of haemorrhagic cyst.

Endometrioma

Endometriomas are formed by extra-uterine functional endometrial tissue involving the ovary. Repeated bleeding every month in response to hormonal stimulation produces thick, concentrated and degraded blood products.

Ultrasound findings. Endometriomas show diffuse, homogeneous low- to medium-level internal echoes giving a ground glass appearance [9] (Figure 8.8). This may appear solid but posterior acoustic enhancement differentiates it from solid masses (Figure 8.9). They are usually unilocular but can be multilocular and may have a thick, fibrous wall. There may be tiny, echogenic foci or small solid areas along the cyst wall (Figure 8.9) [10,11]. These

should not be confused with mural nodules of malignancy. There is no internal vascular flow. Unlike haemorrhagic cysts they do not involute or disappear on follow-up scans. A small percentage (less than 15 per cent) have a less typical appearance, such as anechoic fluid, fluid–fluid level, heterogeneity or calcification [10–12]. Decidualized endometriomas are also uncommon and are characterized by the presence of hyperechoic foci within an otherwise homogeneous cyst, mainly observed in the luteal phase of the menstrual cycle (Figure 8.9b). Doppler signal may be present within these islands. Comparison with previous imaging confirming the presence of an endometrioma and a subsequent scan showing resolution of these changes aids in diagnosis.

> ### Tips and Tricks
>
> Diffuse internal echoes can sometimes be seen in dermoids, haemorrhagic cysts and some ovarian carcinomas [13]. Other features, such as a dermoid plug or solid component, will suggest different diagnoses. An endometrioma is very likely if there are diffuse internal echoes in a cystic mass with no other ultrasound features [10].

Rarely malignancy (endometrioid or clear cell carcinomas) may develop in endometriomas (1 per cent), likely in those larger than 9 cm and in women older than 45 years [14]. Development of a significant solid component with flow on Doppler should raise concern for malignancy.

Clinical significance. Usual presentation is with dysmenorrhoea, dyspareunia and infertility. Treatment is usually by hormonal suppression or surgery.

Dermoid (Mature Cystic Teratoma)

Benign germ cell tumour of the ovary, which occurs during reproductive years, is the most common benign ovarian tumour in women less than 45 years old. It is composed of well-differentiated derivatives of all three germ layers and may be composed of adipose tissue, hair, bone, teeth, cutaneous, bronchial and gastrointestinal tissues. Fat is present in about two-thirds of cases. It is bilateral in 20 per cent of cases.

Ultrasound features. Ultrasound appearance is variable, depending upon histological composition. Demonstration of fat clinches the diagnosis. Characteristic ultrasound appearance is cystic adnexal

103

(a)

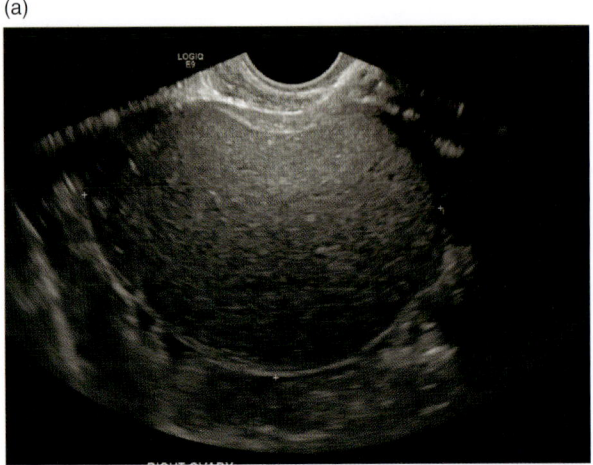

(b)

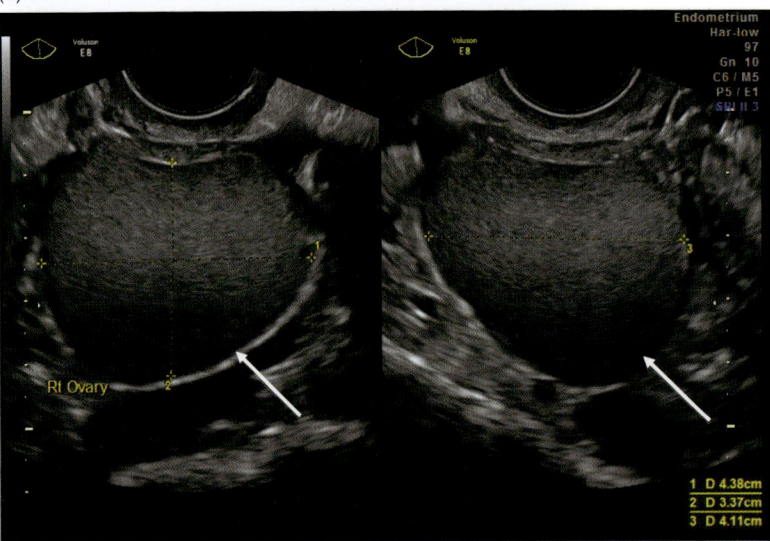

Figure 8.8 (a) An endometrioma in a 34-year-old woman. Homogeneous low-level echoes giving a ground glass appearance. (b) An endometrioma in a different patient, measured in three orthogonal planes. The content is homogeneous, but more hypoechoic in the posterior aspect of the cyst due to attenuation of ultrasound waves (arrows).

mass containing a highly echogenic mural nodule with distal acoustic shadowing (Rokitansky nodule or dermoid plug) (Figure 8.10) [15,16]. The echogenic focus consists of adipose tissue, hair and calcium, which cause posterior acoustic shadowing. Very echogenic focus casting a sharp acoustic shadow is due to the presence of bone or teeth (Figure 8.11).

Other common appearances are:

- Diffusely or partially echogenic mass with distal acoustic shadowing (Figure 8.11). Shadowing may be so marked that only the superficial part of the cyst is seen, called the 'tip of iceberg' sign (Figure 8.12).
- Dermoid mesh: multiple thin echogenic lines and dots caused by hair in the cyst cavity [15,16] (Figure 8.12).

- Floating echogenic globules [17]: multiple echogenic floating globules are present in the cyst cavity, which change position with change in the patient's position (Figure 8.13).
- Fluid–fluid level: more echogenic fluid (sebum) layered on the top of serous fluid [18]. This is opposite to the haemorrhagic cyst, where echogenic blood products are layered at the bottom.

Rarely, a dermoid will have none of these characteristic features [9] (Figure 8.14) and cannot be diagnosed on ultrasound appearance.

Tips and Tricks

Highly reflective area with distal shadowing in a cystic mass is highly predictive of a dermoid. Blood

(a)

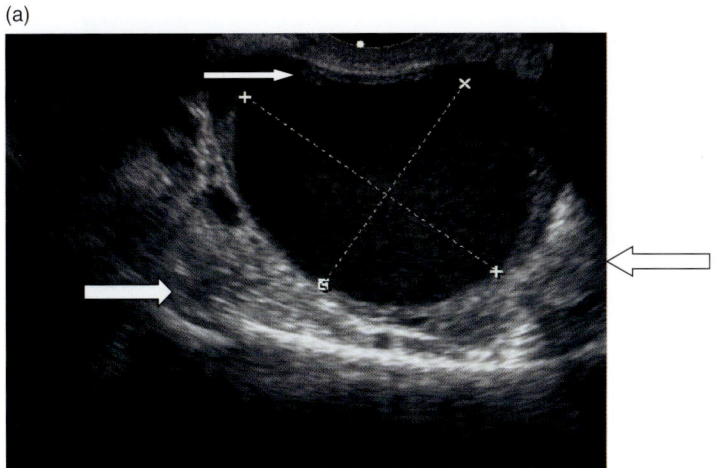

Figure 8.9 (a) An endometrioma (callipers) may appear solid but posterior acoustic enhancement (bold arrow) differentiates it from solid masses. They may show small echogenic nodules in the wall (a and b) (thin arrows). (b) Luteal phase scan; an endometrioma (callipers) with hyperechoic nodules on the periphery (arrows). Vascularity was present on Doppler and comparisons with earlier and subsequent imaging confirmed it was decidualization of the ectopic endometrium.

(b)

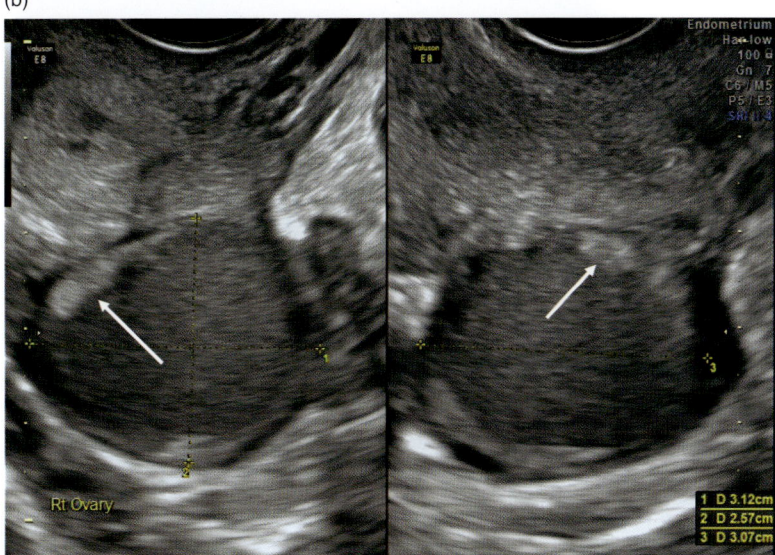

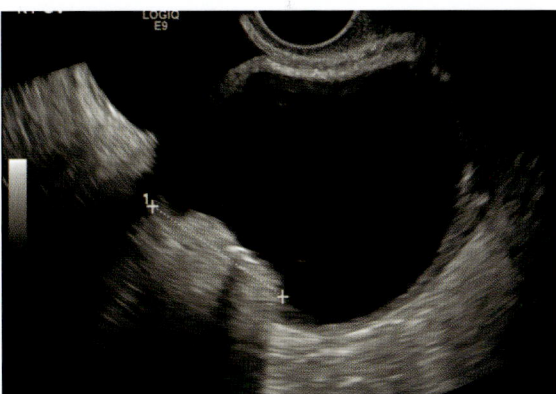

Figure 8.10 Dermoid in a 45-year-old patient. Cystic adnexal mass containing highly echogenic component (marked by callipers) with distal acoustic shadowing (Rokitansky nodule or dermoid plug).

clot in haemorrhagic cyst and solid elements in a complex ovarian cyst can appear echogenic, but these tend to be less echogenic than the fatty component of a dermoid cyst and do not cause shadowing (Figure 8.15). If there is any doubt, CT and MRI can confirm the presence or absence of fat.

Clinical significance. Usually asymptomatic and managed non-surgically if dermoid measures less than 6 cm. Dermoids larger than 7 cm can cause torsion or rupture. Torsion is most common during pregnancy. Surgery involves excision of the dermoid with conservation of ovarian tissue. Malignant transformation is rare and usually occurs in the sixth or seventh decade of life with tumours larger than 10 cm [19]. Squamous cell carcinoma is the most common associated cancer.

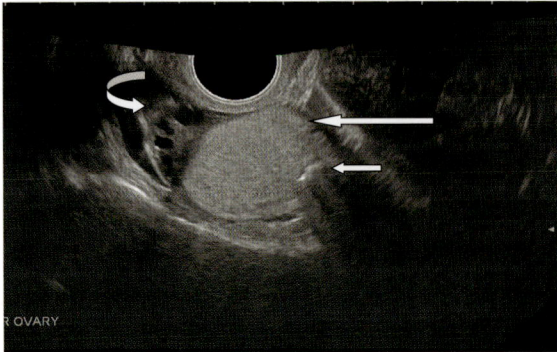

Figure 8.11 Dermoid in a 20-year-old patient. The right ovary shows a well-defined hyperechoic component (long arrow), which did not show any vascular flow. Calcification seen within this mass (short arrow) is even brighter and shows distinct shadowing. Normal ovary is seen (curved arrow) at the periphery.

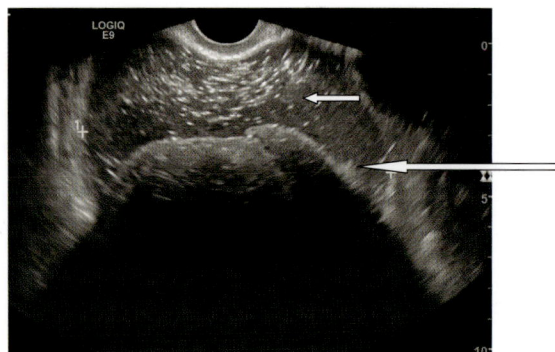

Figure 8.12 Tip of iceberg sign: dermoid with large echogenic component causing marked shadowing (long arrow) and obscuring the posterior part of the dermoid. Hyperechoic dots and lines are termed dermoid mesh (short arrow). There was no blood flow on Doppler.

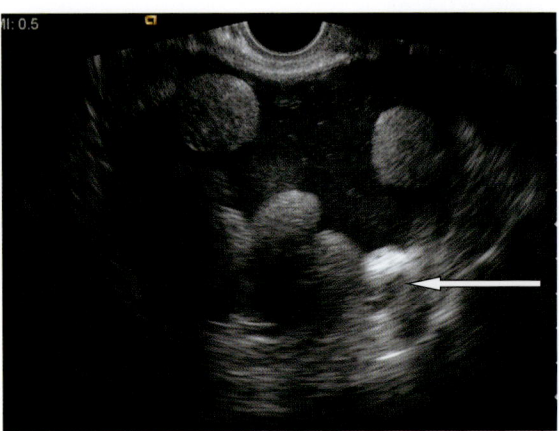

Figure 8.13 Dermoid in a 28-year-old patient. Multiple echogenic floating globules are typical of a dermoid. Small, very echogenic focus with shadowing posteriorly is a calcification (arrow).

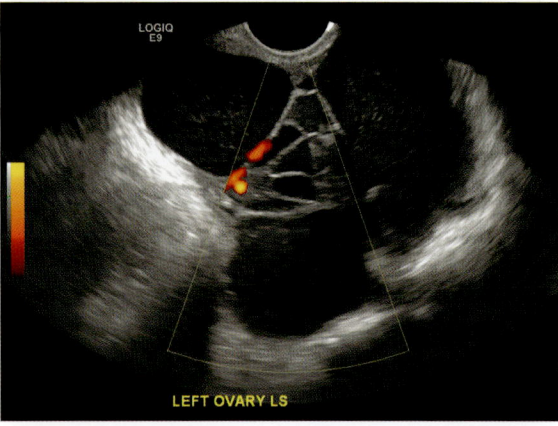

Figure 8.14 Atypical dermoid with septations and colour flow. No typical features of dermoid were seen. The mass was excised and a diagnosis of dermoid was made on histology.

Ovarian Fibroma/Fibrothecoma

A benign solid ovarian neoplasm classified as sex cord-stromal tumour. The spectrum includes fibroma, thecoma and fibrothecoma. These lesions are composed of fibrous tissue and theca cells, which are responsible for the oestrogenic effects of these tumours. They are usually asymptomatic and found incidentally.

Ultrasound features. Well-defined round or oval low-echo solid mass, usually homogeneous with acoustic shadowing (Figure 8.16). Marked acoustic shadowing is a predictive feature that occurs in 18–52 per cent of fibromas [20,21]. With fibromas, shadowing does not arise from an area of increased echogenicity such as dermoid plug or calcification, but due to attenuation of the sound by the mass itself. Calcification can be present. Larger lesion shows cystic change. Generally hypovascular, although may show increased vascularity. Differential diagnosis is pedunculated uterine leiomyoma where a separate ovary is often seen and a pedicle extending to the uterus may be seen. A minority of ovarian fibromas grow exophytically from the ovary [22] and may be difficult to distinguish from a pedunculated uterine fibroid.

Tips and Tricks

A completely solid mass, particularly in a premenopausal woman, is usually a fibroma.

(a)

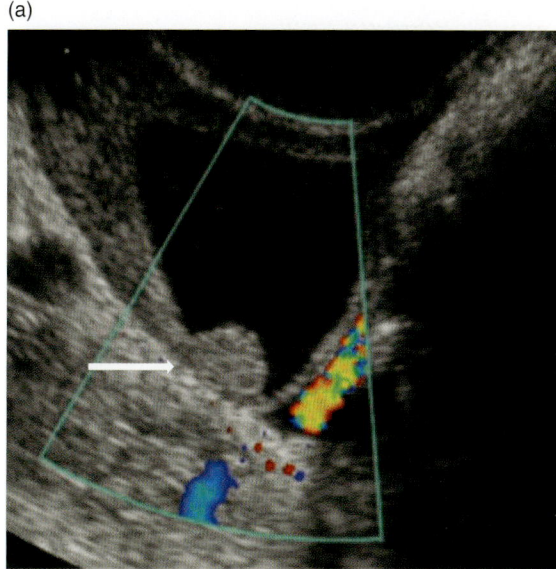

(b)

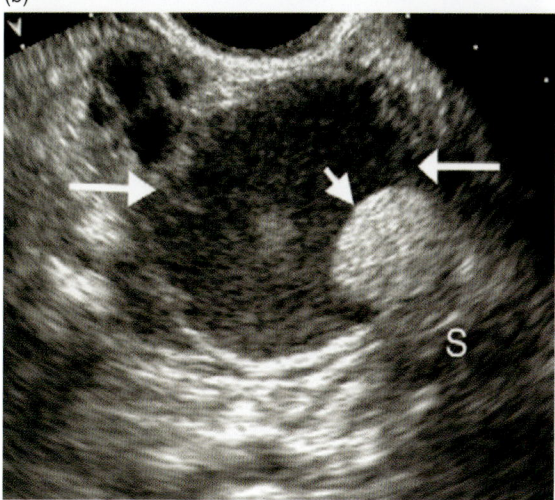

Figure 8.15 Solid elements in a complex ovarian cyst (a) tend to be less echogenic than the fatty component of dermoid (small arrow in (b)) and do not cause shadowing as caused by a dermoid plug (S).

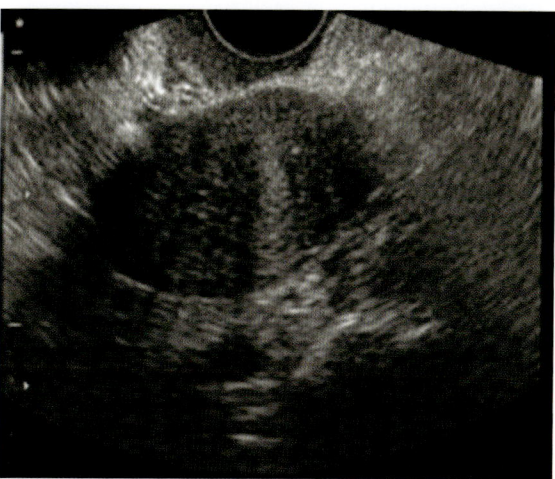

Figure 8.16 Incidental finding of a fibroma in a 42-year-old patient. Well-defined solid mass with posterior shadowing.

of women develop ovarian fibromas which tend to be bilateral, multiple and calcified.

Extra-Ovarian Masses that Can Usually be Diagnosed on Ultrasound

Paraovarian Cyst

Separate from the ovary, it usually arises from peritoneal mesothelium of the broad ligament.

Ultrasound features. Simple unilocular adnexal cyst separate from the ovary. It is thin-walled with no septations or solid elements (Figures 8.17 and 8.18). If the extra-ovarian location is not obvious, the ovary may be separated from the cyst by gentle pressure from the transvaginal probe or the examiner's hand on the lower abdomen.

Clinical significance. Can be symptomatic if large. Almost always benign and no follow-up is required in the vast majority [4].

Hydrosalpinx

A dilated, fluid-filled fallopian tube usually forms owing to obstruction of its ampullary segment. The most common cause is adhesions from pelvic inflammatory disease (PID). It usually contains clear serous fluid. Fluid may be haemorrhagic (haematosalpinx), usually as a result of endometriosis, or purulent (pyosalpinx) as a complication of PID.

Ultrasound features. A normal fallopian tube is usually not visible on an ultrasound. Hydrosalpinx

Clinical significance. Always benign. Excision of affected ovary by laparoscopy for larger lesions. Ovarian thecoma may be associated with endometrial thickening if it secretes oestrogen. One per cent of ovarian fibromas are associated with Meigs syndrome, which consists of ovarian fibroma, ascites and pleural effusion, both of which disappear with excision of the tumour. In Gorlin–Goltz syndrome (rare autosomal dominant syndrome with craniofacial anomalies and multiple basal cell carcinomas of the skin), 25 per cent

107

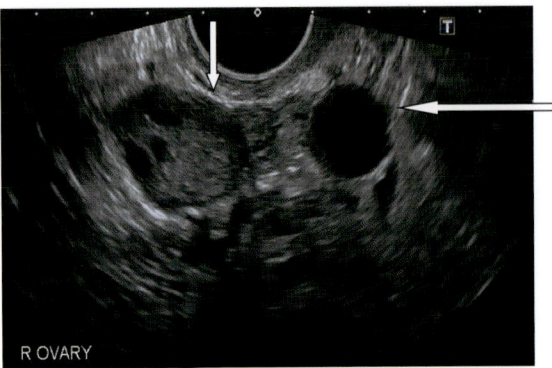

Figure 8.17 Paraovarian cyst in a 41-year-old patient. Simple cyst (long arrow) seen separate to the ovary (short arrow).

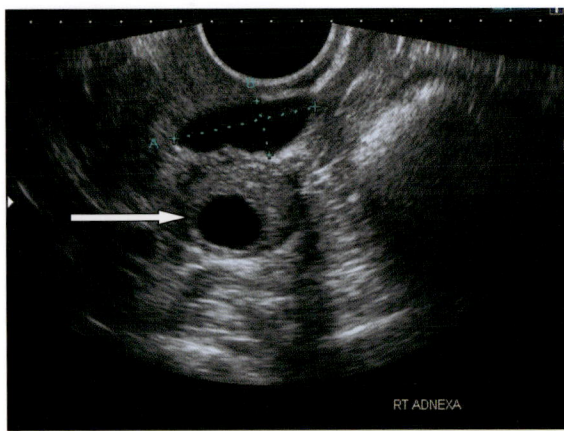

Figure 8.18 Paraovarian cyst in a 29-year-old patient. Simple cyst (callipers) seen separate to the ovary (arrow).

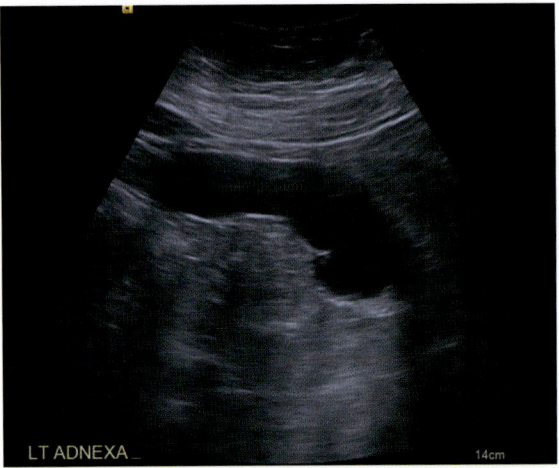

Figure 8.19 Transabdominal scan showing tubular cystic C-shaped structure typical of hydrosalpinx.

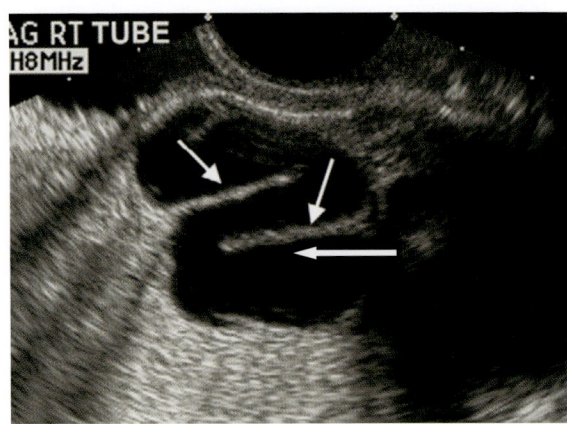

Figure 8.20 Hydrosalpinx in a 25-year-old patient. Tubular tortuous cystic structure with incomplete septations representing endosalpingeal folds (arrows).

is seen as a tubular, thin-walled, fluid-filled structure with a C or S shape, interposed between the uterus and ovary (Figure 8.19). Incomplete septations within the tubular cystic structure represent partially effaced mucosal or submucosal plicae, a finding specific to a hydrosalpinx (Figure 8.20). Thickened endosalpingeal folds can give a 'beads on a string' appearance that consists of small 2–3 mm hyperechoic, short, round projections along the tubal wall [23] (Figure 8.21). The 'waist sign' constitutes indentations of the tube wall directly opposite each other (Figure 8.22), forming a waist [23]. Presence of the 'waist sign' or 'beads on string' sign in a tubular cystic structure is highly predictive of hydrosalpinx [23].

In a haematosalpinx and pyosalpinx, fluid is echogenic and may contain debris (Figure 8.23). In pyosalpinx, the tubal wall is thickened to more than 5 mm and there is increased vascularity and associated fever, pain and raised white cell count. The surrounding pelvic fat is more echogenic and shows increased vascularity due to inflammation. When chronic, the tube has a thick fibrous wall with small lumen and little fluid [24].

Tips and Tricks

Hyperechoic, short, round projections along the tubal wall in hydrosalpinx should not be confused with solid components of a neoplasm, as the solid

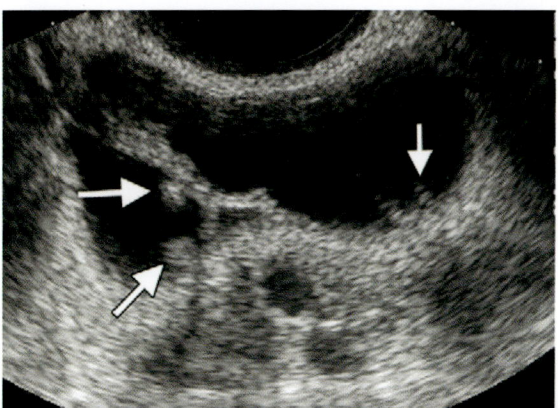

Figure 8.21 'Beads on a string' sign of hydrosalpinx (or cog-wheel appearance) – hyperechoic, short, round projections within the tube (arrows).

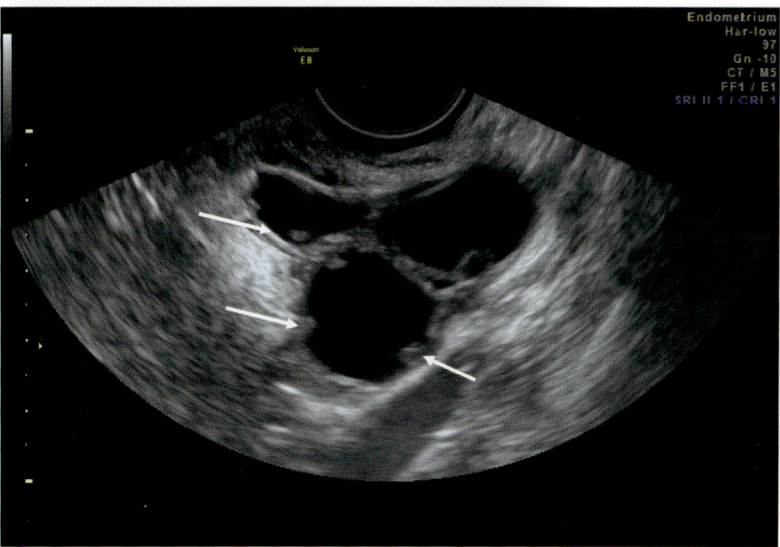

component of the rare fallopian tube carcinoma is usually larger and less numerous than multiple small nodules seen in hydrosalpinx due to thickened endosalpingeal folds.

Clinical significance. Usually asymptomatic. Can present with pelvic pain or infertility. It can be treated by lysis of adhesions and tuboplasty.

Peritoneal Inclusion Cyst

Also referred to as peritoneal pseudocyst, this is a benign non-neoplastic cystic pelvic mass typically seen in premenopausal women with functioning ovaries and pelvic adhesions impairing the absorption of ovarian fluid secreted during ovulation. Almost always, there is a history of pelvic surgery, PID or endometriosis.

Figure 8.22 'Waist sign' of hydrosalpinx. Indentations on the opposite of the tubular cystic structure forming a waist (arrows) are typical of hydrosalpinx.

(a)

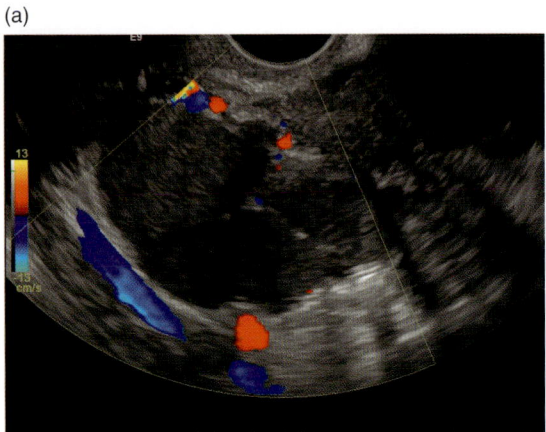

(b)

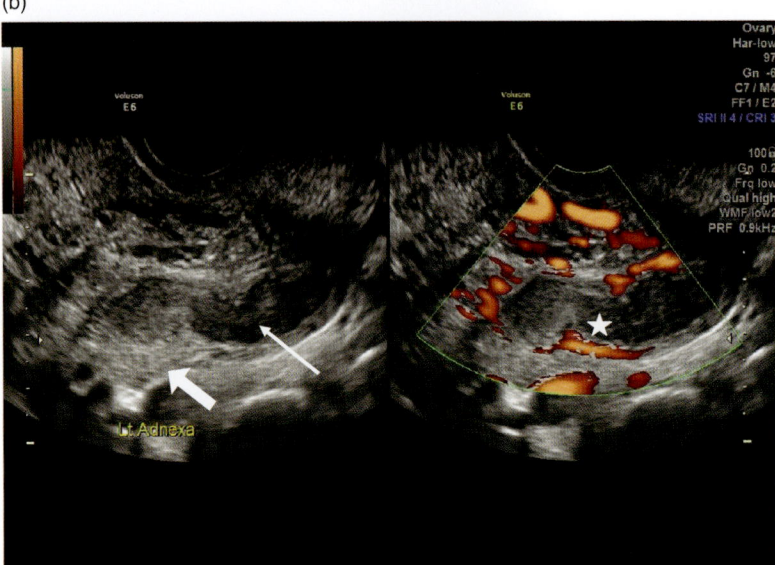

Figure 8.23 (a) Haematosalpinx in a young woman with endometriosis. Tubular C-shaped cystic structure with incomplete septations and internal echoes. (b) Pyosalpinx in a young woman with PID. Note the thick wall of the tube (thick arrow) and particulate content (pus; thin arrow). Power Doppler imaging shows increased vascularity consistent with an inflammatory process (star).

Ultrasound features. Unilocular or multilocular cystic mass conforming to the contours of the peritoneal cavity with a normal-appearing ovary suspended within the mass, either centrally – 'spider in web' appearance – or at the periphery [25] (Figure 8.24). Septations, when present, are usually thin and smooth but may be thick and show colour flow. No solid elements are present. The ovarian contour may be distorted by adhesions. In contrast to septae within true ovarian cysts, the septae in pseudocysts generally move and 'flap' when the cystic area is prodded by the transvaginal ultrasound probe. This has been described as the 'flapping sail sign'.

Tips and Tricks

Key to the recognition of a peritoneal cyst is the demonstration of a normal ovary within or along the periphery of a cystic mass.

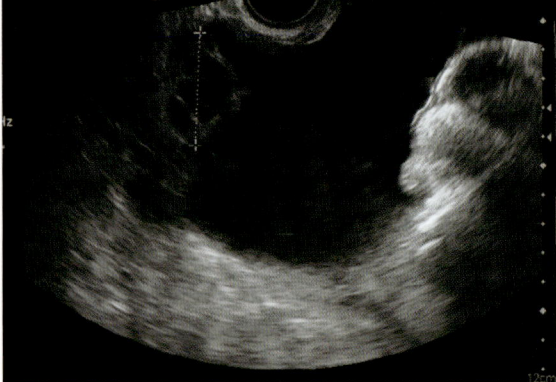

Figure 8.24 Peritoneal inclusion cyst in a 45-year-old woman with a history of pelvic surgery. Unilocular cystic mass conforming to the contours of peritoneal cavity with ovary suspended at the periphery (marked by callipers).

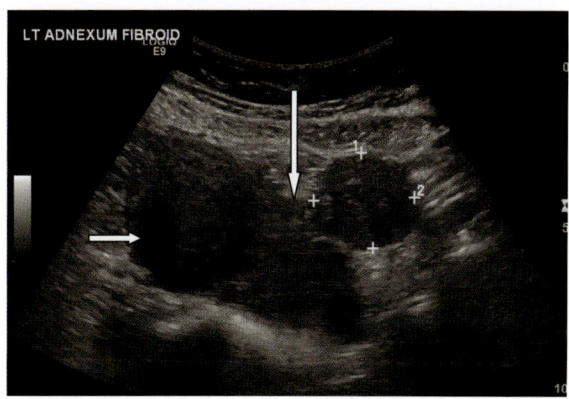

Figure 8.25 Pedunculated uterine fibroid (callipers) in the left adnexum attached to the uterus with a pedicle (long arrow). Uterus also shows an intramural fibroid (short arrow). Left ovary was seen separate to the mass.

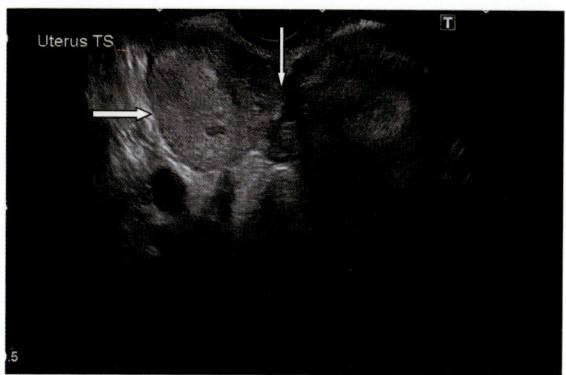

Figure 8.26 Pedunculated uterine fibroid (short arrow) in the right adnexum attached to the uterus with a short pedicle (long arrow).

Clinical significance. Usual presentation is with pelvic pain, discomfort or fullness, although it may be an incidental finding. These are typically treated conservatively as risk of recurrence is high following surgery. Oral contraceptives and gonadotrophin-releasing hormone analogue decrease ovarian fluid production.

Pedunculated Uterine Fibroid

These are solid masses that can be confused with ovarian fibromas if ipsilateral ovary is not seen. Identifying a vascular pedicle ('bridging vascular sign') connecting the mass to the uterus is good evidence of a pedunculated fibroid [26,27] (Figures 8.25 and 8.26). Cystic degeneration can occur.

Benign Adnexal Masses that Are More Challenging to Diagnose on Ultrasound

Tubo-ovarian Abscess

This occurs as a complication of PID, resulting in formation of an inflammatory mass involving both fallopian tube and ovary. It most commonly occurs due to bacterial infection – *Neisseria gonorrhoea* and *Chlamydia trachomatis* are the most common. Rare causes include actinomycosis or tuberculosis (TB).

Ultrasound features. Due to varying ultrasound appearances, tubo-ovarian abscesses can be difficult to diagnose reliably on ultrasound alone. Clinical signs and symptoms consistent with PID are usually necessary to diagnose a tubo-ovarian abscess. Fallopian tube and ovary are usually not seen separately, but together form the tubo-ovarian complex. These tend to be a complex multilocular adnexal mass with varying internal echogenicity (Figure 8.27). Solid-appearing areas may be present. Internal gas is uncommon. When present, gas is seen as echogenic foci with shadowing or 'ringdown' artefact. Adjacent peritoneum is echogenic due to inflammation. There can be reactive thickening of the adjacent bowel wall.

Clinical significance. Occurs in sexually active young women. Most common signs and symptoms are fever, pelvic pain and mucopurulent vaginal discharge. Intrauterine contraceptive devices (IUCD) increase the risk of PID, which tends to occur within the first few months of insertion and there is higher occurrence of actinomycosis.

Adnexal Torsion

This is the rotation of an ovary on its vascular pedicle causing venous congestion and ultimately infarction of the ovary. Venous flow is affected first, followed by arterial. As the fallopian tube is invariably involved in the torsion, adnexal torsion is a more accurate term than ovarian torsion.

Ultrasound features. The ovary is enlarged to more than 4 cm and tends to have a swollen, rounded contour with echogenic stroma and follicles pushed to the periphery due to stromal oedema [28,29] (Figure 8.28–8.30). The affected ovary is often displaced midline, cephalad, anterior to uterine fundus

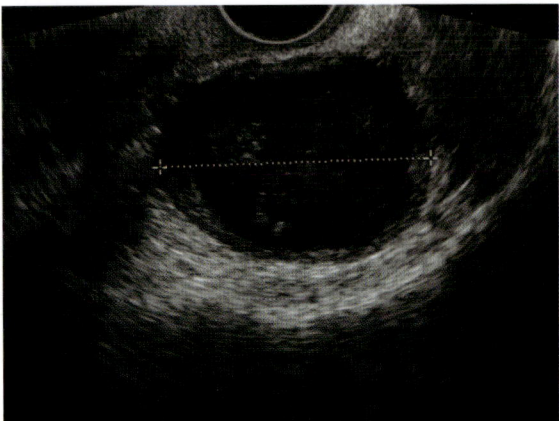

Figure 8.27 Resolving left tubo-ovarian abscess in a 35-year-old patient. There is a thick-walled unilocular complex cystic mass with a large, solid-appearing area. Initial diagnosis was made on CT when she presented with left iliac fossa (LIF) pain and raised inflammatory markers, with diverticulitis suspected clinically. Follow-up ultrasound was performed due to ongoing pain despite antibiotics. Diagnosis of tubo-ovarian abscess was confirmed at surgery.

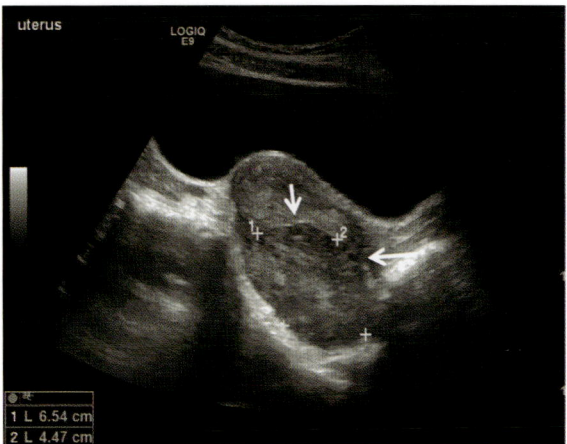

Figure 8.28 Ovarian torsion in a 12-year-old patient with abdominal pain. Enlarged solid ovary (callipers) with small follicles at the periphery (arrows) is seen behind the uterus on transabdominal scan.

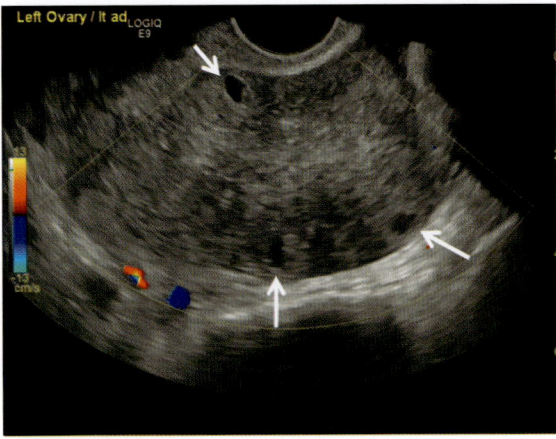

Figure 8.29 Ovarian torsion in a 29-year-old patient. Enlarged echogenic ovary with peripheral follicles (arrows) with no flow on colour Doppler imaging.

or in the pouch of Douglas (Figure 8.28). The uterus tends to deviate towards the side of torsion. Pelvic free fluid may be present. An oedematous fallopian tube may be seen as a heterogeneous tubular structure. A coiled, twisted pedicle is rarely seen on ultrasound and more likely to be seen on CT or MRI. The presence of normal blood flow does not exclude torsion, as twist can be intermittent or incomplete. The presence of venous flow indicates a viable ovary. If no flow is seen, the ovary is infracted (Figure 8.29). Visualization of blood vessels in the ovarian pedicle with the aid of colour Doppler imaging may reveal a whirlpool arrangement, indicating the position of torsion. Comparison of the ultrasound appearance and flow of the contralateral ovary may aid significantly in diagnosis.

In adults, the majority of women will have an ovarian mass that serves as the lead point for torsion (Figure 8.30). Large follicular or corpus luteal cysts followed by dermoid are the most common masses serving as the lead point for torsion. Infants and children rarely have adnexal masses and torsion is caused due to long mesosalpinx causing hypermobility.

Clinical significance. Ovarian torsion is most common in the first three decades of life and more common in pregnancy. Women undergoing ovarian stimulation are at increased risk. Patients present with severe acute pelvic pain, which may be intermittent due to torsion/detorsion. Surgical untwisting can preserve the ovary if non-infracted. The mass serving as the lead point should be removed. Salpingo-oophrectomy is undertaken for an infarcted ovary.

Tips and Tricks

Absent venous flow in an enlarged echogenic ovary with prominent peripheral follicles is the earliest reliable sign to diagnose ovarian torsion. Presence of normal blood flow does not exclude torsion.

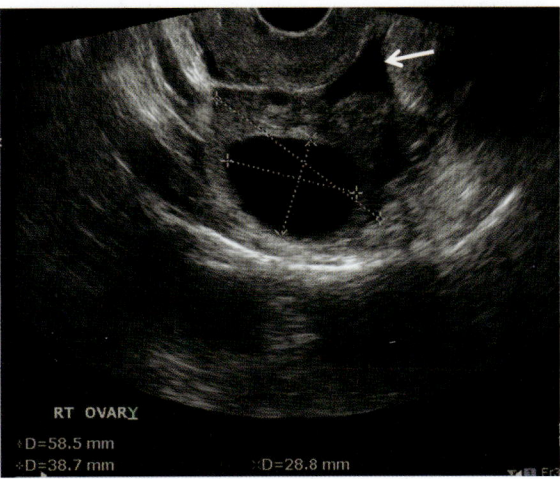

Figure 8.30 Ovarian torsion in a 24-year-old patient with acute pelvic pain. The ovary is enlarged (long callipers) with small follicles seen at the periphery and trace of fluid surrounding the ovary (arrow). There is a 3.8 cm follicular cyst (short callipers) within the ovary, considered to be the lead point for torsion.

Uncommon Benign Non-gynaecological Pelvic Masses

It should be borne in mind that non-gynaecological causes can present as pelvic cysts and masses. Tarlov (peri-neural) cyst should be considered when a cystic mass is seen posteriorly separate from the ovaries. Appendiceal mucocele can be seen as a cystic mass with internal echoes in the right iliac fossa. Following pelvic surgery, cystic masses can be lymphoceles or haematomas. Pelvic lymph nodes are seen as well-defined solid masses separate from the ovaries.

Ovarian Neoplasms

Ovarian neoplasms are classified histologically as epithelial, germ cell, sex cord-stromal and metastatic neoplasms [30]. Ninety per cent of ovarian cancers are epithelial in origin [31]. All epithelial ovarian neoplasms can be classified as benign, borderline (i.e. having a low potential for malignancy and more favourable prognosis) or malignant. The two most common types of epithelial neoplasms are serous and mucinous tumours, others being clear cell, endometrioid, Brenner, and undifferentiated tumours. Epithelial tumours are rare before puberty; their prevalence increases with age and peaks in the sixth and seventh decades of life [32]. The most common type of ovarian malignancy is serous carcinoma (approximately 70 per cent of cases). The

vast majority of epithelial ovarian malignancies are cystic in nature and very rarely entirely solid [33,34]. Ovarian cancers most commonly present as complex cystic adnexal masses on imaging.

When ultrasound features of an adnexal mass do not fit into a common benign pathology, these are considered indeterminate and potentially malignant. Determination of a degree of suspicion for malignancy is the most critical next step after identification of the mass. The degree of suspicion for malignancy in a given mass is based largely on imaging appearance, but other factors such as serum CA-125 level and menopausal status must also be considered. This stratification of risk becomes particularly important when conservative management is being considered. Expedited referral of patients with suspicious masses to a gynaecological oncology team for definitive staging with laparotomy correlates with better survival rates [3].

Ultrasound Features

A septum is defined as a thin strand of tissue running across the cyst cavity from one internal surface to the contralateral side [19]. An incomplete septum runs across the cyst cavity from one internal surface to the contralateral side without being complete in some scanning planes [35]. If a cyst has more than one complete septum, it is classified as multilocular. A cyst with no complete septum is classified as unilocular. Septations can be described as thin (less than 3 mm) (Figures 8.31 and 8.32) or thick (greater than 3 mm) (Figure 8.33), and smooth or irregular.

A solid component can be described as papillary projections, excrescence or nodule. Solid nodules that protrude 3 mm or more from the cyst wall should be considered as papillary projections (Figure 8.34). Diffuse wall thickening of a cyst, ovarian stroma, blood clots, fat and regular septa are not regarded as solid tissue [9,35]. The presence of Doppler flow in solid components is suspicious for malignancy. Other ultrasound features, such as size of the mass and wall thickness, are less useful findings to predict malignancy.

There is a general trend towards low-resistance and high-velocity flow in malignant neoplasms. There is, however, substantial overlap in the spectral Doppler indices between benign and malignant disease and it is not reliable in differentiating the two. Spectral Doppler is useful in a situation in which distinct vessels are not seen on colour or power Doppler and only a few scattered pixels are seen,

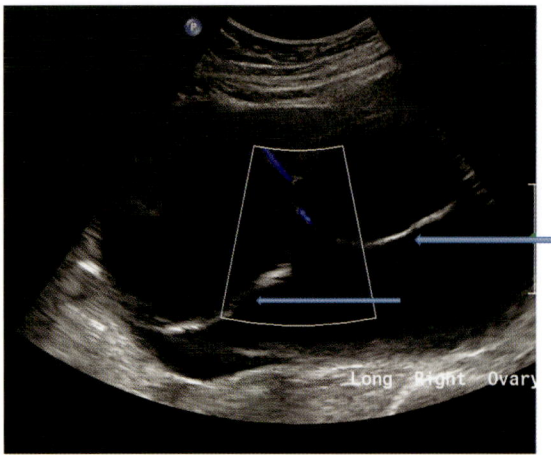

Figure 8.31 Multilocular cystic mass showing a few smooth, thin septations with flow on Doppler in a 62-year-old patient. No solid component is present. It was a mucinous cystadenoma on histology.

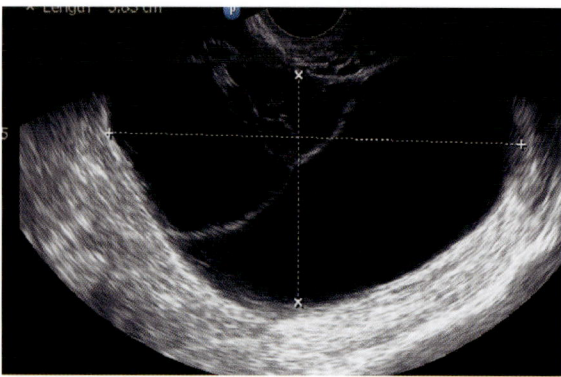

Figure 8.32 Multilocular cystic mass with multiple thin septations in a 67-year-old patient. No solid nodules or colour flow were seen. It was a mucinous cystadenoma on histology.

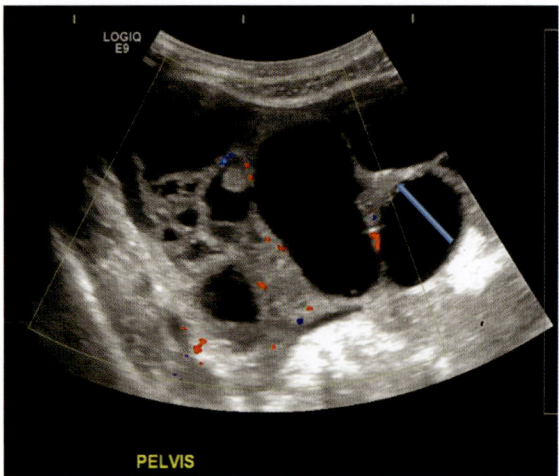

Figure 8.33 Multilocular cystic mass with thick septations and large solid component showing colour flow in a 63-year-old woman. Serous cystadenocarcinoma was demonstrated on histology.

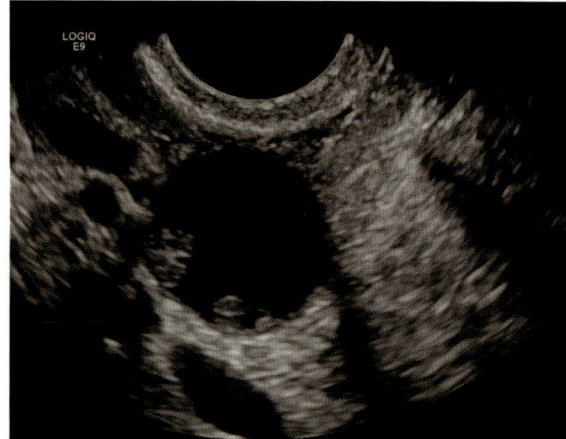

Figure 8.34 Unilocular cystic mass with small papillary projections showing no flow in a 66-year-old. Histology confirmed serous cystadenoma.

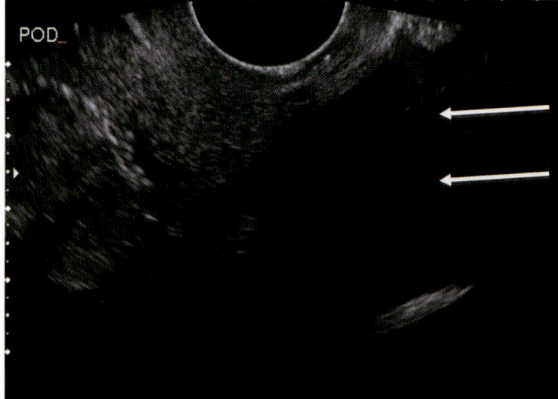

Figure 8.35 Free fluid with internal echoes were seen in the pouch of Douglas (arrows) in the same patient as in Figure 8.34.

making it difficult to determine if they are artefacts from noise or whether real blood flow is present.

Ancillary findings that are strong indicators of malignancy are: ascites (Figure 8.35), peritoneal metastasis and abdominal lymphadenopathy. Ascites occurs with peritoneal spread of malignancy and may allow peritoneal implants to be seen. It should be borne in mind that no single ultrasound finding differentiates categorically between benign and malignant ovarian masses unless there is evidence of metastatic spread.

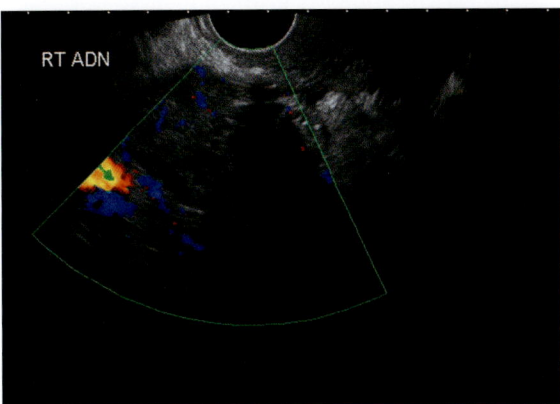

Figure 8.36 Complex solid cystic mass showing avid flow in the solid areas in a 71-year-old patient. Histology revealed mucinous adenocarcinoma.

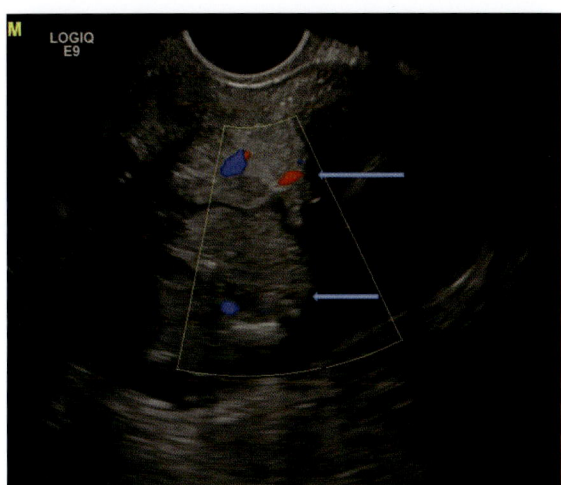

Figure 8.37 Cystic mass with large solid components with Doppler flow in a 46-year-old woman. On histology, this was grade 1 endometrioid adenocarcinoma.

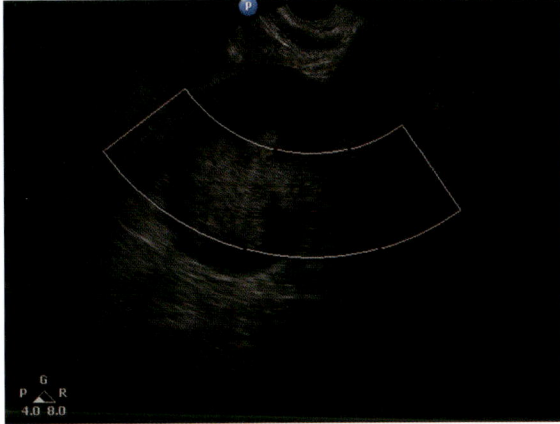

Figure 8.38 Unilocular cystic mass with large solid component showing no vascular flow in a 30-year-old woman. It was a borderline serous tumour on histology.

Multiple thin septations or a solid nodule without detectable flow is suggestive of benign neoplasm (Figures 8.31, 8.32 and 8.34). Thick, irregular septations and solid elements with significant blood flow are worrisome for malignant neoplasms (Figures 8.33, 8.36 and 8.37).

Although cystic mass with solid component is an indicator of malignancy, solid components can be seen in benign as well as borderline epithelial tumours [2,36] (Figures 8.38 and 8.39). The presence of flow increases concern for malignancy but benign neoplasms can also show vascularity. Borderline tumours tend to show more proliferation (papillary projections) than cystadenomas; there

are, however, no reliable ultrasound features to differentiate borderline tumours from invasive or benign tumours.

There are some ultrasound features to differentiate between serous and mucinous tumours, but this differentiation is not always reliable on imaging features. Serous tumours tend to be unilocular, have serous fluid and papillary projections. Mucinous ovarian tumours tend to be very large, multiloculated (Figures 8.31 and 8.32) and often have variable signal intensity in the loculi due to proteinaceous or mucinous contents and haemorrhage.

Tips and Tricks

Thick, irregular septa, papillary projections and solid elements with increased blood flow are highly indicative of malignant neoplasm. Features that are more suggestive of benign cystic neoplasm include unilocular cysts, minimal thin septations, and absence of papillary projections.

Risk Assessment for Malignancy

Various models have been described in the literature to assess the risk of malignancy in complex ovarian masses based on ultrasound characteristics. At present, the Risk of Malignancy Index (RMI) [37] is the most widely used model. A systematic

115

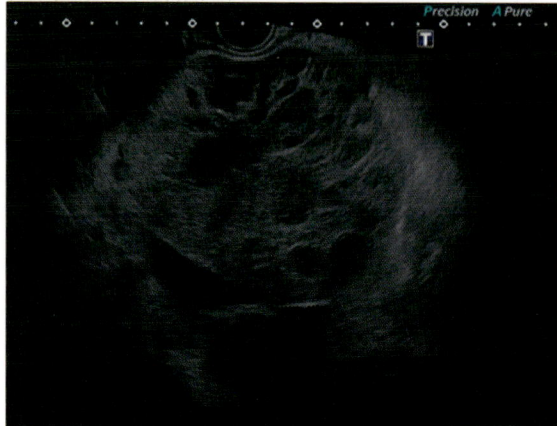

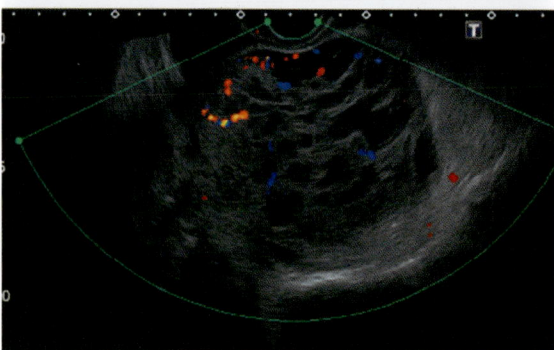

Figure 8.39 This 28-year-old, six-weeks-pregnant lady presented with abdominal pain. Ultrasound showed a 20 cm very complex solid cystic mass in the left adnexum showing avid blood flow. Left salpingo-oophorectomy showed a borderline seromucinous tumour.

review of diagnostic studies concluded that the RMI score was the most effective for women with suspected ovarian malignancy [38]. The National Institute for Health and Care Excellence (NICE) guidelines on ovarian cancer [39] recommend an RMI score to guide management for women with suspected ovarian malignancy. RMI combines three pre-surgical features: serum CA-125 (CA-125), menopausal status (M) and ultrasound score (U):

$$RMI = U \times M \times CA\text{-}125 \, (IU/ml)$$

- The ultrasound result is scored 1 point for each of the following characteristics: multilocular cysts, solid areas, metastases, ascites and bilateral lesions.
- The menopausal status is scored as 1 for premenopausal and 3 for postmenopausal status.

- The classification of 'postmenopausal' is a woman who has had no period for more than 1 year or a woman over 50 who has had a hysterectomy.
- Serum CA-125 is measured in IU/ml and can vary between 0 and hundreds or even thousands of unit.

U score

  0 = no features of malignancy on ultrasound

  1 = one feature of malignancy on ultrasound

  3 = more than one feature of malignancy on ultrasound

M score

  1 = premenopausal

  3 = postmenopausal

- RMI score greater than 200: high risk, referral to specialist gynaecological cancer service, and staging CT advised.
- RMI score 25–200: intermediate risk, MRI may be recommended to further evaluate the lesion.
- RMI score of less than 25: low risk, with repeat clinical assessment advised.

Recent studies have shown a specific model of ultrasound parameters, the ultrasound 'rules' derived from the International Ovarian Tumor Analysis (IOTA) Group, to have increased performance when differentiating benign or malignant ovarian masses compared to that of RMI (sensitivity 90–96 per cent, specificity 74–79 per cent, versus 67 per cent sensitivity and 91 per cent specificity for IOTA and RMI, respectively) [40]. The Royal College of Obstetricians and Gynaecologists (RCOG) in the UK have included the Simple Rules in their guidelines on the assessment and management of ovarian masses in premenopausal women [1]. These Simple Rules [34] are based on a set of five ultrasound features indicative of a benign tumour (B features) and five ultrasound features indicative of a malignant tumour (M features).

Ultrasound features of the Simple Rules are shown in Table 8.1.

Simple Rules

Rule 1: if one or more M features are present in absence of B feature(s), the mass is classified as malignant.

Table 8.1 Ultrasound features of the Simple Rules

B features	M features
B1 unilocular cyst	M1 irregular solid tumour
B2 solid components present, but <7 mm	M2 ascites
B3 acoustic shadows	M3 at least four papillary structures
B4 smooth multilocular tumour, largest diameter <100 mm	M4 irregular multilocular-solid tumour, largest diameter ≥100 mm
B5 no blood flow; colour score 1	M5 very strong flow; colour score 4

Rule 2: if one or more B features are present in absence of M feature(s), the mass is classified as benign.

Rule 3: if both M features and B features are present, or if no B or M features are present, the result is inconclusive and a second-stage test is recommended.

Solid Ovarian Neoplasms

Completely solid (100 per cent solid) solitary adnexal masses are usually benign and most commonly represent pedunculated uterine leiomyoma or an ovarian fibroma [22,41]. Most epithelial ovarian malignancies have a cystic component and are rarely completely solid. Ovarian malignancies that are most likely to manifest as solid or nearly completely solid masses include metastasis, lymphoma, neoplasms of sex cord-stromal group and other rare malignancies such as malignant teratomas or dysgerminomas [31,42]. When a patient has a known malignancy with a propensity to metastasize to the ovaries such as breast or GI carcinomas, the presence of bilateral solid masses should raise concern for ovarian metastasis [6] (Figure 8.40).

Tips and Tricks

An adnexal mass on ultrasound can be approached by following these steps:

- When an adnexal mass is identified, look for the ovaries to determine whether the mass is ovarian or extra-ovarian.
- Consider if ultrasound features are typical of a common benign ovarian (such as simple cyst, haemorrhagic cyst, endometrioma or dermoid) or extra-ovarian abnormality (such as hydrosalpinx, peritoneal inclusion cyst, pedunculated fibroid).

- If features are not typical of common benign pathology, consider the mass indeterminate and potentially malignant.
- Indeterminate lesions must be further categorized as low risk or high risk based on the ultrasound features, menopausal status and CA-125 levels. A scoring system like RMI or Simple Rules by IOTA can be used for risk stratification.
- Further management can include follow-up ultrasound, MRI for further characterization or surgical excision. All potentially malignant masses should be referred to the gynaecological oncology multidisciplinary team.

Follow-Up Ultrasound

Follow-up ultrasound may be considered when findings suggest benign disease or diagnosis is uncertain. Simple/haemorrhagic cysts bigger than 5 cm in premenopausal and more than 1 cm in postmenopausal women are followed up [4], although there is no consensus about optimum follow-up interval. First follow-up ultrasound in four months seems reasonable as slow growth will not be appreciated on follow-up scans done too soon. Further follow-up ultrasound intervals can be at four months or adjusted according to the degree of change noted on the first follow-up scan.

When ultrasound appearances are not suspicious but exact diagnosis is uncertain, a follow-up ultrasound is appropriate and may be done earlier than 4–6 months. Typically, a suspected haemorrhagic cyst but with some atypical features can be followed up at a six-week interval as this will allow time for the cyst to resolve and also provides the opportunity to scan in a different phase of the menstrual cycle. Known benign lesions such as endometriomas, dermoids and hydrosalpinges can be followed up on serial ultrasounds as per clinical needs.

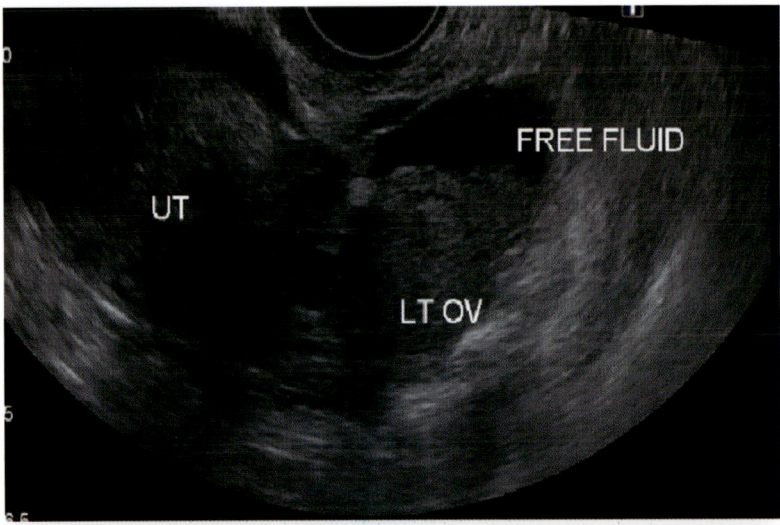

Figure 8.40 Progressively enlarging solid ovaries with surrounding fluid in a 45-year-old woman with known breast carcinoma. As there was no metastatic disease elsewhere, these were excised and confirmed histologically to be metastasis from breast carcinoma.

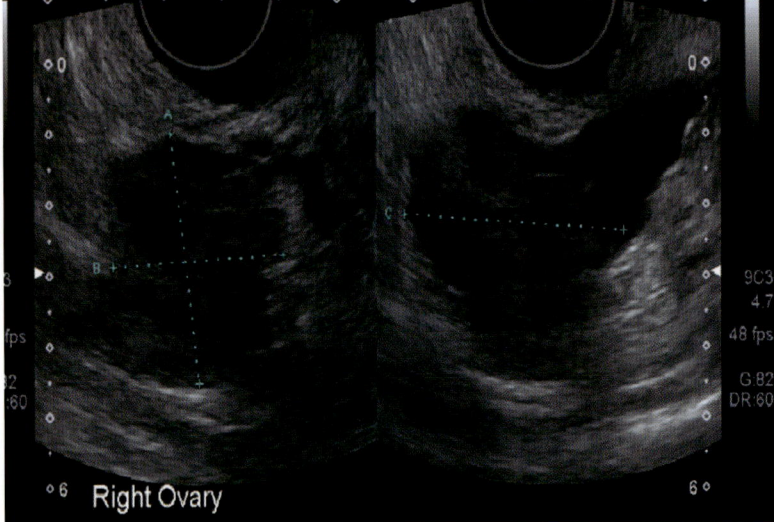

Alternative Imaging Modalities

A small number of ovarian and adnexal masses which are indeterminate on ultrasound are best characterized further by MRI due to its high soft tissue resolution and high predictive value for identifying blood products and fat. Several benign lesions have characteristic features on MRI that allow differentiation from ovarian cancers.

Computed tomography (CT) scanning is used for showing extra-ovarian spread and hence staging of ovarian cancers. Apart from demonstrating macroscopic fat in dermoid, CT has little role to play in characterization of adnexal masses. It is also useful in suspected tubo-ovarian abscesses as it is superior to ultrasound for revealing contiguous inflammatory changes and involvement of adjacent organs.

References

1. RCOG/BSGE. *Management of Suspected Ovarian Masses in Postmenopausal Women.* Green-top Guideline No. 62. RCOG/BSGE 2011.

2. Valentin L, Ameye L, Jurkovic D, et al. Which extrauterine pelvic masses are difficult to correctly classify as benign or malignant on the basis of ultrasound findings and is there a way of making a correct diagnosis? *Ultrasound Obstet Gynecol* 2006;**27**:438–44.

3. Vernooij F, Heintz P, Witteveen E, et al. The outcomes of ovarian cancer treatment are better when provided

by gynecologic oncologists and in specialized hospitals: a systematic review. *Gynecol Oncol* 2007;**105**:801–12.

4. Levine D, Brown DL, Andreotti RF, et al. Management of asymptomatic ovarian and other adnexal cysts imaged at US: Society of Radiologists in Ultrasound Consensus Conference Statement. *Radiology* 2010;**256** (3):943–54.

5. Modesitt SC, Pavlik EJ, Ueland FR, et al. Risk of malignancy in unilocular ovarian cystic tumors less than 10 centimeters in diameter. *Obstet Gynecol* 2003;**102**:594–9.

6. Brown DL. A practical approach to the ultrasound characterization of adnexal masses. *Ultrasound Q* 2007;**23**:87–105.

7. Durfee SM, Frates MC. Sonographic spectrum of the corpus luteum in early pregnancy: gray-scale, color, and pulsed Doppler appearance. *J Clin Ultrasound* 1999;**27**:55–9.

8. Jain KA. Sonographic spectrum of hemorrhagic ovarian cysts. *J Ultrasound Med* 2002;**21**:879–86.

9. Valentin L. Use of morphology to characterize and manage common adnexal masses. *Best Pract Res Clin Obstet Gynaecol* 2004;**18**:71–89.

10. Patel MD, Feldstein VA, Chen DC, et al. Endometriomas: diagnostic performance of ultrasound. *Radiology* 1999;**210**:739–45.

11. Asch E, Levine D. Variations in appearance of endometriomas. *J Ultrasound Med* 2007;**26**:993–1002.

12. Bhatt S, Kocakoc E, Dogra VS. Endometriosis: sonographic spectrum. *Ultrasound Q* 2006;**22**:273–80.

13. Patel D. Practical approach to the adnexal mass. *Radiol Clin North Am* 2006;**44**:879–99.

14. Kobayashi H, Sumimoto K, Kitanaka T, et al. Ovarian endometrioma: risk factors of ovarian cancer development. *Eur J Obstet Gynecol Reprod Biol* 2008;**138**:187–93.

15. Caspi B, Appelman Z, Rabinerson D, et al. Pathognomonic echo patterns of benign cystic teratomas of the ovary: classification, incidence and accuracy rate of sonographic diagnosis. *Ultrasound Obstet Gynecol* 1996;**7**:275–9.

16. Patel MD, Feldstein VA, Lipson SD, et al. Cystic teratomas of the ovary: diagnostic value of sonography. *Am J Roentgenol* 1998;**171**:1061–5.

17. Saba L, Guerriero S, Sulcis R, et al. Mature and immature ovarian teratomas: CT, US and MR imaging characteristics. *Eur J Radiol* 2008;**72** (3):454–63.

18. Kim HC, Kim SH, Lee HJ, et al. Fluid–fluid levels in ovarian teratomas. *Abdom Imaging* 2002;**27**:100–5.

19. Park JY, Kim DY, Kim J, et al. Malignant transformation of mature cystic teratoma of the ovary: experience at a single institution. *Eur J Obstet Gynecol Reprod Biol* 2008;**141**:173–8.

20. Conte M, Guariglia L, Panici PB, et al. Ovarian fibrothecoma: sonographic and histologic findings. *Gynecol Obstet Invest* 1991;**32**:51–4.

21. Bazot M, Ghossain MA, Buy JN, et al. Fibrothecomas of the ovary: CT and US findings. *J Comput Assist Tomogr* 1993;**17**:754–9.

22. Oh SN, Rha SE, Byun JY, et al. MRI features of ovarian fibromas: emphasis on their relationship to the ovary. *Clin Radiol* 2008;**63**:529–35.

23. Patel MD, Acord DL, Young SW. Likelihood ratio of sonographic findings in discriminating hydrosalpinx from other adnexal masses. *Am J Roentgenol* 2006;**186**:1033–8.

24. Timor-Tritsch IE, Lerner JP, Monteagudo A, et al. Transvaginal sonographic markers of tubal inflammatory disease. *Ultrasound Obstet Gynecol* 1998;**12**:56–66.

25. Sohaey R, Gardner TL, Woodward PJ, et al. Sonography diagnosis of peritoneal inclusion cysts. *J Ultrasound Med* 1995;**14**:913–17.

26. Kim SH, Sim JS, Seong CK. Interface vessels on color/power Doppler US and MRI: a clue to differentiate subserosal uterine myomas from extrauterine tumors. *J Comput Assist Tomogr* 2001;**25**:36–42.

27. Madan R. The bridging vascular sign. *Radiology* 2006;**238**:371–2.

28. Albayram F, Hamper UM. Ovarian and adnexal torsion: spectrum of sonographic findings with pathologic correlation. *J Ultrasound Med* 2001;**20** (10):1083–9.

29. Graif M, Shalev J, Strauss S, et al. Torsion of the ovary: sonographic features. *Am J Roentgenol* 1984;**143** (6):1331–4.

30. Scully RE. Classification of human ovarian tumors. *Environ Health Perspect* 1987;**73**:15–24.

31. Koonings PP, Campbell K, Mishell DR, et al. Relative frequency of primary ovarian neoplasms: a 10-year review. *Obstet Gynecol* 1989;**74**:921–6.

32. Chen VW, Ruiz B, Killeen JL, et. al. Pathology and classification of ovarian tumors. *Cancer* 2003;**97**:2631–42.

33. Granberg S, Norstrom A, Wikland M. Tumors in the lower pelvis as imaged by vaginal sonography. *Gynecol Oncol* 1990;**37**:224–9.

34. Timmerman D, Testa AC, Bourne T, et al. Simple ultrasound-based rules for the diagnosis of ovarian cancer. *Ultrasound Obstet Gynecol* 2008;**31**:681–90.

35. Timmerman D, Valentin L, Bourne TH. Terms, definitions and measurements to describe the sonographic features of adnexal tumors: a consensus opinion from the International Ovarian Tumor Analysis (IOTA) Group. *Ultrasound Obstet Gynecol* 2000;**16**:500–5.

36. Ekerhovd E, Wienerroith H, Staudach A, et al. Preoperative assessment of unilocular adnexal cysts by transvaginal ultrasonography: a comparison between ultrasonographic morphologic imaging and histopathologic diagnosis. *Am J Obstet Gynecol* 2001;**184**:48–54.

37. Jacobs I, Oram D, Fairbanks J, et al. A risk of malignancy index incorporating CA 125, ultrasound and menopausal status for the accurate preoperative diagnosis of ovarian cancer. *Br J Obstet Gynaecol* 1990;**97**:922–9.

38. Geomini P, Kruitwagen R, Bremer GL, et al. The accuracy of risk scores in predicting ovarian malignancy: a systematic review. *Obstet Gynecol* 2009;**113**:384–94.

39. National Institute for Health and Care Excellence. *Ovarian Cancer: The Recognition and Initial Management of Ovarian Cancer.* NICE Clinical Guideline 122. NICE; 2011.

40. Testa A, Kaijser J, Wynants L, et al. Strategies to diagnose ovarian cancer: new evidence from phase 3 of the multicentre international IOTA study. *Br J Cancer* 2014;**111**:680–8.

41. Barney SP, Muller CY, Bradshaw KD. Pelvic masses. *Med Clin North Am* 2008;**92**:1143–61.

42. Valentin L, Ameye L, Testa A, et al. Ultrasound characteristics of different types of adnexal malignancies. *Gynecol Oncol* 2006;**102**:41–8.

Sonographic Assessment of Pelvic Endometriosis

Tom Holland

Introduction

Endometriosis is a common gynaecological problem, affecting approximately 5 per cent of women [1]. The diagnosis can take many years [2] and the condition can cause debilitating pain and infertility. The disease can be found in many sites throughout the pelvis, in particular the ovaries, pelvic peritoneum, pouch of Douglas (POD), rectum, rectosigmoid, rectovaginal septum (RVS), uterosacral ligaments (USLs), vagina and urinary bladder. Mapping of deeply infiltrating disease is essential to enable the correct counselling regarding treatment modalities (medical or surgical) and risks of surgery, triaging to the correct surgical centre, informing the surgeon in order to correctly plan surgery and enabling other specialities, such as colorectal or urology support, to be organized in advance. Magnetic resonance imaging (MRI) has been used as the main pre-operative imaging modality, but with the correct training and experience transvaginal ultrasound can perform the same role [3]. Vaginal digital examination has been shown to be inferior diagnostically to transvaginal scanning (TVS) [4].

Before undertaking any ultrasound examination it is vital to first assess and clearly document the symptoms that have led to the examination. The history should include general gynaecological history and features specific to endometriosis, including: parity; menstrual period; previous surgery including laparoscopic or open; family history of endometriosis; previous non-surgical treatment for endometriosis (type, duration, effect); subfertility including duration; treatment for infertility and outcome of fertility treatment; pain (dysmenorrhoea, dyspareunia, dysuria, dyschezia, non-cyclic pelvic pain). The onset and duration of symptoms should be noted and the intensity of the pain symptoms should be objectively assessed using a 1–10 visual analogue score. Cyclic haematochezia and/or haematuria associated with menstruation are of particular significance.

Transvaginal Ultrasound Examination

A systematic approach to thoroughly assessing all the pelvic organs is necessary and should be followed for all patients with suspected endometriosis. It is helpful to ask women to empty their bladder before starting the examination so that the bladder is empty or minimally filled.

First, the uterus should be assessed in the transverse and sagittal planes, paying particular attention to the features of adenomyosis [5,6]. Next, the adnexa are assessed; the ovaries are found and their size measured in three orthogonal planes. Ovarian cysts are diagnosed as endometriomas when they appear as well-circumscribed, thick-walled cysts that contain low-level, homogeneous internal echoes ('ground glass') [7] (Figure 9.1). Measurements are recorded from the inside of the cyst wall in three orthogonal planes. The adnexa are also systematically examined for the presence of tubal dilation and, if present, the type of fluid should be documented, as haematosalpinx is often found with severe disease.

Ovarian mobility is important and can be assessed by a combination of gentle pressure with the vaginal probe and abdominal pressure with the examiner's free hand, as in a bimanual examination. The ovary is deemed to be completely free when all of its borders can be seen sliding across the surrounding structures. Ovarian adhesions can be identified as the inability to slide the ovary against its surrounding structures. Ovarian endometriomas are almost always associated with adhesions, and this should be documented clearly [8] (Figure 9.2).

If the tubes are dilated, their mobility should be documented in a similar fashion. Normal fallopian tubes are difficult to identify in the absence of background fluid in the pelvis. It is difficult to see filmy

(a)

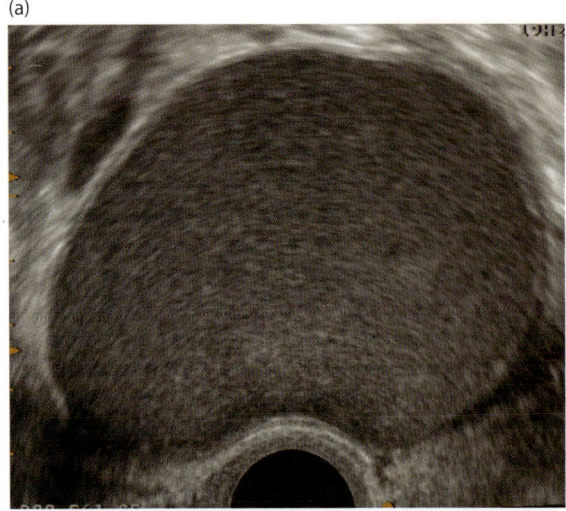

(b)

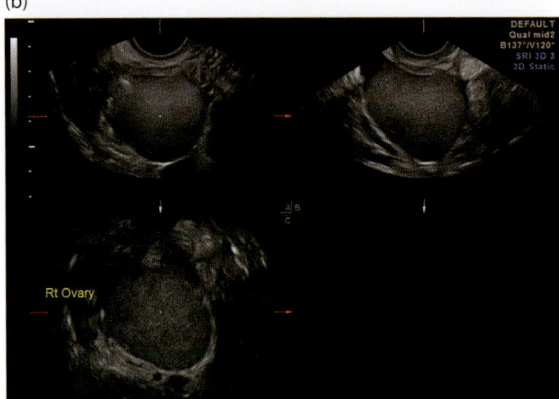

Figure 9.1 (a) Transvaginal ultrasound image of an ovarian endometrioma with the typical ground glass appearance. (b) Three-dimensional ultrasound of an ovarian endometrioma (multiplanar view). Note the homogeneous appearance of the cyst content on all planes.

adhesions on TVS unless there is fluid entrapped within the adhesions, giving rise to the 'flapping sail sign' [9] and peritoneal pseudocysts.

Anterior Pelvic Structures

The probe is positioned in the anterior vaginal fornix. It should be possible to gently push the bladder away from the anterior aspect of the uterus. If the bladder cannot be separated from the uterus with ease, this should raise the suspicion of adhesions between the bladder and uterus (more common after Caesarean section) which may be due to endometriosis in this location. The bladder should be examined throughout in the sagittal

plane. The presence of a hypoechoic or isoechoic thickening (nodule) of the bladder wall or a nodule with a heterogeneous echotexture containing numerous anechoic ('bubble-like') areas within the bladder wall is considered indicative of bladder endometriosis [10]. This is normally located where the bladder comes into contact with the uterus, but bladder dome endometriosis is also possible (Figure 9.3).

Ureteric and Renal Assessment

Endometriosis can, in very severe cases, involve the ureter and cause ureteric stenosis, hydroureter and eventually hydronephrosis. For this reason, the ureters should be routinely examined. It is possible to visualize the ureters in the following way, which is a modification of the technique first described by Pateman et al. in 2013 [11]. The urethra is found in the mid-sagittal plane. The probe is then moved laterally until the ureteral meatus can be seen as a ridge in the internal wall of the bladder. The intra-vesical portion of the ureter can then be followed until it exits the bladder at the vesico-ureteric junction. The extravesical ureter can then be followed caudally until it reaches the iliac vessels. If severe endometriosis is suspected, it is important to wait for peristalsis as this confirms ureteric patency [12]. Any evidence of ureteric dilation, abnormal bending or discrepancy in peristalsis frequency should raise the suspicion of a stricture. In women with evidence of partial (Figure 9.4) and complete (Figure 9.5) ureteric obstruction, the distance from the stricture to the ureteric orifice should be measured (Figure 9.6).

After the posterior pelvic structures are assessed (see the next section) the examination is completed by performing an abdominal ultrasound scan to assess the kidneys using a 3.5–5 MHz probe. For examination of the left kidney, the patient lies in the right lateral decubitus position with the probe placed in the lower intercostal space on the posterior axillary line. For examination of the right kidney, the patient lies supine and the probe is placed in the right lower intercostal space in the midaxillary line. Both entire kidneys are scanned through obtaining longitudinal (long axis) and transverse (short axis) views.

Hydronephrosis is diagnosed and graded using a generally accepted ultrasound criteria [13]. Any dilated ureter is followed abdominally to the level of

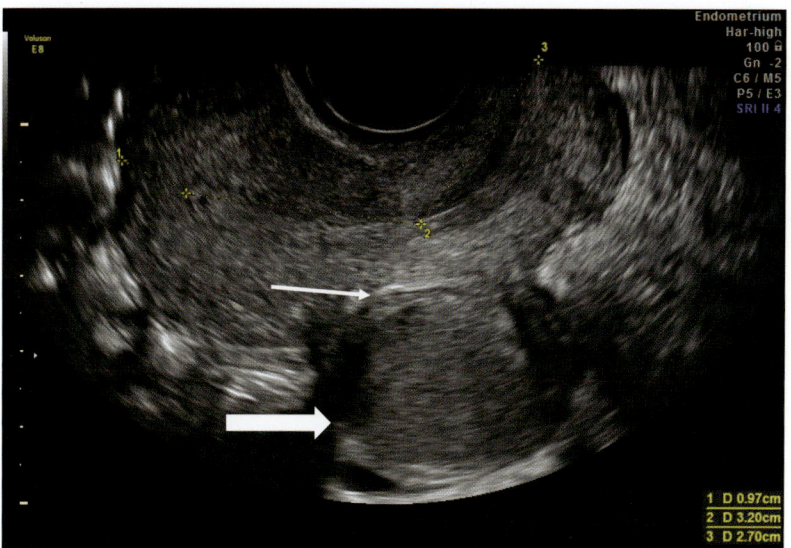

Figure 9.2 Transvaginal scan of a patient with extensive pelvic endometriosis. The ovary is adherent to the posterior aspect of the uterus and there is no mobility of the structures when pressure is applied via the ultrasound transducer. There are thick, hyperechoic plaques (thin arrow) which further raise suspicion of a frozen pelvis. The ovary is also distended by an endometrioma (large arrow).

obstruction if not already seen vaginally. Renal cysts are classified using the Bosniak classification [14].

Posterior Pelvic Structures

The presence of adhesions in the POD is assessed next. The uterus is gently mobilized by a combination of pressure on the cervix with the ultrasound probe alternating with pressure on the fundus from the examiner's free hand on the abdominal wall. The aim is to watch the interface of the posterior uterine serosa and the bowel behind to ensure that the two structures are sliding easily across one another. If these two surfaces are completely free of one another, this is assessed as there being no adhesions present. Obliteration of the POD is assessed as the absence of any sliding between the serosa on the posterior surface of the cervix or uterus and the bowel behind (Figure 9.2).

Endometriotic nodules or deeply invasive endometriosis (DIE) are typically visualized as stellate hypoechoic or isoechogenic solid masses with irregular outer margins [15] which are tender on palpation and fixed to the surrounding pelvic structures. They are usually located in the USLs, rectosigmoid colon, vagina and urinary bladder (Figure 9.3). Endometriotic nodules located in the wall of the rectosigmoid colon tend to appear as hypoechoic thickenings of bowel muscularis propria (Figures 9.7 and 9.8), which sometimes protrude into the lumen of the bowel [16]. These lesions should be measured in three orthogonal planes [17]. To find lesions in the rectosigmoid colon it is helpful to withdraw the vaginal probe to the lower part of the vagina, where the anal muscle sphincter can be identified posteriorly. The muscle layer (muscularis propria) can then be followed cranially as it runs parallel to the vagina. In women with normal anatomy the rectum diverges posteriorly from the vaginal wall at the lower part of the POD and is no longer straight, but follows a more tortuous route. It is necessary to continue to follow it left and right as higher sigmoid nodules are possible. If this technique is used, it is normally relatively straightforward to find thickened nodules of endometriosis in the rectal wall. This technique will also place the probe in the posterior fornix, which is the ideal position to assess for any hypoechoic vaginal thickening and uterosacral thickening [17]. In the sagittal plane, track left and right in the posterior fornix to find thickening of the USLs and posterior vagina. Normal USL cannot be visualized with TVS; however, DIE involving the USL can be visualized as hyperechoic thickening which is usually located at the point of insertion into the cervix. The *torus uterinus* is the bridge of connective tissue across the back of the cervix, which links the two USLs. This can also be a common site for DIE with or without bowel involvement.

Conclusions

TVS in the hands of well-trained and experienced staff is a good method to detect ovarian and deeply infiltrating endometriosis. A systematic approach is necessary to assess all the possible areas that can be affected. A good knowledge of normal pelvic anatomy is essential to finding DIE.

(a)

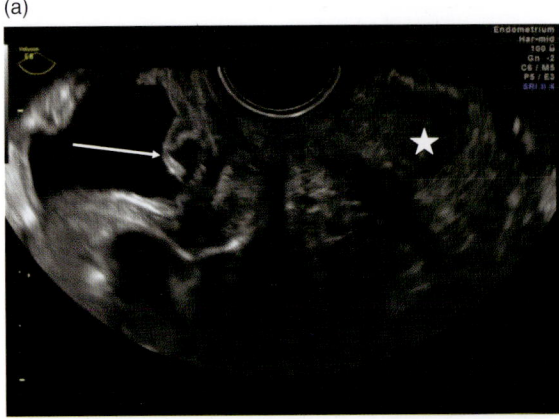

(b)

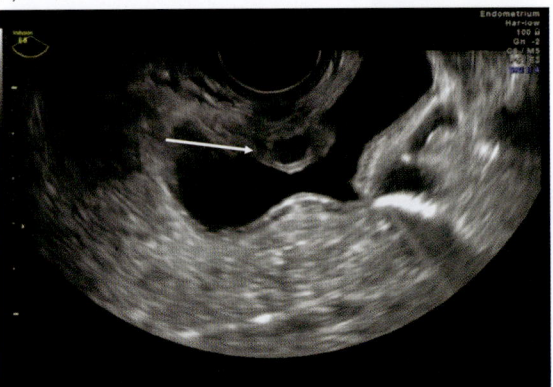

(c)

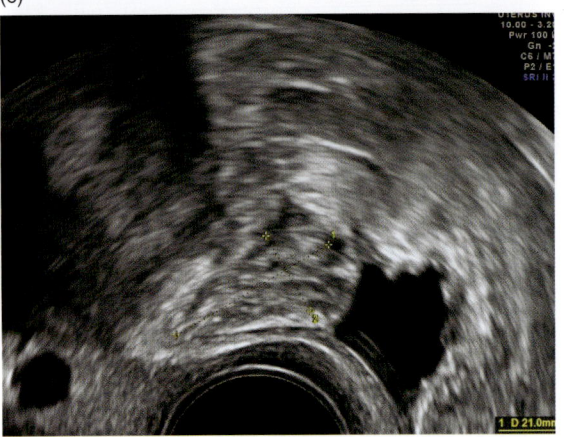

Figure 9.3 Transvaginal scan of an endometriotic bladder nodule. (a) sagittal section, (b) transverse view. Moderately filled bladder allows for good visualization of the bladder wall. The cervix is located to the right of the screen (star). The endometriotic nodule (arrows) indenting the bladder wall is hypoechogenic ((a) and (b)) or hyperechoic ((c), callipers). Cystoscopy and a biopsy may be needed to exclude bladder malignancy.

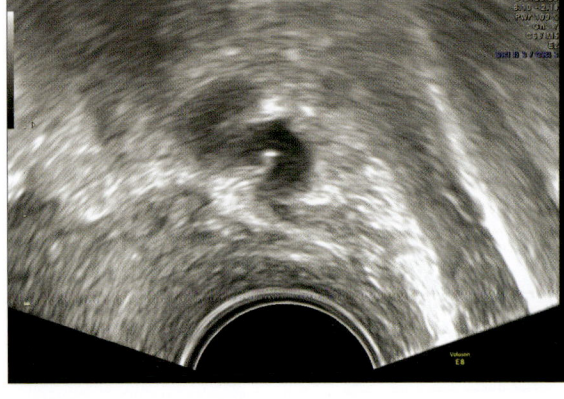

Figure 9.4 Partially obstructed ureter.

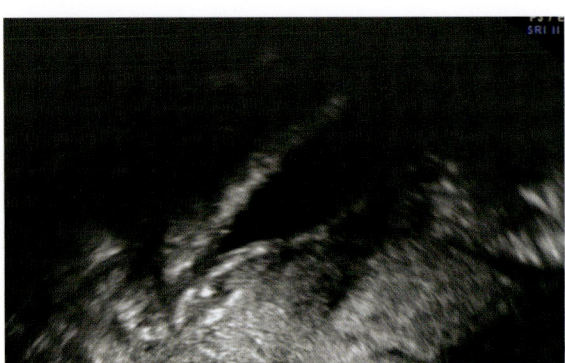

Figure 9.5 Completely obstructed ureter.

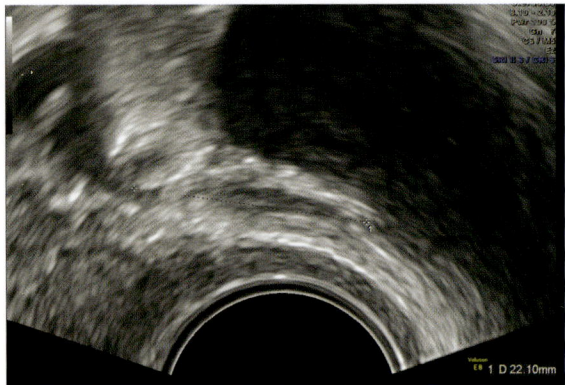

Figure 9.6 Distance from level of stricture to ureteral orifice.

Tips and Tricks

- Always follow a systematic approach.
- Have a thorough understanding of normal anatomy, which will facilitate recognizing abnormality.

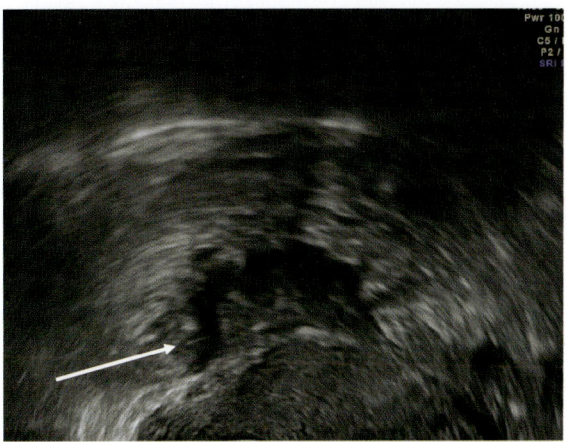

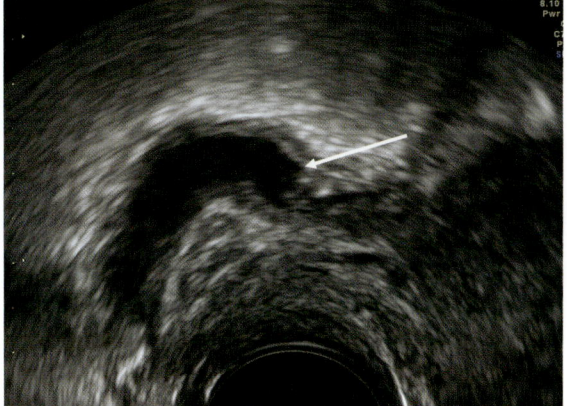

Figure 9.7 Two transvaginal ultrasound images of hypoechoic thickening of the muscularis layer (arrows) of the rectum due to deeply infiltrating endometriosis.

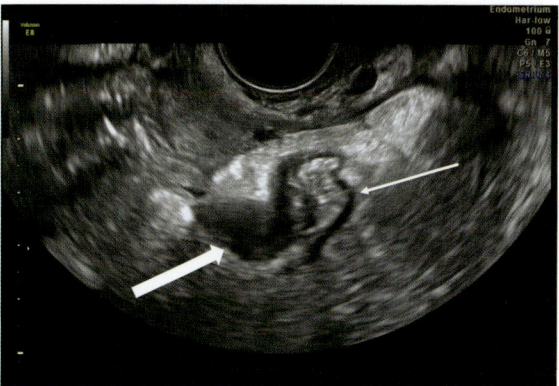

Figure 9.8 Transvaginal ultrasound of deep infiltrating endometriosis of the sigmoid colon. Note the thickening of the muscularis propria (thick arrow) in comparison to the normal layer (thin arrow).

- Look for the way organs move across one another to assess for mobility.
- Use your non-probe hand suprapubically and abdominally to assess for mobility, in addition to gentle pressure with the probe.
- In the sagittal plane, track left and right in the posterior fornix to find thickening of the uterosacral ligaments and posterior vagina.

References

1. Ferrero S, Arena E, Morando A, Remorgida V. Prevalence of newly diagnosed endometriosis in women attending the general practitioner. *Int J Gynaecol Obstet* 2010;**110**:203–7.

2. Hadfield R, Mardon H, Barlow D, et al. Delay in the diagnosis of endometriosis: a survey of women from the USA and the UK. *Hum Reprod* 1996;**11** (4):878–80.

3. Bazot M, Lafont C, Rouzier R, et al. Diagnostic accuracy of physical examination, transvaginal sonography, rectal endoscopic sonography, and magnetic resonance imaging to diagnose deep infiltrating endometriosis. *Fertil Steril* 2008;**92**:1825–33.

4. Hudelist G, Ballard K, English J, et al. Transvaginal sonography vs. clinical examination in the preoperative diagnosis of deep infiltrating endometriosis. *Ultrasound Obstet Gynecol* 2011;**37**:480–7.

5. Naftalin J, Hoo W, Pateman K, et al. How common is adenomyosis? A prospective study of prevalence using transvaginal ultrasound in a gynaecology clinic. *Hum Reprod* 2012;**27**(12):3432–9.

6. Naftalin J, Hoo W, Nunes N, et al. Association between ultrasound features of adenomyosis and severity of menstrual pain. *Ultrasound Obstet Gynecol* 2016;**47** (6),779–83.

7. Tailor A, Jurkovic D, Bourne TH, Collins WP, Campbell S. Sonographic prediction of malignancy in adnexal masses using an artificial neural network. *Br J Obstet Gynaecol* 1999;**106**:21–30.

8. Holland TK, Yazbek J, Cutner A, et al. The value of transvaginal ultrasound in assessing the severity of pelvic endometriosis. *Ultrasound Obstet Gynecol* 2010;**36**:241–8.

9. Savelli L, de Iaco P, Ghi T, et al. Transvaginal sonographic appearance of peritoneal pseudocysts. *Ultrasound Obstet Gynecol* 2004;**23**:284–8.

10. Savelli L, Manuzzi L, Pollastri P, et al. Diagnostic accuracy and potential limitations of transvaginal sonography for bladder endometriosis. *Ultrasound Obstet Gynecol* 2009;**34**:595–600.

11. Pateman K, Mavrelos D, Hoo WL, et al. Visualization of ureters on standard gynecological transvaginal scan: a feasibility study. *Ultrasound Obstet Gynecol* 2013;**41**:696–701.

12. Pateman K, Holland TK, Knez J, et al. Should a detailed ultrasound examination of the complete urinary tract be routinely performed in women with suspected pelvic endometriosis? *Hum Reprod* 2015;**30**:2802–7.

13 Block B. *The Practice of Ultrasound: a Step-By-Step Guide to Abdominal Scanning*. 2nd ed. Thieme Medical Publishers, 2011.

14. Bosniak MA. The Bosniak renal cyst classification: 25 years later. *Radiology* 2012;**262**:781–5.

15. Fedele L, Piazzola E, Raffaelli R, Bianchi S. Bladder endometriosis: deep infiltrating endometriosis or adenomyosis? *Fertil Steril* 1998;**69**:972–5.

16. Koga K, Osuga Y, Yano T, et al. Characteristic images of deeply infiltrating rectosigmoid endometriosis on transvaginal and transrectal ultrasonography. *Hum Reprod* 2003;**18**:1328–33.

17. Guerriero S, Condous G, Van den Bosch T, et al. Systematic approach to sonographic evaluation of the pelvis in women with suspected endometriosis, including terms, definitions and measurements: a consensus opinion from the International Deep Endometriosis Analysis (IDEA) group. *Ultrasound Obstet Gynecol* 2016;**48**(3):318–32.

Sonographic Assessment of Fallopian Tubes and Tubal Pathologies

Sonal Panchal and Chaitanya Nagori

Introduction

While the uterus, cervix and ovaries can be well assessed by transvaginal ultrasound, normal fallopian tubes are not visible on ultrasound. Therefore, evaluation of the fallopian tubes needs special consideration. Tubal disease accounts for a significant proportion of female infertility and pelvic pain [1]. The fallopian tubes may be damaged, most commonly due to pelvic inflammatory disease (PID), but endometriosis, previous pelvic surgery, fibroids, and pelvic tuberculosis may also be seen as frequent causes for tubal damage [2]. Prior uterine surgeries like surgical or medical termination of pregnancy and myomectomy may predispose to subclinical inflammation or infection leading to tubal damage. Tubal patency may also be affected due to polyps, myomas or *salpingitis isthmica nodosa*, though the latter is not very commonly seen and not very confidently diagnosed on ultrasound. These pathologies may lead to obstruction, stenosis, dilation, and impaired peristaltic function of the tubes [3]. Tubal function may also be affected by changes in the tubal mucosal lining, muscular wall or any pathology external to the tube. Proximal tubal involvement is more in the form of muscular spasm, stromal oedema, amorphous debris, mucosal agglutination and viscous secretions causing obstruction. Mid-tubal disease causes stenosis or occlusion, typically with bulbous termination due to scarring and fibrosis. Fimbrial end involvement may lead to hydrosalpinx.

Functional Anatomy of the Fallopian Tubes

Fallopian tubes are tubal structures extending from the lateral end of the uterus towards the ovaries and are about 10–12 cm in length. These can be divided into five parts (Figure 10.1): the intramural or interstitial part is the part of the tube in the muscular uterine wall and is 1 cm long; the isthmic part following the interstitial part is 2 cm; the following 5 cm is the ampullary part, which has a variable length; this is followed by the infundibulum – the wide part before the fimbria – and then the fimbria. The inner diameter of the tube is barely 1 mm. Fallopian tubes play an important role in the transport of sperm and egg, sperm capacitation, fertilization and embryo transport [4]. It is essential that the fallopian tubes are patent for the tubo-ovarian relationship to be normal. The fimbrial condition should be good and accommodative to envelop the ovary, and the cilia should be functional to guide the passage of ovum and embryo towards the uterus and guide the passage of sperm towards the ovum.

Assessment of the Tubes

Assessment of the tubes is done to check the patency and to rule out pathologies. Tubal patency cannot be assessed on a routine pelvic transvaginal ultrasound, although a fluid distended tube (hydrosalpinx) can be diagnosed reliably. It is essential to use fluid as a contrast to visualize the normal tubal lumen on ultrasound. Assessment of the tubal patency can be done under x-ray guidance (hysterosalpingogram; HSG), ultrasound guidance (saline infusion sonography; SIS) and hystero-contrast sono-salpingography

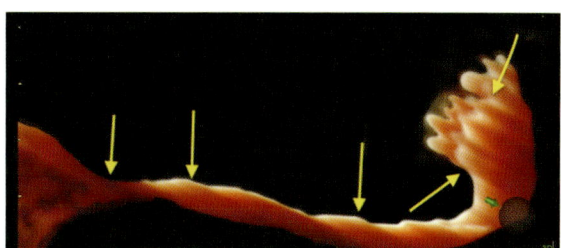

Figure 10.1 Fallopian tube as seen on 3D hystero-contrast sonosalpingography (HyCoSy), demonstrating normal anatomy of the tube: from left to right the arrows indicate the intramural, isthmic, ampullary, infundibular and fimbrial parts of the tube.

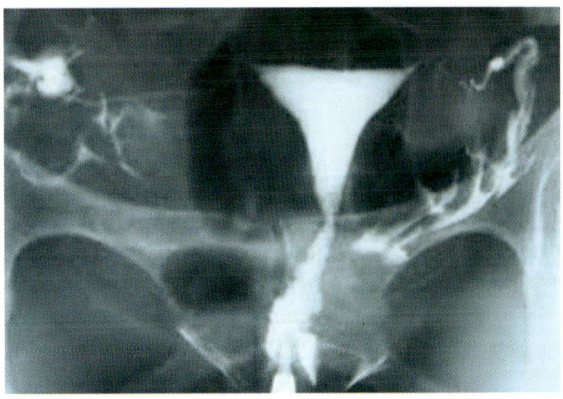

Figure 10.2 Hysterosalpingogram showing filling of the normal endometrial cavity and both fallopian tubes with free spill on both sides.

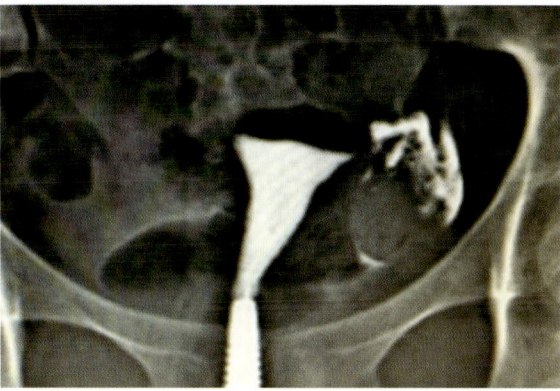

Figure 10.3 Hysterosalpingogram showing normal endometrial cavity with free spill from the left fallopian tube and non-filling of the right tube, suggestive of right cornual block.

(HyCoSy) or surgically by laparoscopic guidance. HSG, SIS and HyCoSy are less invasive and associated with less serious risks than surgical techniques like laparoscopy and the dye test (chromopertubation), although the latter is considered the gold standard for assessment of tubal patency and pathology.

HSG is widely used for tubal evaluation in subfertile women. This method is fairly accurate in detecting proximal tubal disease, is safe, inexpensive and may potentially be associated with increased pregnancy rates [5]. HSG provides optimal delineation of the fallopian tubes, tubal patency, lumen irregularity and peritubal disease. The radio-opaque solution (contrast) is injected in the minimal required dose. Under fluoroscopic guidance, filling of the uterine cavity and passage with the radio-opaque solution into the tubes and its spill from the fimbrial end is observed and documented in the form of x-rays (Figure 10.2). HSG also allows for a study of the endometrial cavity, diagnosing some Mullerian abnormalities and endometrial lesions (Figure 10.3).

However, the main disadvantages include exposure to radiation, use of iodinated contrast, severe pain and high false-negative rates. The procedure is to be done in the radiology environment, where neither the gynaecologist nor the patient feels very comfortable, though that may not be an important issue. It gives a static image, and the tubo-ovarian relation that is vital for fertility cannot be fully evaluated. Further, tubal block seen on HSG will be confirmed by laparoscopy in only 38 per cent of women

[6], with pooled estimates of sensitivity and specificity for HSG as a test for tubal obstruction of 0.65 (95 per cent CI 0.50–0.78) and 0.83 (95 per cent CI 0.77–0.88), respectively [7].

The ultrasound-guided tubal patency test avoids the risk of radiation as well as the risk of potential adverse reaction to iodinated contrast, but provides information similar to that obtained by HSG. The ultrasound-guided tubal patency test is commonly referred to as sonohysterosalpingography, but this is a group of investigations and the method of each varies a little depending on the contrast agent and the ultrasound technology used. The variations are:

1. SIS
2. SIS with pulsed wave Doppler
3. SIS with colour Doppler
4. saline and air infusion salpingography
5. SIS with 3D power Doppler
6. HyCoSy
7. hystero-foam salpingography (HyFoSy).

Saline Infusion Salpingography

Sonographic evaluation of tubes was initially described by various authors [8–10], who performed abdominal sonography following intracervical injection of fluid, but was reported first by Richman. For this procedure, 200 ml of saline was injected transvaginally. Fluid would fill the uterine cavity and pass through the tubes into the pelvic cavity. Retrouterine fluid documented on abdominal ultrasound was

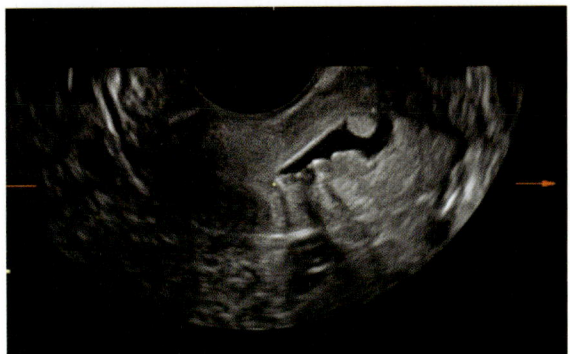

Figure 10.4 Saline infusion HSG: saline filled in the endometrial cavity appears anechoic and allows clear demonstration of multiple polyps as solid projections against the anechoic saline.

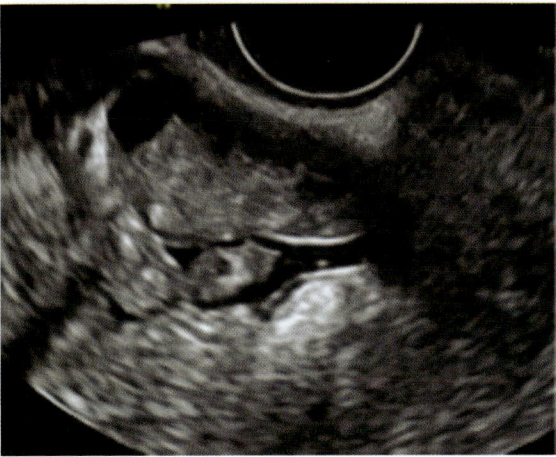

Figure 10.5 Saline infusion salpingography on B-mode ultrasound shows anechoic fluid collection posterior to the ovary due to the fluid spill from the normal tube.

accepted as a criterion for patency. Tufekci reported use of isotonic saline with transvaginal ultrasound for assessment of tubal patency in 1992 [11]. Deichert was the first to report on transvaginal sonographic evaluation of tubal patency, following transcervical injection of echogenic ultrasonic contrast fluid [12].

Technique

Saline infusion salpingography is ideally done in the mid-proliferative phase (days 6–10 of a typical 28-day cycle), after menstruation stops but before ovulation occurs. Oral analgesic, ibuprofen 400 mg and/or paracetamol 500–1000 mg, may be given 1–2 hours before the procedure. Pre-procedural screening for infections like chlamydia and/or prophylactic oral antibiotics are recommended. Strict asepsis is essential. A detailed transvaginal ultrasound scan is done to assess the position of the pelvic organs and to rule out any pathologies, which would get in the way of visualization of the uterus and ovaries. Moreover, any free fluid in the pelvis is also checked for, as this may interfere with the observation for tubal patency.

The probe is removed and Cusco's speculum is placed in the vagina to visualize the cervix. The cervix is cleaned with an antiseptic solution. If required, the cervix is fixed with tenaculum forceps and manipulated to align it with the uterus. A size 5–8 Fr balloon HSG or SIS catheter is used. It is attached to a 10–20 ml syringe prefilled with saline. The catheter is introduced through the cervix into the uterus. The balloon is placed just beyond the internal os and is distended with 1–2 ml of distilled water or normal saline. Alternatives to this catheter are paediatric feeding tubes or intrauterine insemination (IUI) catheters.

A catheter with a balloon has the advantage of preventing any reflux of saline or contrast media through the cervical canal. Once the catheter is fixed, the speculum (and tenaculum if used) are removed and a transvaginal probe is introduced into the vagina for further assessment.

Saline is injected through the catheter slowly. Scanning is done to assess the uterine cavity that is distended by saline and also the passage of saline (fluid) seen through the tubes. When the uterine cavity is filled with saline, endometrial pathologies like polyps, synechiea and hyperplasia can be demonstrated and diagnosed (Figure 10.4). Spill of saline from the fimbrial end is seen as fluid flow surrounding the ovary and subsequently appears as a collection in the pelvis on B-mode scanning (Figure 10.5). The latter is seen more confidently when the uterus and ovary are seen in the transverse axis, on the same image.

Absence of spill may indicate blockage. At times, when there is unilateral blockage, it is difficult to judge the side of the blockage. In patients with bilateral block, distension of the uterine cavity causes severe pain. Once the procedure is completed, the catheter is removed after deflating the balloon. The patient is informed that she might get some pelvic cramping or spotting, but this is short term and expected.

The procedure is generally safe without any major complications. The risk of pelvic infection and associated peritonitis is approximately 1 per cent. Other

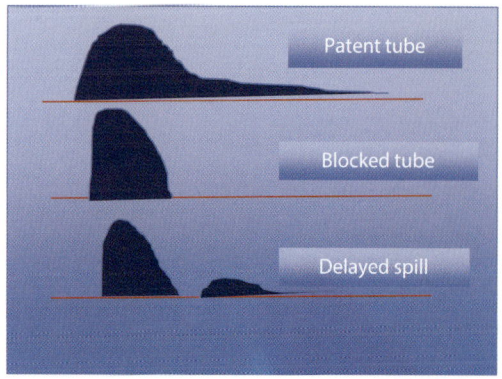

Figure 10.6 Diagrammatic presentation of fluid flow in patent, partially obstructed and obstructed tube on pulse Doppler assessment for tubal patency [19].

risks include nausea or vomiting, vasovagal syncope and pain during or immediately after the procedure. The reported prevalence of the latter three risks combined is 8.8 per cent [13]. Failure to perform or complete the procedure was documented in 7 per cent in a meta-analysis of 24 studies and 2278 procedures [14]. The accuracy of SIS compared to laparoscopic chromopertubation varies from 81.82 per cent [15] to 100 per cent [16,17].

The shortcoming of the procedure is that even when patency of individual tubes can be confirmed, it does not give any information about the site of the blockage, the condition of the lumen or the tubo-ovarian relationship. Some variations in this technique were created to overcome those limitations.

SIS Using Pulse Doppler

If examination during conventional ultrasound reveals evidence suggesting tubal occlusion or if a small segment of the tube measuring less than 2 cm is not visualized, a pulse Doppler examination can be performed [18], although is not routinely done. A Doppler gate is placed where the block is expected. This is exactly the point beyond which the tube is not filled with saline or colour flow is not seen on injection of saline when examination is done with colour Doppler. The gate is reduced to the width of the tube. Brief injections of fluid/saline lasting for 5 s are done while Doppler signals are observed [19]. Patent tube is indicated by a short filling phase with rapid, steep increase in Doppler shift followed by slow, uniform fall in Doppler shift. Obstruction presents

as short, steep Doppler shift with no subsequent noise signals (Figure 10.6).

SIS Using Colour Doppler

Under ultrasound guidance, the tip of the catheter is placed close to either cornu, one by one. First, the colour box is placed on the transverse section of the uterus. Colour signals in the uterine cavity confirm the passage of fluid in the uterus. The field of vision is immediately changed over to the ovary and adnexa, by spanning the probe from the transverse section of the uterus, laterally. While injecting saline in short jets, the colour box is placed to visualize the adnexa and ovary. Filling the box with colour signals immediately after colour signals are seen in the uterus indicates patency of the tube; absence of such signals indicates blockage [20] (Figure 10.7). The same procedure is repeated on the opposite side. A detailed evaluation for any pathology is important immediately prior to performing the procedure as hydrosalpinx may create turbulence in the fluid present in the tube and give a false impression of a patent tube.

In a study by Peters and Coulam of 129 infertile patients, Doppler SIS showed complete agreement with HSG in 81 per cent of cases. When compared with chromopertubation, Doppler SIS showed agreement in 86 per cent of cases, while HSG agreed with chromopertubation only in 75 per cent of cases [21]. In another small study by Kupesic et al., 91.5 per cent agreement was seen between colour Doppler SIS and chromopertubation [16]. Correlation of colour Doppler SIS and HSG with chromopertubation was 81 per cent versus 60 per cent, respectively, in another study [13].

SIS Using Saline with Air

When air is mixed with saline, bubbles are formed and this produces hyperechoic shadows which help better outline the tubal lumen. This can be done either by agitating air and saline or by injecting air after saline has already been pushed in to fill the uterine cavity and tubes (Figure 10.8). This technique was described by Jeanty et al. and showed a 79.4 per cent agreement with results of chromopertubation and a sensitivity of 85.7 per cent and specificity of 77.2 per cent for tubal patency [21].

SIS with 3D Power Doppler

Transvaginal three-dimensional saline infusion sono-hysterosalpingography provides good visualization of

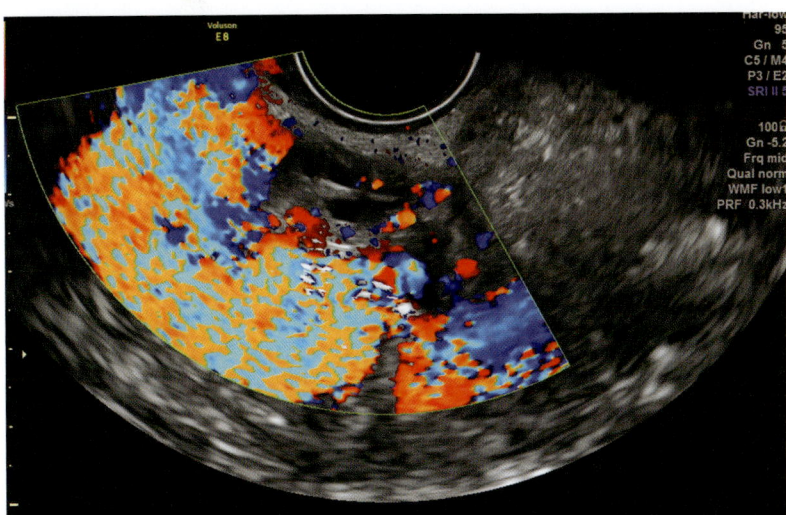

Figure 10.7 Saline infusion salpingography with colour Doppler shows filling of the colour box with colour due to spill of saline from the fimbrial end of the normal tube.

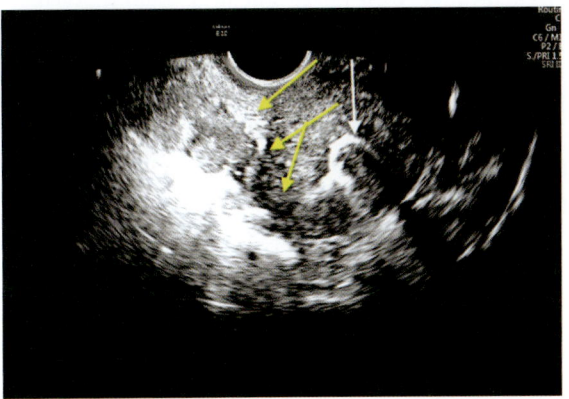

Figure 10.8 Salpingography with saline and air. Air is seen as hyperechoic contrast filling the uterus (white arrow) and the tube with the spill (yellow arrows).

the uterine cavity and myometrial walls in three orthogonal planes. However, it does not diagnose tubal occlusion or depict architecture of the fallopian tube as accurately as x-ray HSG. Although the distal fallopian tube and fimbria are seen with real-time imaging, the proximal tube is not satisfactorily imaged even with 3D power Doppler. This technique may be reserved as an initial screening test to evaluate the uterine cavity and to test tubal patency. Patients at high risk for tubal disease by history or with suspected tubal occlusion on 3D saline infusion HSG should be evaluated by either x-ray HSG or laparoscopy with chromopertubation [22].

Kiyokawa et al. reported that when 3D was added to saline salpingography, the positive predictive value, negative predictive value, sensitivity and specificity of predicting tubal patency were 100, 33.3, 84.4 and 100 per cent, respectively. Over and above this, this method also has the advantage of assessing the shape of the uterine cavity. The complete contour of the uterine cavity was depicted in 96 per cent of cases using 3D HyCoSy and 64 per cent by x-ray HSG [23].

Hystero-Contrast Salpingography

While intra-cavitary lesions are clearly delineated by anechoic media, very small hollow cavities, such as normal tubes, are not always easily visualized using SIS [24]. Demonstration of the lumen of tubes requires visualization of movement of fluid using a highly echogenic medium [25]. Hyperechogenic contrast medium enhances echo signals and allows detection of the flow, both by B-mode and Doppler ultrasound. Experimental and clinical data suggest that insonation of echo-enhancing contrast agents with high acoustic power produces disintegration of microbubbles, resulting in a phenomenon called stimulated acoustic emission (SAE). It is based on this principle that the positive ultrasound contrast media are developed [26]. A cheap and cost-effective option is the use of saline mixed with air, which produces a high-contrast fluid due to the presence of air bubbles, as discussed earlier. However, these bubbles exist only for a very short period and therefore tubal patency assessment may become practically difficult.

Commercially available contrast media consist of microbubbles that can exist for a longer time, including Echovist and Levovist (Schering AG, Berlin), which

131

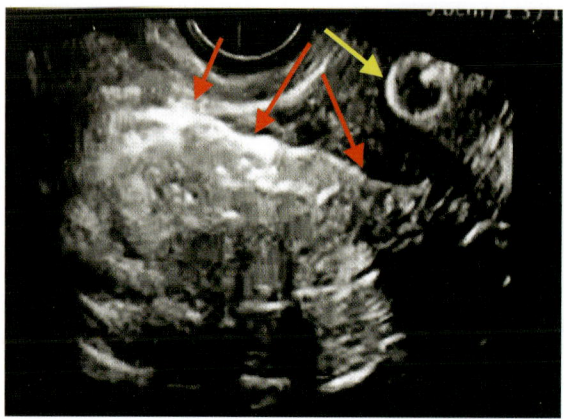

Figure 10.9 HyFoSy: B-mode image of hysterosalpingo-foam sonography (HyFoSy) showing hyperechoic shadows in the endometrial cavity (yellow arrow) and the tube with the spill (red arrows).

consist of a suspension of microbubbles made of special galactose microparticles. These are suspended either in galactose solution, as in Echovist, or in sterile water, as in Levovist. Just before use, these solutions are constituted by mixing and vigorously shaking the microparticles with the solvent and remain stable for 5–10 min. These solutions completely dissolve in the body within about 30 min. The use is unrestricted, except for patients with galactosaemia. Non-embryo toxic gel (ExEm-gel® Gynaecologiq BV, Delft, the Netherlands), containing hydroxyethylcellulose and glycerol, has also been used as an intrauterine medium for sonohysterography as an alternative to saline [27].

Gel instillation offers more stable filling of the uterine cavity. This gel and its compounds have been tested extensively and may be used safely. The foam contrast is reconstituted by mechanically mixing 10 ml of ExEm-gel and 10 ml of sterile water [28]. When the gel is pushed rigorously through small openings in syringes or tubes, turbulence causes local pressure drop, resulting in air dissolving in the solution, and yielding foam that is stable for several minutes. ExEm-gel (containing 88.25 per cent purified water), however, is rather viscous for passing into the fallopian tubes. Therefore, 10 ml of ExEm-gel is diluted with 10 ml of purified water (to give a mixture containing 94.12 per cent water) and mixed to create foam. The mixture at this ratio creates foam that is sufficiently stable to show echogenicity for at least 5 min and sufficiently fluid to pass through patent tubes. The viscosity of this foam (270 cP) is comparable to that of Echovist (400 cP) [29]. The foam is

slowly injected into the endometrial cavity through the GIS catheter, or similar catheter, in repeated small (0.5–1 ml) boluses while observing for antegrade flow through the uterine cornua on the transverse plane using B-mode. Distal flow of contrast is followed through each tube until peritoneal spill is visualized (Figure 10.9). It is easier to visualize spill of the foam into the peritoneal cavity after locating the ovaries [28].

According to some studies it can maintain echogenicity for about 7 min, allowing it to be used as a contrast medium for HyFoSy [30]. The foam usually maintains its echogenicity long enough to allow acquisition of 3D volume images.

A positive contrast agent that is more easily available in most countries is Sonovue (Bracco, Italy). This contrast agent consists of sulphur hexafluoride microparticles and 5 ml of solvent in a prefilled syringe. After reconstitution it makes 5 ml of solution. For assessment of tubal status, 1 ml of Sonovue is diluted with 4 ml of normal saline and agitated to create a foam for injection through the cervix into the uterus. This contrast is safe for intravascular use also. It is used as an ultrasound contrast agent for vascular studies and for diagnosis of malignancy.

The scanning technique is the same as that for SIS. Using positive contrast, it is possible to delineate the whole tube along with the uterine cavity even on B-mode scanning (Figure 10.9).

There is ultrasound equipment with contrast mode (contrast-tuned imaging technology based on harmonics). The advantage is that it enhances the contrast and makes visualization of tubes even better (Figure 10.10). Using a contrast mode with positive contrast makes it easier to view the spill from the fimbrial end if the tube is patent. If the tube is not patent, the contrast column in the tube can identify the site of the blockage.

Technique

The procedure for HyCoSy is the same as for SIS. As delineation of the tube is better with HyCoSy, the total amount of contrast needed is as little as 2–3 ml per tube. For diagnosis of tubal patency, two or three observation phases per tube are needed, with an observation period of continuous flow of about 10 s. Visualization of long segments of tube beyond the intramural part of the tube usually indicates patency, though the whole tube

(a) (b)

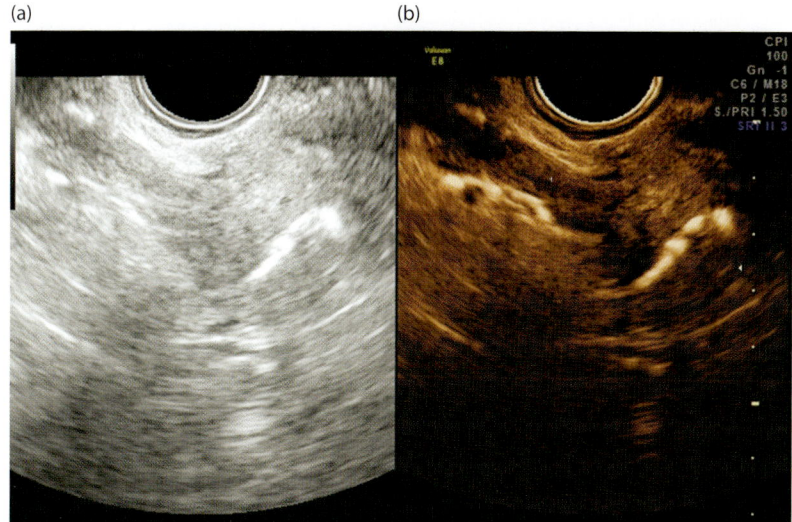

Figure 10.10 HyCoSy showing hyperechoic uterus and tube on B-mode (a) and contrast mode (b).

must be observed and spill should be confirmed. Appearance or increase in the fluid in the pouch of Douglas may be an indirect sign of tubal patency, the same as for SIS.

HyCoSy is usually performed within the fertility unit. HyCoSy has several advantages over SIS in that it helps to provide clearer visualization of the uterine cavity, better assessment of tubal lumen and fimbriae, clearer visualization of spill and a more exact localization of the site of blockage. HyCoSy with contrast is more efficient than with saline solution in determining fallopian tube patency and is as efficient as HSG and can be used instead of HSG for screening infertile patients [28]. The test shows good concordance with lap-and-dye (chromopertubation) (80.4–92.5 per cent) and HSG (83.8–90.5 per cent) [31]. The main disadvantage of HyCoSy is that it is more operator-dependent compared to HSG and has a high false occlusion rate [32].

In a study comparing HyCoSy and chromopertubation, there was a high degree of correlation in assessing tubal patency, with sensitivity, specificity, positive predictive value (PPV) and negative predictive value (NPV) of 100, 55.6, 80 and 100 per cent, respectively [31]. HyCoSy is accurate in determining tubal patency and evaluating the uterine cavity and can supplant HSG as the first-line diagnostic test in an infertility work-up [33]. Compared to conventional HSG, HyCoSy provides a simultaneous ultrasound evaluation of the pelvis and a more cost-effective evaluation of tubal pathology and can be successfully

used as a first-line non-invasive screening method [34]. In a diagnostic accuracy study of HyCoSy performed with air and saline (Hydro-HyCoSy) and with contrast media (SonoVue-HyCoSy) considering HSG and/or chromopertubation as reference tests, SonoVue-HyCoSy has been found to be more accurate than Hydro-HyCoSy for the assessment of fallopian tubes [31]. While the sensitivity, specificity, PPV and NPV of Hydro-HyCoSy were 91, 71, 55 and 95 per cent, respectively, they were 87, 84, 69, and 94 per cent respectively for SonoVue-HyCoSy. The diagnostic accuracy of Hydro-HyCoSy and of SonoVue-HyCoSy were 77 and 85 per cent, with a Cohen's kappa of 0.52 and 0.66, respectively. In another small study comparing HyCoSy and chromopertubation, there was a high degree of correlation in assessing tubal patency, with sensitivity, specificity, PPV and NPV of 100, 55.6, 80 and 100 per cent, respectively [28].

Moreover, the amount of contrast agent required for adequate examination was also less with positive contrast. Mean volumes of contrast injections were 35.3 ml of saline, 14.4 ml of Infoson, and 13.8 ml of Iopamiron 370. Infoson-enhanced HyCoSy provided a significantly larger ($p = 0.006$) number of correct diagnoses (20/22 fallopian tubes) than did saline HyCoSy (12/24 fallopian tubes), and the same number as that achieved by HSG [33].

Yet another study has shown that HSG and HyCoSy demonstrated a high concordance with laparoscopy (83 and 80 per cent, respectively).

The two methods had a high NPV for tubal disease (HSG, 94 per cent; HyCoSy, 88 per cent), and the PPVs were 47 and 75 per cent, respectively [35]. A study by Exacoustos et al. has also shown that HSG and HyCoSy had the same high concordance as laparoscopy, at 86.7 and 86.7 per cent, respectively [36]. The study concluded that HyCoSy proved to be superior to conventional HSG in evaluating adjacent myometrial structures, adnexa and degree of follicular maturation, was equal to HSG in visualizing the passage of the contrast medium into the peritoneum, but inferior to HSG in imaging the fallopian tubes owing to their tortuosity [36]. Conversely, Balen et al. found that both SIS and HyCoSy are insufficiently accurate and inferior to HSG [37]. They quoted a false-positive rate of 9 per cent and false-negative rate of 20 per cent for HyCoSy. This is because fallopian tubes are tortuous and usually not confined to a single plane. Moreover, distal parts of the tube may be obscured by bowel gas.

There are many factors that can give rise to a false occlusion result. First, the tubal lumen may be temporarily occluded by a mucous plug, blood clot, myometrial spasm or mucosal oedema [38]. The proximal segment, being the narrowest part of the fallopian tube, is especially prone to this, resulting in a diagnosis of a cornual block. Second, technical difficulties can arise for multiple reasons. Contrast leakage or cervical stenosis can occur, resulting in failure to achieve adequate pressure of hydrotubation [35]. Tubal convolution or distorted anatomy from pelvic adhesions can lead to difficulty in tracing the course of the tubes.

Modifications of HyCoSy

Three-dimensional power Doppler helps to visualize the whole tube and spill. This technique has been shown to be superior to conventional HyCoSy with free spill from fallopian tubes demonstrated in 91 per cent of tubes using 3D power Doppler (3D-PD) as compared to only 46 per cent by conventional HyCoSy, and the contrast agent required was almost half for 3D-PD in this study [37].

The advantages of 3D-PD HyCoSy techniques are that it allows simultaneous visualization of the uterine cavity and whole tube, has a short procedure time and reduced patient discomfort, requires less contrast and allows storage of the 3D volume, which allows offline review and reassessment.

Technique of 3D HyCoSy

Patient preparation, catheter placement and preparation of contrast media are done according to the method described earlier. Scanning is performed using a 3D ultrasound machine (e.g. Voluson E8 Expert BT 12; GE Medical Systems). A high-frequency transvaginal transducer (6–9 MHz) is used for pelvic evaluation. Contrast mode is switched on. As the contrast is slowly injected through the balloon catheter into the uterus, the transvaginal probe is oriented such that uterine cornu and ovaries are seen on the same plane. Having defined the contrast filling in the tubes, 3D is switched on and volumes are independently acquired for each side (Figure 10.11).

Rendering is done in the front–back viewing direction. Surface enhanced mode is used. The threshold is set to make the contrast path more obvious. Magicut (electronic scalpel) is then used to cut all shadows other than the contrast path. Then the HDLive rendering mode is switched on and the direction of the light is adjusted to best visualize the fimbriae and spill. After the final picture is ready, both halves are matched and put together to form a complete picture of the uterus and both tubes (Figure 10.12).

In a series of 65 subfertile women in whom we performed 3D HyCoSy followed by a laparoscopy and dye test to evaluate the diagnostic accuracy, the results of 3D HyCoSy were consistent with those of laparoscopy, except in two women. One of these two patients had unilateral tubal block on HyCoSy, but the tube was patent at laparoscopy with injection of methylene blue dye with pressure. In the other patient, the fimbrial end of the tube was not clearly visualized on 3D HyCoSy and was thought to be blocked, but at laparoscopy the distal tubal portion was buried behind the ovary due to endometriosis and the tube was patent.

This technique is more informative and reliable than 2D HyCoSy. The whole extent of the tubal lumen and fimbrial condition can be visualized. The relation of the fimbrial end of the tube to the ovary can also be defined. The site of the blockage can be identified (Figure 10.13).

HyCoSy with automated 3D technology retains the advantages of conventional 2D HyCoSy while overcoming the disadvantages. Two-dimensional HyCoSy is highly observer-dependent and is only accurate in the hands of experienced investigators; by obtaining a volume of the uterus and tubes, automated 3D volume acquisition permits visualization of the tubes in the coronal view and of the tubal course in 3D space, and should allow less experienced operators

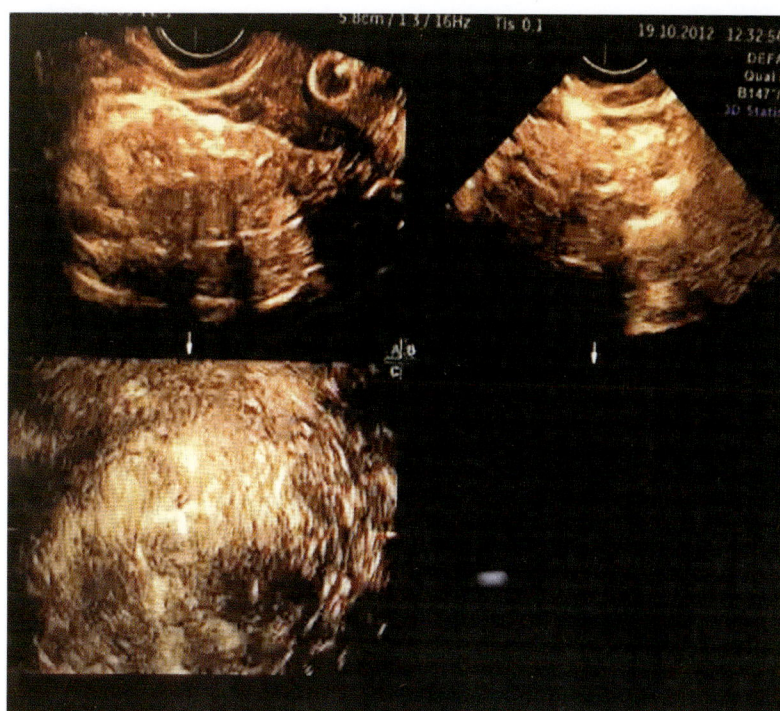

Figure 10.11 3D volume of the HyCoSy.

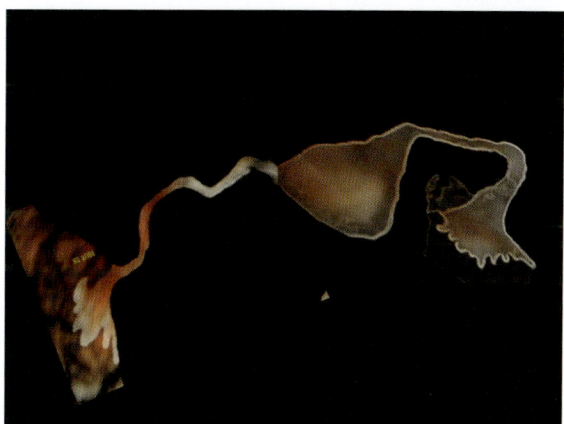

Figure 10.12 3D reconstructed volume of the uterus and the tube on HyCoSy.

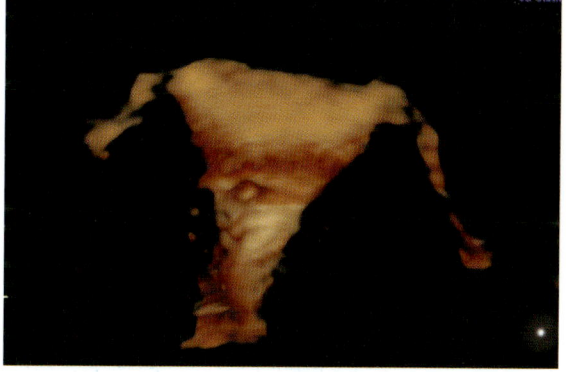

Figure 10.13 3D reconstructed volume of the uterus and tubes on HyCoSy with bilateral mid-tubal block.

to evaluate tubal patency status relatively easily [39]. But 3D HyCoSy should be regarded as complementary and cannot fully replace 2D HyCoSy.

Large studies have reported that 3D HyCoSy is highly accurate, with 100 per cent sensitivity, 67 per cent specificity, 89 per cent PPV and 100 per cent NPV for tubal patency and concordance rate with laparoscopy of 91 per cent [40]. In a study by Kupesic et al., 3D HyCoSy (sensitivity, specificity, PPV and NPV of 97.9, 100, 97.9 and 100 per cent, respectively) was found to be marginally superior to 2D HyCoSy (sensitivity, specificity, PPV and NPV of 93.6, 97.3, 98.2 and 97.3 per cent, respectively) for tubal assessment [41]. It has been shown in another study that for detecting tubal patency among the 150 fallopian tubes assessed, 3D SonoVue-HyCoSy had a sensitivity of 93.5 per cent, specificity of 86.3 per cent, positive and negative predictive values of 87.8 and 92.6 per cent, respectively, and diagnostic accuracy of 90.0 per cent. The test-positive rates of 3D SonoVue-HyCoSy versus lap-and-dye were not significantly different (82/150 versus 77/150, $p > 0.05$) [42].

Yet another study by Chan et al. has shown that the sensitivity of 3D HyCoSy for detecting tubal patency was 100 per cent, with a specificity of 67 per cent. The positive and negative predictive values were 89 and 100 per cent, respectively; the concordance rate was 91 per cent. The mean duration ($\pm$ SD) for 3D HyCoSy was 13.4 ± 5.5 min [43].

Colour-coded 3D-PD imaging (PDI) with surface rendering allows visualization of the flow of contrast through the entire tubal length and free spill of contrast can be clearly identified in the majority of cases. The 3D-PDI method appears to have advantages over the conventional HyCoSy technique, especially in terms of visualization of spill from the distal end of the tube, which has been achieved twice as often with the 3D technique. The 3D-PDI technique allows better storage of information for re-analysis and archiving than conventional HyCoSy. The mean duration of the imaging procedure is less with 3D-PDI, but the operator time, including post-procedure analysis of the stored information, is similar. A significantly lower volume of contrast medium (5.9 ± 0.6 ml) is used for 3D-PDI in comparison with that (11.2 ± 1.9 ml) used for conventional 2D HyCoSy [41]. A recent systematic review [44] reported that 3D HyCoSy offers high diagnostic accuracy with a pooled sensitivity of 98 per cent and pooled specificity of 90 per cent.

In spite of all the sophisticated imaging technologies, the gold standard is still endoscopy. If any abnormality is found in the tubes on imaging, confirmation by endoscopy is required. Endoscopy consists of hysteroscopy to assess the cornual end of the tube and laparoscopy to observe the fimbrial end of the tube. However, while lap-and-dye enables direct visualization of external tubal morphology, assessment of the internal architecture of the tube is not permitted and it is not always possible to identify the site of tubal occlusion.

Summarizing Tubal Patency Evaluation by Ultrasound

Tubal evaluation is an essential step in subfertile patients. HSG has been used for a long time for assessment of tubal patency. Saline infusion sonosalpingography has been proven to be a fairly reliable technique for tubal evaluation. Its diagnostic accuracy can be improved by the use of pulse Doppler and colour Doppler. Introduction of ultrasound contrast media and HyCoSy have improved the visibility of the tubal lumen. HyCoSy is accurate in determining tubal patency and evaluating the uterine cavity, suggesting it could supplant HSG as the first-line diagnostic test in an infertility work-up [45]. Evaluative studies of HyCoSy showed good statistical comparability and concordance with HSG and laparoscopy combined with dye [39]. HyCoSy is well tolerated and can be a suitable alternative outpatient procedure [46]. HyCoSy using contrast agent appears to be more efficient than saline solution in detecting tubal obstruction [47].

HyCoSy is as efficient as HSG in assessing tubal patency and has the advantage of simultaneous pelvic evaluation for pelvic pathology and ovarian reserve. It can, therefore, be considered as a first-line investigative tool in low-risk women who are not known to have any reproductive co-morbidities. HyCoSy combined with 3D ultrasound has the ability to increase diagnostic accuracy, but this technique is not widely used because of limited availability of 3D ultrasound.

The Royal College of Obstetricians and Gynaecologists (RCOG) recommends that where appropriate expertise is available, screening for tubal occlusion using HyCoSy should be considered because it is an effective alternative to HSG for women who are not known to have co-morbidities. Women who are thought to have co-morbidities should be offered laparoscopy and dye so that tubal and other pelvic pathology can be assessed at the same time. Because of the good degree of statistical comparability and concordance of conventional HyCoSy with HSG and laparoscopy and dye test, the National Institute for Health and Care Excellence (NICE) has recommended HyCoSy as a suitable outpatient procedure for tubal patency assessment in women who are not known to have any co-morbidities such as pelvic inflammatory disease (PID), previous ectopic pregnancy or endometriosis [46,48].

HyCoSy is well tolerated by women and associated risks are minimal, with the risk of pelvic infection being 1 per cent. Recommendations by the American Society of Reproductive Medicine (ASRM) state that all available methods for evaluation of tubal factors have technical limitations that must be considered when any

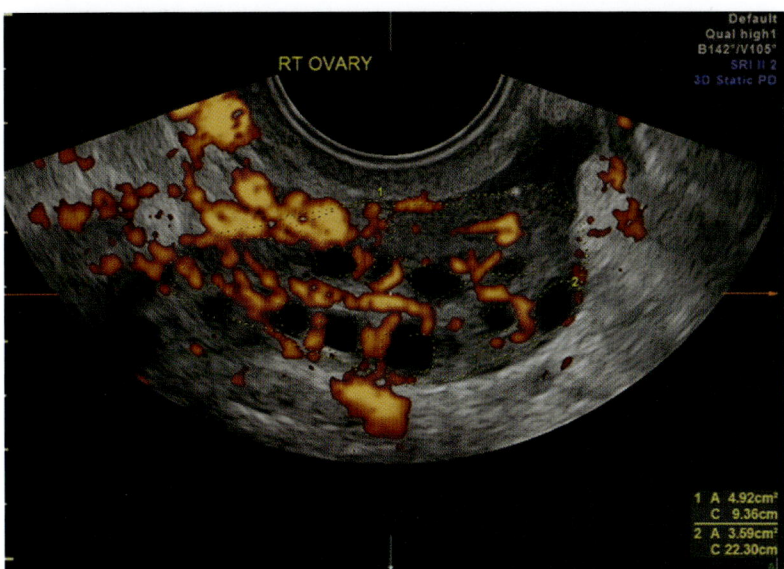

Figure 10.14 Hypoechoic hypervascular ovarian stroma in a case of oophoritis.

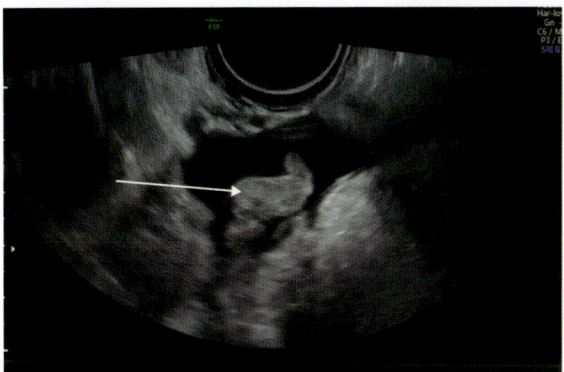

Figure 10.15 Free fluid seen in the pelvis with floating thickened tube (arrow) on B-mode ultrasound due to acute inflammation of the tube and PID.

one technique yields abnormal results. Further evaluation with a second, complementary method is prudent whenever the specific diagnosis or best treatment strategy is uncertain [49].

Tubal Pathologies

Common tubal pathologies include inflammation, tubal block due to endometriosis, infection or previous surgery, tubal pregnancy and tubal neoplasms.

Inflammation is the commonest pathology affecting tubal patency and tubal function. Inflammation of the tube (salpingitis) is most commonly due to PID. Patients present with pelvic pain, tenderness and signs

of acute inflammation in severe cases. The chronic cases more often present with subfertility, or chronic salpingitis may be diagnosed incidentally.

The propagating function of the fallopian tubes, as has been discussed earlier, is due to peristalsis and also mucosal ciliary movement. Infection and inflammation may lead to mucosal damage, thus affecting the tubal function. This may not compromise the patency of the tube but surely increases the risk of tubal ectopic pregnancy. Oedema caused by acute inflammation leads to obliteration of tubal lumen and tubal block.

This phase of inflammation is often difficult to diagnose on ultrasound, though some patients may typically show thickened adnexal soft tissue band and tenderness on probe pressure. Acute salpingitis is very commonly associated with oophoritis. Oophoritis on ultrasound presents as hypoechoic ovarian stroma with low resistance and abundant blood flow in the ovary (Figure 10.14).

Acute inflammation may often show associated fluid in the pelvis. When fluid collection is present, a thick fimbrial end of the tube floating in the fluid may be visualized (Figure 10.15). Fluid collection may often show septations or low-level internal echogenicities due to the infective pathology (Figure 10.16).

Involvement of the fimbrial end in the inflammatory process leads to fimbrial adhesions and hydrosalpinx (dilation of the tube with fluid collection in the lumen).

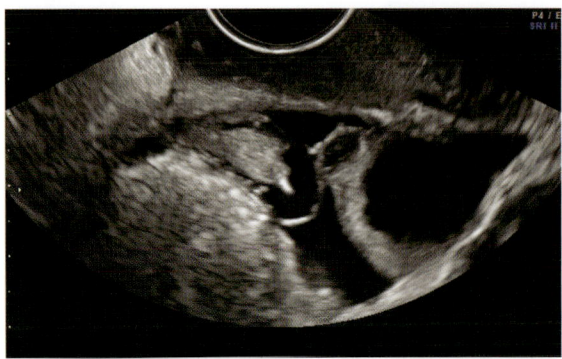

Figure 10.16 Pelvic inflammatory disease showing free fluid and septations in the pelvis.

The walls of the cystic lesion are thick and appear irregular due to the thickened oedematous haustra in acute inflammatory hydrosalpinx (Figure 10.19), whereas in chronically inflamed tubes the walls may appear thinner and show adhesions with the surrounding tissues and with the ovaries; tubo-ovarian masses are more common in chronic salpingitis.

It is often difficult to identify the tubal and ovarian structures separately in these masses (Figure 10.20a), especially when the structures are grossly damaged due to inflammation. If infection in such a mass is still active and the content is purulent, it is termed a tubo-ovarian abscess (Figure 10.20b). *Chlamydia trachoma-*

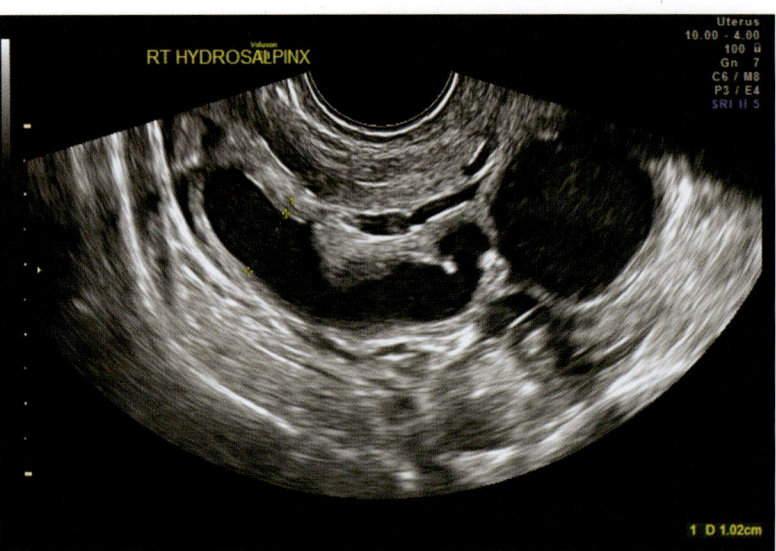

Figure 10.17 Tubular cystic lesion on B-mode ultrasound with thin walls, anechoic contents, partial septum and posterior acoustic enhancement.

Hydrosalpinx can be seen and diagnosed on ultrasound as a cystic extra-ovarian lesion in the adnexa. Its cystic nature is identified by thin walls, anechoic contents in the lumen and posterior acoustic enhancement (Figure 10.17). Sometimes the contents may show low-level echogenicity representing blood or pus in the lumen; in those cases it is called haematosalpinx or pyosalpinx, respectively (Figure 10.18). Though on ultrasound alone it is difficult to differentiate between the two, the relevant clinical history and presentation may point towards haematosalpinx, which is common in patients as a consequence of ectopic pregnancy. Patients with pyosalpinx may present with systemic signs of severe infection, but this is not a rule.

tis and tuberculosis are the two commonest infections causing this and both have a very similar presentation.

Tuberculous involvement of the tube can be mild, with damage to the tubal lining, or more severe, with tubal scarring, rigidity, fibrosis, stenosis or occlusion, hydrosalpinx, and peritubal and pelvic adhesions. Because of thick, rigid tubal walls it may often show only a mildly dilated tube and might be difficult to differentiate from the blood vessels on a still image (Figure 10.21).

It is therefore very important to evaluate any lesion in the adnexa in at least two orthogonal planes (by rotating the probe 90°). Any extra-ovarian cystic lesion that changes shape on rotation of the probe should be

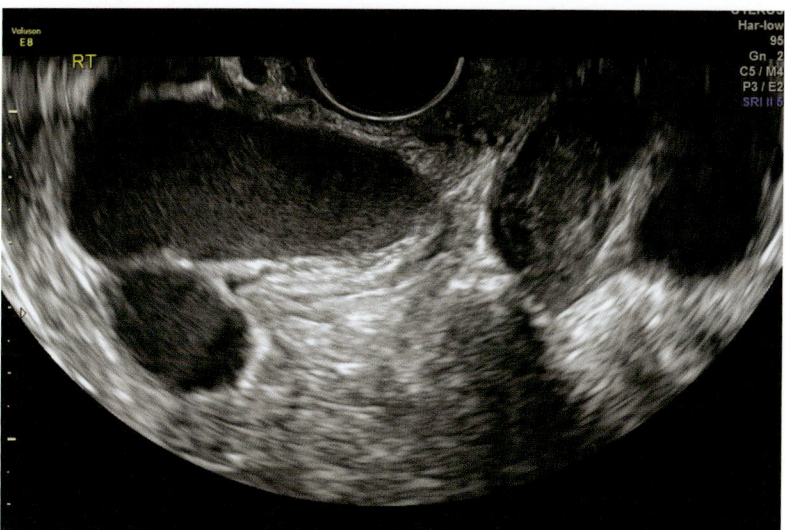

Figure 10.18 Two cystic lesions close to each other, possibly two loops of dilated tube with low-level echoes due to viscous fluid within.

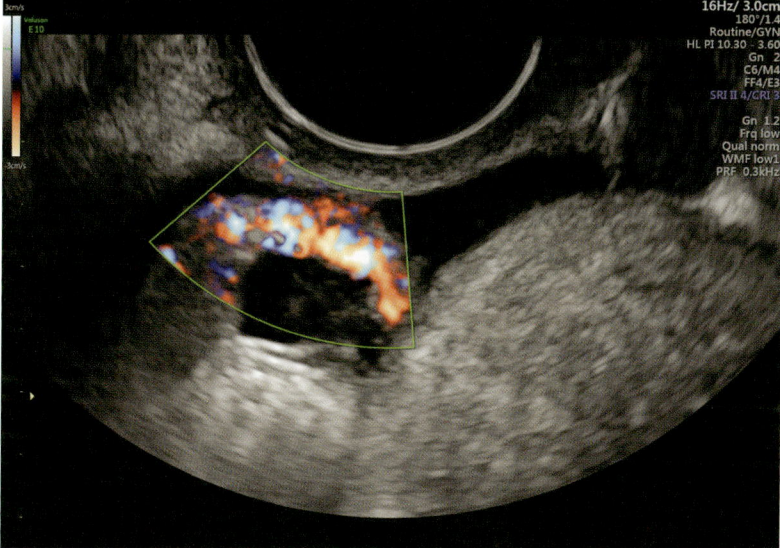

Figure 10.19 Thickened tube with free fluid and increased vascularity of acute salpingitis.

considered as hydrosalpinx, unless proved otherwise. At times this change in shape may typically show a cystic round lesion becoming typically tubular or sausage shaped, but often may be only slightly elongated or may show a small beak-like projection or tapering of one of the ends of the elongated tubular cystic lesion (Figure 10.22).

The two structures that may behave the same are the blood vessels and the bowel loops. These can be differentiated from hydrosalpinx by using colour Doppler that shows colour in the case of a blood vessel and by observing peristalsis in a bowel loop. Hydrosalpinges may typically show incomplete septa on longitudinal sections and this has been considered as one of the most diagnostic signs on ultrasound for hydrosalpinx. On the transverse section, especially acute hydrosalpinx may show a typically described, cog-wheel appearance due to thick walls and oedematous haustra (Figure 10.23).

Endometriosis may at times involve the fimbrial end of the tube independently or as an extension of ovarian endometriosis. This leads to adhesions of the

139

(a)

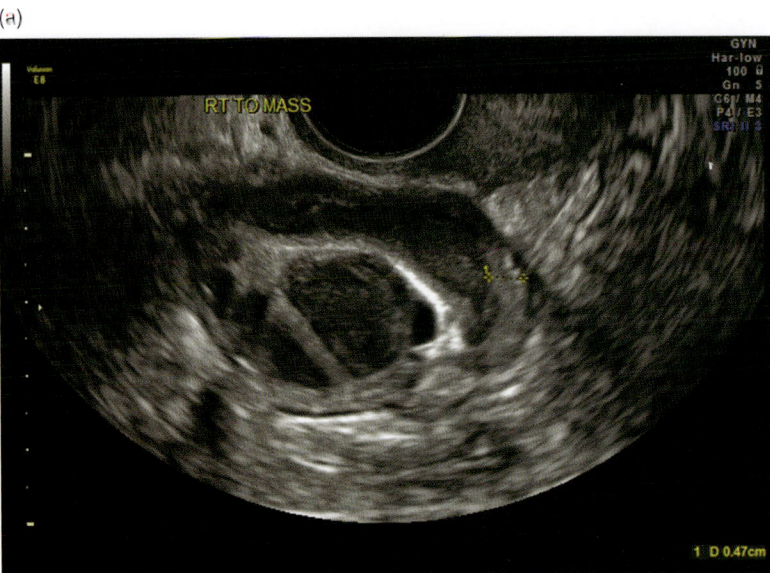

(b)

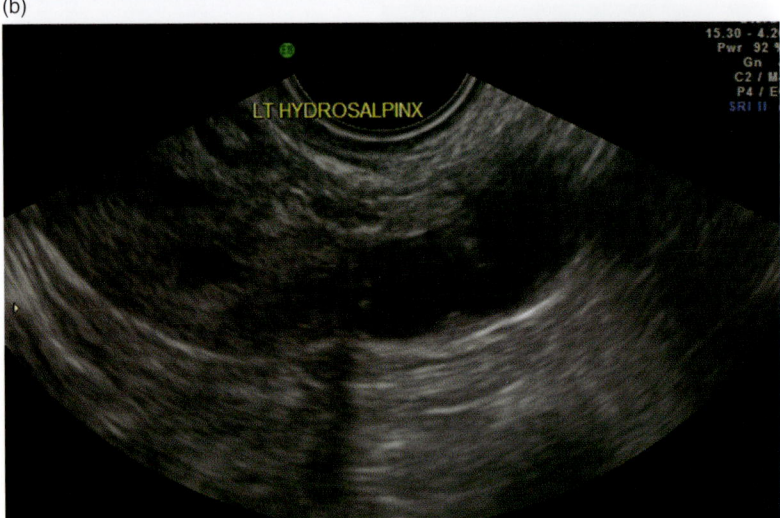

Figure 10.20 B mode ultrasound shows tubo-ovarian mass (a) and tubo-ovarian abscess (b).

fimbrial end of the tube and therefore may lead to hydrosalpinx. The ultrasound presentation is the same as hydrosalpinx due to the inflammatory process.

Tubal ectopic pregnancy is discussed separately in Chapter 14.

Tubal Neoplasms

Tubal neoplasms are rare. They account for approximately 0.14–1.8 per cent of all female genital malignancies [50]. Tubal neoplasms are most commonly primary fallopian tube carcinoma or adenocarcinoma. Both are uncommon. Primary fallopian tube carcinoma (PFTC) is a rare tumour that histologically and clinically resembles epithelial ovarian cancer. Nulliparous women appear to be at a higher risk for developing PFTC [51]. Intermittent hydrosalpinx, with watery vaginal discharge or bleeding, may be a common clinical presentation.

On ultrasound, this lesion appears similar to ovarian epithelial tumours, presenting as a complex adnexal extra-ovarian mass, usually multicystic and solid. The solid components have irregular margins

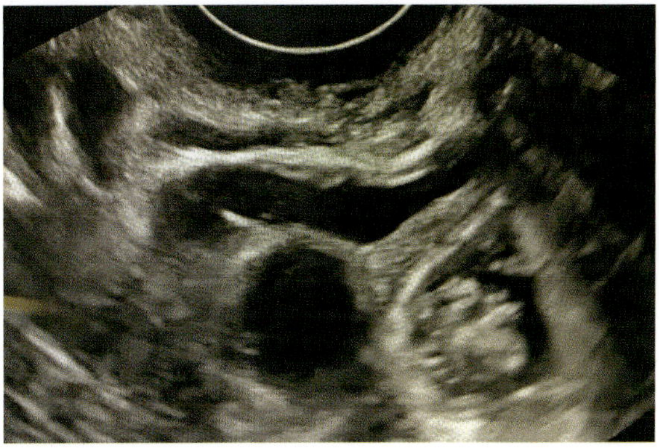

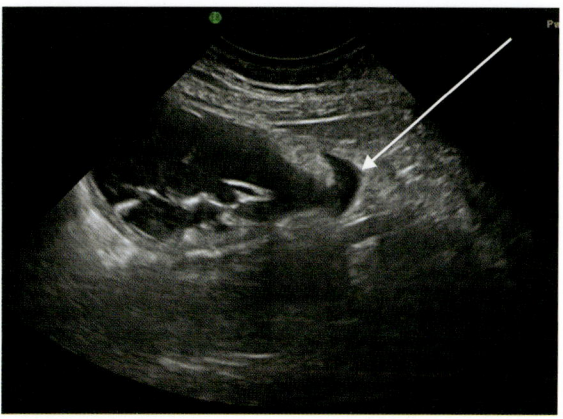

Figure 10.21 B-mode ultrasound showing dilated rigid fallopian tube secondary to tuberculosis.

Figure 10.22 Hydrosalpinx with beak-like projection (arrow) on B-mode ultrasound.

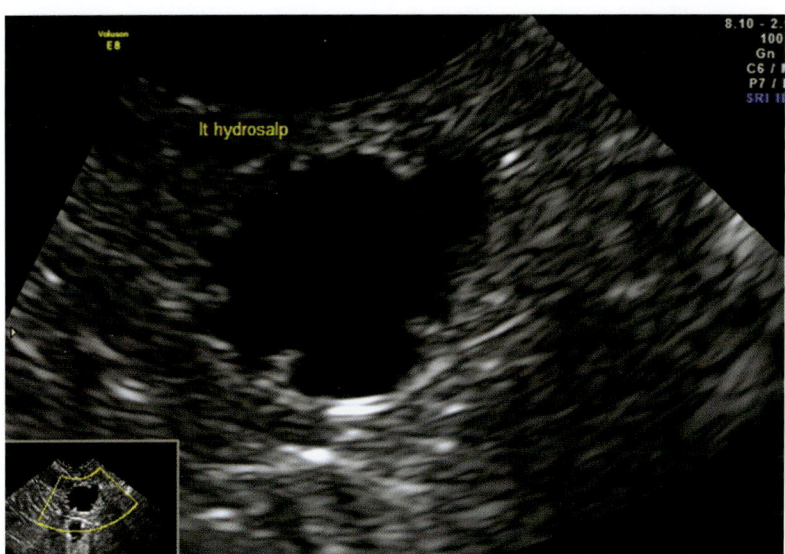

Figure 10.23 Transverse section of hydrosalpinx on B-mode ultrasound: cog-wheel appearance.

and show abundant low-resistance vascularity. The heterogeneous echogenicity, irregular shape of the solid components, heterogeneously increased vascular density and irregular calibre of the blood vessels may be the signs that indicate the malignant nature of the neoplasm (Figure 10.24).

Though extra-ovarian, it is often difficult to confirm its extra-ovarian origin because it is usually diagnosed late, when it may become adherent to the ovary due to ovarian invasion. Primary fallopian tube carcinoma has a worse prognosis than ovarian cancer as it is not routinely suspected and so treatment may be

delayed. It is usually managed in the same manner as ovarian cancer [52].

Conclusion

Tubal patency evaluation is essential for the work-up of any subfertile patient. Ultrasound-guided tubal patency evaluation is a patient- and clinician-friendly procedure. It can be done using negative or positive contrast. Both may be done using various ultrasound modalities such as B-mode ultrasound, Doppler and 3D ultrasound. However, hystero-laparoscopy with dye test is still considered as the

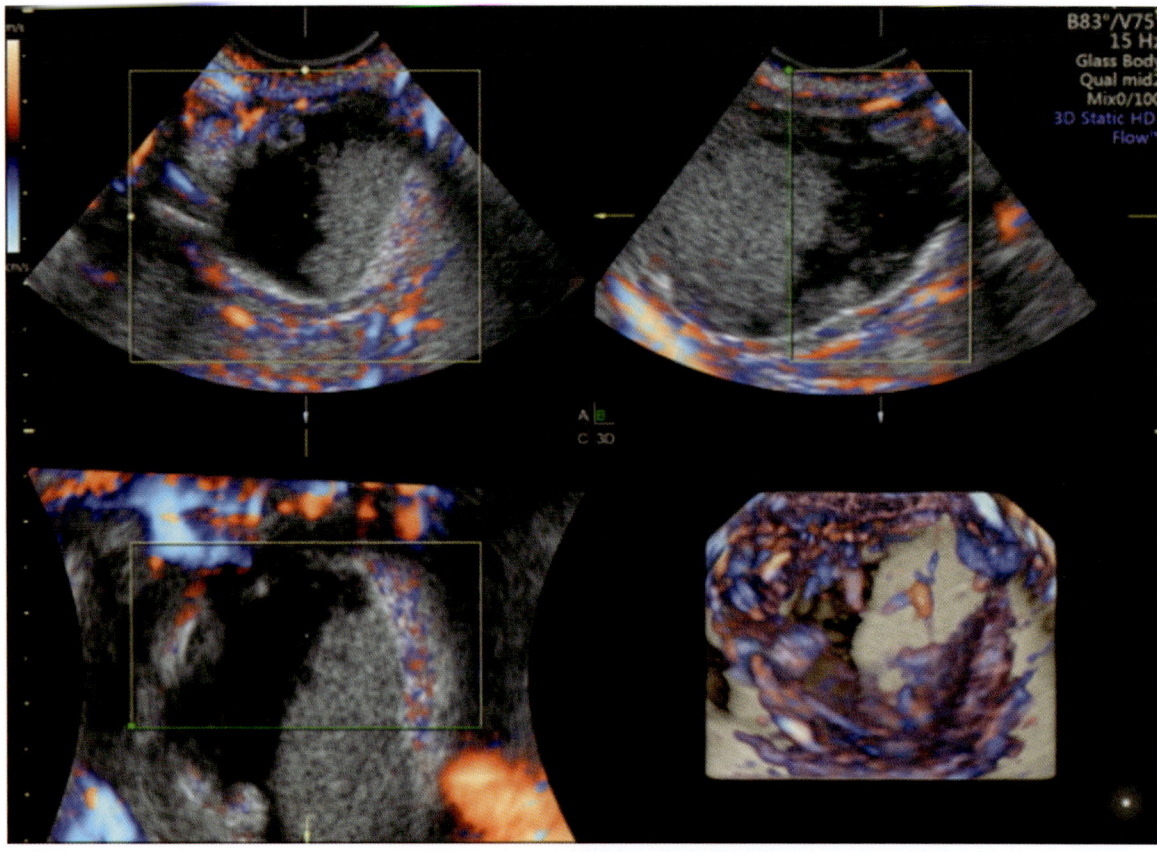

Figure 10.24 Cystic malignant mass with irregular solid component and grossly increased vascularity.

gold standard method. Among tubal pathologies, inflammation is the commonest and may have variable ultrasound picture. Endometriosis may affect the fimbrial end of the tube and lead to hydrosalpinx. Tubal neoplasms are uncommon and are difficult to differentiate confidently from ovarian neoplasm. However, ultrasound still remains the modality of choice for diagnosis of all tubal pathologies.

Tips and Tricks

- Tubal patency tests should be carried out in the early follicular phase to avoid disruption of potential pregnancy.
- Utilization of all possible ultrasound modalities (colour, power or gated Doppler) allows for more accurate assessment of tubal patency.
- In the absence of newer contrast media or foam, agitated saline is a good alternative.
- Slow administration of small volumes of contrast media makes the procedure less uncomfortable.

- Antibiotic prophylaxis is good practice before tubal patency testing.
- Addition of 3D ultrasound allows for simultaneous assessment of the endometrial cavity and congenital or acquired anomaly.

References

1. Serafini P, Batzofin J. Diagnosis of female infertility: a comprehensive approach. *J Reprod Med* 1989;**34** (1):29–40.

2. Dun EC, Nezhat CH. Tubal factor infertility: diagnosis and management in the era of assisted reproductive technology. *Obstet Gynecol Clin North Am* 2012;**39** (4):551–66.

3. Patil M. Assessing tubal damage. *J Hum Reprod Sci* 2009;**2**(1):2.

4. Gordts S, Campo R, Rombauts, Brosens I. Endoscopic visualization of the process of fimbrial ovum retrieval in the human. *Hum Reprod* 1998;**13** (6):1425–8.

5. Johnson N, Vandekerckhove P, Watson A, et al. Tubal flushing for subfertility. *Cochrane Database Syst Rev* 2003; **3**:CD003718.

6. Belisle S, Collins JA, Burrows EA, Willan AR. The value of laparoscopy among infertile women with tubal patency. *J Soc Obstet Gynaecol Can* 1996;**18**:326–36.

7. Watrelot A, Dreyfus JM, Andine JP. Evaluation of the performance of fertiloscopy in 160 consecutive infertile patients with no obvious pathology. *Hum Reprod* 1999;**14**:707–11.

8. Nanini R, Chelo E, Branconi F, et al. Dynamic echohysteroscopy: a new diagnostic technique in the study of female infertility. *Acta Eur Fertil* 1981;**12** (2):165–71.

9. Richman TS, Visconi GN, deChurney A, et al. Fallopian tubal patency assessed by ultrasound fluid injection: work in progress. *Radiology* 1984;**152**(2):507–10.

10. Randolph JR, Ying YK, Maier DB, et al. Comparison of real time ultrasonography, hysterosalpingography and laparoscopy/hysteroscopy in the evaluation of uterine abnormalities and tubal patency. *Fertil Steril* 1986;**46** (5):828–32.

11. Tufekci EC, Girit S, Bayirli MD, et al. Evaluation of tubal patency by transvaginal sonosalpingography. *Fertil Steril* 1992;**57**:336–40.

12. Deichert U, Schlief R, van de Sandt M, et al. Transvaginal hysterosalpingo-contrast sonography (Hy-Co-Sy) compared with conventional tubal diagnostics. *Hum Reprod* 1989;**4**(4):418–24.

13. Dessole S, Farina M, Rubattu G, et al. Side effects and complications of sonohysterosalpingography. *Fertil Steril* 2003;**8**(3):620–4.

14. de Kroon CD, de Bock GH, Dieben SW, Jansen FW. Saline contrast hysterosonography in abnormal uterine bleeding: a systematic review and meta-analysis. *BJOG* 2003;**110**(10):938–47.

15. Stern J, Peters AJ, Coulam CB. Colour Doppler ultrasonography assessment of tubal patency: a comparison study with traditional techniques. *Fertil Steril* 1992;**58**(5):897–900.

16. Kupesic S, Kurjak A. Gynecological vaginal sonographic interventional procedures: what does colour add? *Gynecol Perinatol* 1994;**3**:57–60.

17. Deichert U, Schlief R, van de Sandt M, et al. Transvaginal hysterosalpingo-contrast sonography for the assessment of tubal patency with gray scale imaging and additional use of pulsed wave Doppler. *Fertil Steril* 1992;**57**(1):62–7.

18. Deichert U, van de Sandt M. Transvaginal hysterosalpingo-contrast sonography(Hy-Co-Sy). The assessment of tubal patency and uterine abnormalities by contrast enhanced sonography. *Adv Echo-Contrast* 1993;**2**:55–8

19. Kleinkauf-Houcken A, Huneke B, Lindner Ch, Braendle W. Combining B mode ultrasound with pulsed wave Doppler for assessment of tubal patency. *Hum Reprod* 1997;**12**(11):2457–60.

20. Peters AJ, Coulam CB. Hysterosalpingography with colour Doppler sonography. *Am J Obstet Gynecol* 1991;**164**(6 Pt 1):1530–2.

21. Jeanty P, Besnard S, Arnold A, et al. Air-contrast sonohysterography as a first step assessment of tubal patency. *J Ultrasound Med* 2000;**19**(8):519–27.

22. Sankpal RS, Confino E, Matzel A, Cohen LS. Investigation of the uterine cavity and fallopian tubes using three-dimensional saline sonohysterosalpingography. *Int J Gynaecol Obstet* 2001;**73**(2):125–9.

23. Kiyokawa K, Masuda H, Fuyuki T, et al. Three-dimensional hysterosalpingo-contrast sonography (3D-HyCoSy) as an outpatient procedure to assess infertile women: a pilot study. *Ultrasound Obstet Gynecol* 2000;**16**(7):648–54.

24. Davison GB, Leeton J. A case of female fertility investigated by contrast-enhanced echo-gynecography. *J Clin Ultrasound* 1988;**16** (1):44–7.

25. Bonilla-Musoles F, Simon C, Sampaio M, et al. An assessment of hysterosalpingosonography as a diagnostic tool for uterine cavity defects and tubal patency. *J Clin Ultrasound* 1992;**20**(3):175–81.

26. Prefumo F, Serafini G, Martinoli C, et al. The sonographic evaluation of tubal patency with stimulated acoustic emission imaging. *Ultrasound Obstet Gynecol* 2002;**20**(4):386–9.

27. Emanuel MH, Exalto N. Hysterosalpingo-foam sonography (HyFoSy): a new technique to visualize tubal patency. *Ultrasound Obstet Gynecol* 2011;**37** (4):498–9.

28. Emanuel MH, van Vliet M, Weber M, Exalto N. First experiences with hysterosalpingo-foam sonography (HyFoSy) for office tubal patency testing. *Hum Reprod* 2012;**27**(1):114–17.

29. Boudghene FP, Bazot M, Robert Y, et al. Assessment of fallopian tube patency by HyCoSy: comparison of a positive contrast agent with saline solution. *Ultrasound Obstet Gynecol* 2001;**18**(5):525–30

30. Van Schoubroeck D, Van den Bosch T, Meuleman C, et al. The use of a new gel foam for the evaluation of tubal patency. *Gynecol Obstet Invest* 2013;**75**(3):152–6.

31. Campbell S, Bourne TH, Tan SL, Collins WP. Hysterosalpingo contrast sonography (HyCoSy) and its future role within the investigation of infertility in Europe. *Ultrasound Obstet Gynecol* 1994;**4**(3):245–53.

32. Tanawattanachaeron S, Suwajanakorn S, Uerpairojkit B, Boonkasemsamti W, Virutamasen P.

Transvaginal hystero-contrast sonography (HyCoSy) compared with chromolaparoscopy. *J Obstet Gynecol Res* 2000;**26**(1):71–5.

33. Lucaino DE, Exacoustos C, Johns DA, et al. Transabdominal saline contrast sonohysterography: can it replace hysterosalpingography in low resource countries? *Am J Obstet Gynecol* 2011;**204**(1):79.el–5.

34. Korell M, Seehaus D, Strowitzki T, Hepp H. Radiologic versus ultrasound fallopian tube imaging: painfulness of the examination and diagnostic reliability of hysterosalpingography and hysterosalpingo-contrast-ultrasonography with Echovist. *Ultraschall Med* 1997;**18**(1):3–7.

35. Lanzani C, Savasi V, Leone FP, Ratti M, Ferrazzi E. Two-dimensional HyCoSy with contrast tuned imaging technology and a second-generation contrast media for the assessment of tubal patency in an infertility program. *Fertil Steril* 2009;**92**(3):1158–61.

36. Exacoustos C, Zupi E, Carusotti C, et al. Hysterosalpingo-contrast sonography compared with hysterosalpingography and laparoscopic dye perturbation to evaluate tubal patency. *J Am Assoc Gynecol Laparosc* 2003;**10**(3):367–72.

37. Balen FG, Allen CM, Gardener JE, Siddle NC, Lees WR. 3-dimensional reconstruction of ultrasound images of the uterine cavity. *Br J Radiology* 1993;**66**,588–91.

38. Exacoustos C, Di Giovanni A, Szabolcs B, et al. Automated sonographic tubal patency evaluation with three-dimensional coded contrast imaging (CCI) during hysterosalpingo-contrast sonography (HyCoSy) *Ultrasound Obstet Gynecol* 2009;**34**(5):609–12

39. Sladkevicius P, Ojha K, Campbell S, et al. Three dimensional power Doppler imaging in the assessment of fallopian tube patency. *Ultrasound Obstet Gynecol* 2000;**16**(7):644–7.

40. Exacoustos C, Di Giovanni A, Szabolcs B, et al. Automated three-dimensional coded contrast imaging hysterosalpingo-contrast sonography: feasibility in office tubal patency testing. *Ultrasound Obstet Gynecol* 2013;**41**(3):328–35.

41. Kupesic S, Plavsic MB. 2D and 3D hysterosalpingocontrast-sonography in the assessment of uterine cavity and tubal patency. *Eur J Obstet Gynecol Reprod Biol* 2007;**133**(1):64–9.

42. Zhou L, Zhang X, Chen X, et al. Value of three-dimensional hysterosalpingo-contrast sonography with SonoVue in the assessment of tubal patency. *Ultrasound Obstet Gynecol* 2012;**40**(1):93–8.

43. Chan CC, Ng EH, Tang OS, et al. Comparison of three-dimensional hysteron-contrast-sonography and diagnostic laparoscopy with chromopertubation in the assessment of tubal patency for the investigation of subfertility. *Acta Obstet Gynecol Scand* 2005;**84**(9):909–13.

44. Alcázar JL, Martinez-Astorquiza Corral T, Orozco R, et al. Three-dimensional hysterosalpingo-contrast-sonography for the assessment of tubal patency in women with infertility: a systematic review with meta-analysis. *Gynecol Obstet Invest* 2016;**81**(4):289–95.

45. Boudghene FP, Bazot M, Robert Y, et al. Assessment of fallopian tube patency by HyCoSy: comparison of a positive contrast agent with saline solution. *Ultrasound Obstet Gynecol* 2001;**18**(5):525–30.

46. Tanahatoe S, Hompes PG, Lambalk CB. Accuracy of diagnostic laparoscopy in the infertility work-up before intrauterine insemination. *Fertil Steril* 2003;**79**:361–6.

47. Dijkman AB, Mol BW, van der Veen F, Bossuyt PM, Hogerzeil HV. Can hysterosalpingocontrast-sonography replace hysterosalpingography in the assessment of tubal subfertility? *Eur J Radiol* 2000;**35**:44–8.

48. Volpi E, De Grandis T, Sismondi P, et al. Transvaginal salpingo-sonography (TSSG) in the evaluation of tubal patency. *Acta Eur Fertil* 1991;**22**(6):325–8.

49. Practice Committee of the American Society for Reproductive Medicine. Diagnostic evaluation of the infertile female: a committee opinion. *Fertil Steril* 2015;**103**(6):e44–50.

50. Riska A, Leminen A, Pukkala E. Sociodemographic determinants of incidence of primary fallopian tube carcinoma, Finland 1953–97. *Int J Cancer* 2003;**104**:643–5.

51. King A, Seraj IM, Thrasher T, Slater J, Wagner RJ. Fallopian tube carcinoma: a clinicopathological study of 17 cases. *Gynecol Oncol* 1989;**33**:351–5.

52. Kosary C, Trimble EL. Treatment and survival for women with fallopian tube carcinoma: a population-based study. *Gynecol Oncol* 2002;**86**:190–1.

Role of Ultrasound in Assisted Reproductive Treatment

Lukasz Polanski, Mamata Deenadayal and Aarti Deenadayal Tolani

Introduction

Assisted reproductive treatment (ART) has become the only hope for biologically own children for numerous infertile couples. It is estimated that 1.7–4.0 per cent of children born in developed countries are the result of assisted conception [1,2]. As a minimally invasive diagnostic tool, ultrasound is used readily throughout ART – starting with the pre-treatment assessment of pelvic organs, through cycle monitoring, oocyte collection and embryo replacement, to diagnosis of complications and outcome monitoring.

In this chapter, we will cover the application of ultrasound in assisted reproduction.

The Pre-treatment Scan

This scan, carried out before embarking on ART, serves multiple purposes. First, it serves to identify any pathology that might have contributed to infertility, or which may affect the outcome of the treatment (hydrosalpinx or uterine anomaly). Findings of the pre-treatment scan help to predict the response to ovarian stimulation by assessing the antral follicle count (AFC) and help guide dosing of gonadotrophins, provide a guide to endometrial receptivity and inform on the ease of access to the ovaries during oocyte collection.

Antral follicle count and anti-Mullerian hormone levels (AMH) are the best predictors of oocyte yield and stimulation response in ART, with an ongoing debate as to the superiority of one test over another [3]. Ultrasound-based AFC measurement can be performed with ease using 2D and 3D ultrasound modalities (the exact method is described in Chapter 7) (Figure 11.1). Typically, AFC assessment is carried out at the beginning of the menstrual cycle, as the follicles of interest are 2–10 mm in diameter [4–6]. Scanning later in the menstrual cycle could underestimate the value due to exclusion of the dominant follicle(s) as these are >10 mm in diameter; however,

some evidence indicates that accuracy of AFC is not affected when scanned at any stage of the menstrual cycle [7]. Antral follicle count produces instant results and, as such, has the advantage over AMH. There are, however, limitations of the test, and these are related to variations between centres, differences in ultrasound equipment, training and the timing of scanning [3]. Three-dimensional ultrasound scanning may be able to overcome the inconsistencies when assessing AFC; however, the technology is not in routine use.

In juvenile women, a transvaginal ultrasound scan may be inappropriate, limiting the use of AFC as a predictor of ovarian reserve [8]. Obesity may also affect the AFC due to the poor image quality when carrying out the scan, as well as due to reported significant inter-cycle variability of AFC in this population [9–11].

In order to obtain the most reliable information from the AFC scan, the process has to be standardized and consistent. It is recommended that the procedure be carried out between days 2 and 4 of a natural menstrual cycle or of a contraceptive pill cycle; only follicles measuring 2–10 mm should be included and appropriate training should be provided with the use of standard ultrasound settings and equipment [4,12]. Identification and characterization of ovarian cysts must be carried out during the scan. Details of ovarian assessment are described in Chapters 2 and 8.

Assessment of the uterus and endometrium, as well as of the adnexa, is a component of the pre-treatment scan. The endometrial and myometrial assessment for the presence of endometrial polyps, submucosal and intramural fibroids, and adenomyosis are described in Chapters 4 and 6.

In order to exclude the presence of endometrial polyps, the scan ideally should be carried out in the late follicular phase or mid-cycle. Endometrial polyps distort the triple-layer appearance and are easily distinguishable as hyperechoic structures distorting the midline echo with generally a single

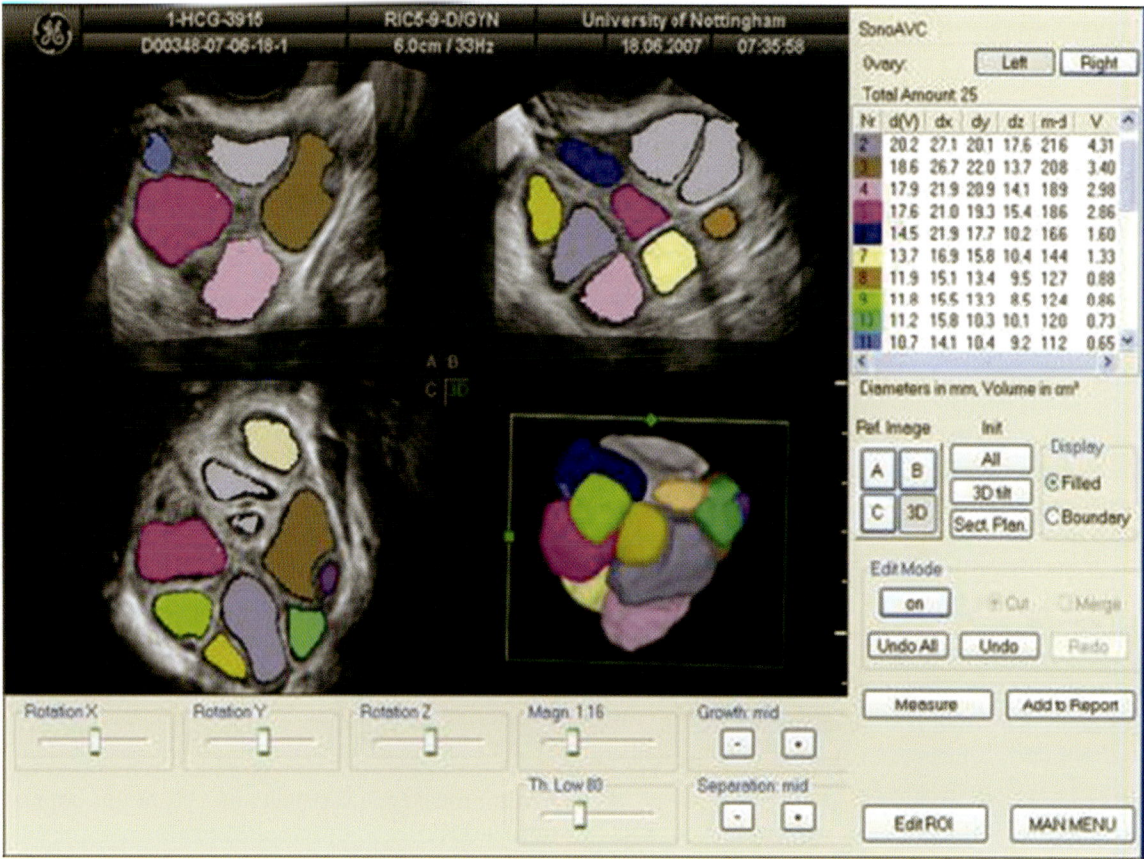

Figure 11.1 SonoAVC of an ovary during controlled ovarian hyperstimulation, with follicles represented by different colours. Use of SonoAVC allows for automated measurement of volume and the average diameter of each follicle on the output seen to the right of the SonoAVC image. It shows the total number of follicles, lists each follicle number and its relaxed sphere diameter (d(V)), three orthogonal diameters (dx, dy and dz), mean diameter of dx, dy and dz (m-d) and follicle volume (V) in millilitres.

feeding blood vessel (Figure 11.2). Scanning early in the cycle may cause confusion as the endometrial cavity may be distended by sloughed cells and blood clots produced during menstrual shedding. Doppler imaging may help to differentiate these structures, with Doppler signal present in polyps and fibroids and absent in the menstrual material (Figure 11.3). Adenomyosis within the myometrium is most clearly visible in the luteal phase of the menstrual cycle due to decidual reaction of the ectopic endometrium. The adenomyotic islands appear hyperechogenic compared to the myometrium and are similar in appearance to the endometrium (Figure 11.4). Hyperechoic and thick endometrium, as seen in the luteal phase, allows for better outline of the endometrial cavity, thus increasing the chances and accuracy of congenital uterine anomaly diagnoses. This is detailed in Chapter 5.

Adnexal lesions, mainly hydrosalpinges, may be present at the pre-treatment scan, and may also develop during controlled ovarian stimulation. A detailed scan of the adnexal region is essential in every gynaecological scan (see Chapter 8), and even more so in the ART setting, as the presence of a distended fallopian tube significantly decreases the chances of success [13]. Ultrasound-guided aspiration of hydrosalpinx may be considered (see Chapter 12); however, salpingectomy offers the best chance of favourable ART outcome [13].

Cycle Monitoring

Ultrasound assessment throughout the natural menstrual cycle or controlled ovarian hyperstimulation (COH) serves the purpose of assessment of follicular maturity and endometrial receptivity [14].

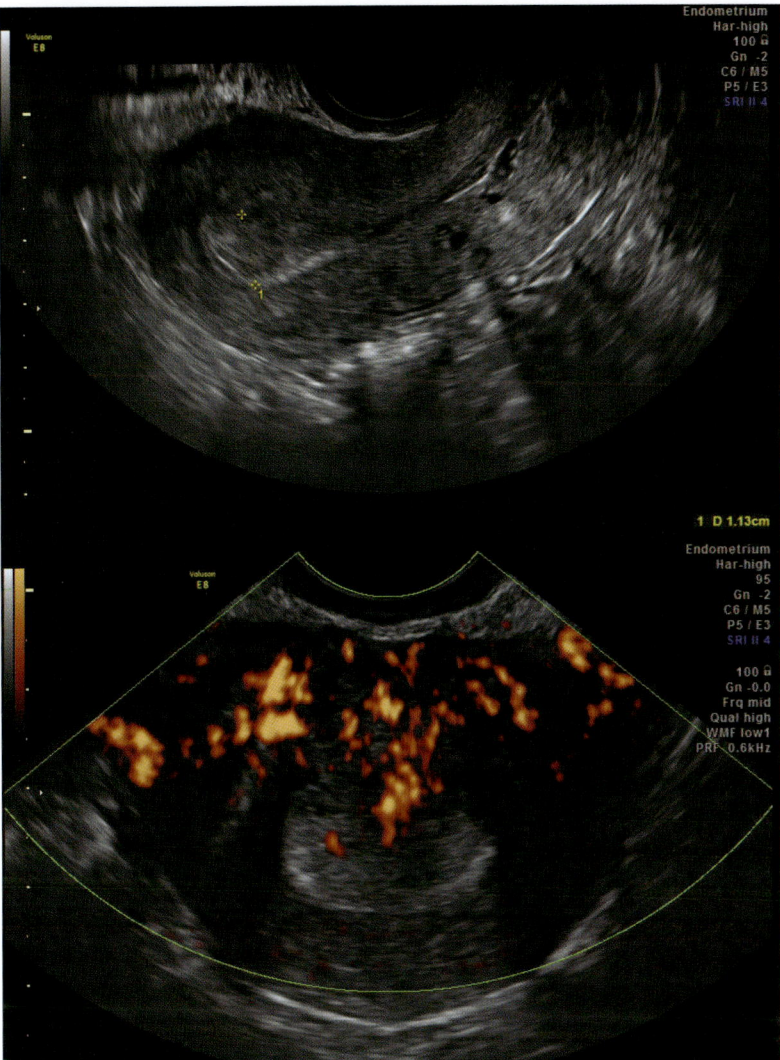

Figure 11.2 Endometrial polyp displacing the midline endometrial echo. Doppler modality demonstrates a single feeding blood vessel.

Endometrial assessment comprises description of the appearance and thickness, as detailed in Chapters 2 and 6. Follicular assessment aims to measure the response to treatment in the form of linear measurements of follicular growth, often combined with measurements of serum estradiol, luteinizing hormone (LH) and progesterone [15].

In a natural menstrual cycle, the follicle grows at a rate of 2 mm per day until approximately 20–25 mm, when ovulation is expected to occur (Figure 11.5) [14]. It is occasionally possible to visualize the *cumulus oophorus* prior to ovulation, represented as an irregularity on the internal wall of the leading follicle. Shortly prior to ovulation, the uniform walls of the follicle loose cohesion and appear blurred on ultrasound scan (Figure 11.6), which is followed by the presence of free fluid in the pouch of Douglas. After ovulation occurs, the follicle undergoes rapid changes and transforms into a *corpus luteum*. Sonographically, the appearance of this structure varies greatly, but most commonly has an irregular, thick-walled structure with heterogeneous content and very intense blood flow on the periphery, as demonstrated by Doppler ultrasound (Figure 11.7) [15]. Rarely, rupture does not occur and the follicle still undergoes luteinization in a rare condition known as luteinized unruptured follicle syndrome (LUFS) (Figure 11.8).

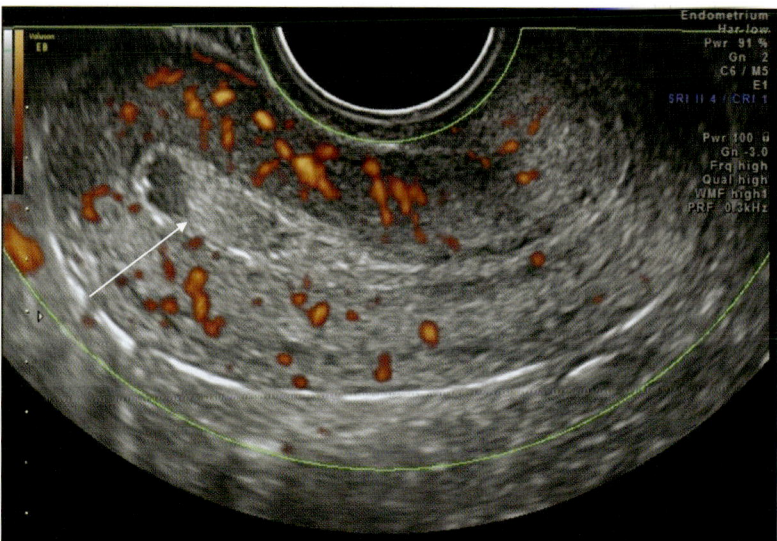

Figure 11.3 Menstrual debris as demonstrated by fluid level (arrow) within the endometrial cavity and no Doppler signal.

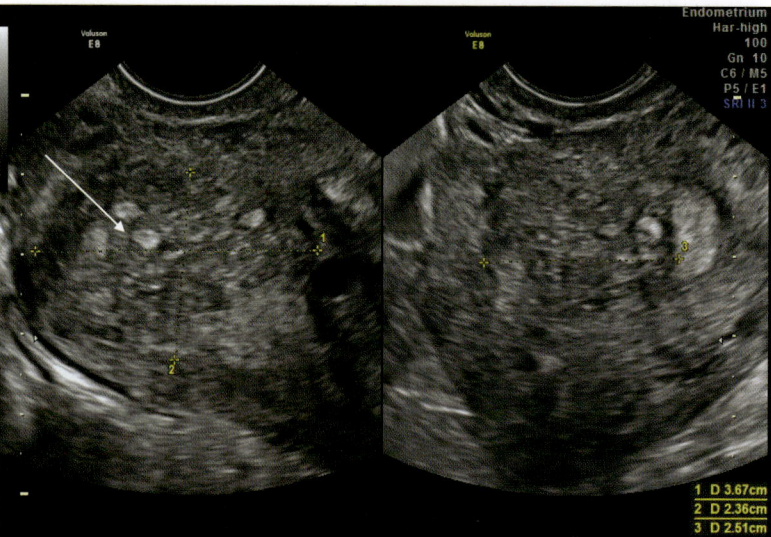

Figure 11.4 Adenomyosis. Hyperechoic islands of ectopic endometrium (arrow) are widespread throughout the bulky uterus.

In the *in vitro* fertilization (IVF) setting, ultrasound scan is used to monitor the ovarian response to gonadotrophins in order to obtain a large number of mature oocytes safely, minimizing the risk of ovarian hyperstimulation syndrome (OHSS) and to time administration of the final oocyte maturation trigger. Most IVF centres aim to achieve at least three follicles measuring 17–18 mm in diameter before the maturation trigger is administered. The likelihood of obtaining a mature oocyte increases with the size and volume of the follicle. An oocyte recovery rate of 83.5 per cent may be achieved when aspirating follicles of 18–20 mm in diameter (equivalent to 3–4 ml of fluid), but a high cleavage rate of 92 per cent may be achieved when oocytes are obtained from follicles measuring 23–24 mm (6–7 ml) [16]. Follicle tracking may be carried out using 2D and 3D ultrasound modalities, with a live or offline analysis. There is no uniform standard recommending follicular diameter measurements [17] with some measuring the single largest diameter and others measuring the mean of two or three diameters obtained from one or two planes, respectively. Automated measurement of

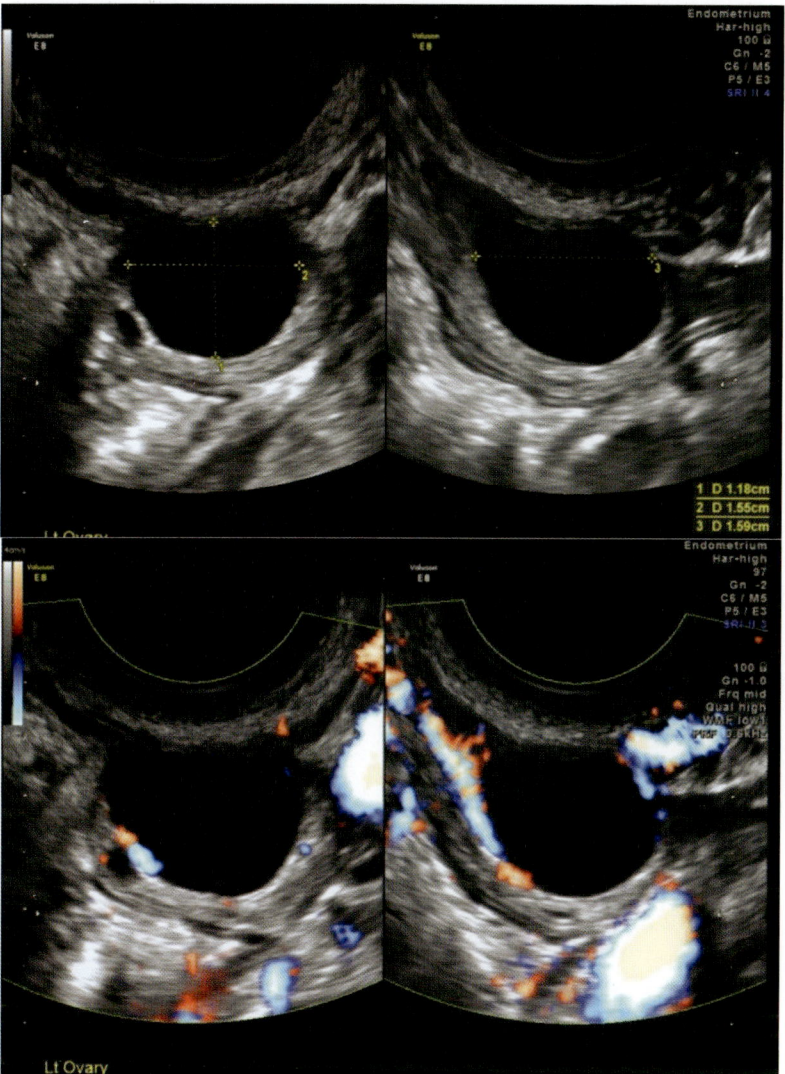

Figure 11.5 Dominant follicle on day 7 of a natural menstrual cycle. Measurements obtained in all three orthogonal planes. Minimal Doppler signal present on the periphery of the follicle.

follicular size using SonoAVC, while speeding up the analysis, does not translate to an improved ART outcome [18] (Figure 11.9). Three-dimensional assessment of follicular size does, however, correlate closely with actual volume of aspirated follicular fluid [19,20] and number of mature oocytes [20,21] (Figure 11.1).

Endometrial assessment forms an integral component of US cycle monitoring as it allows for a minimally invasive and non-disruptive indirect assessment of the organ. In the most basic and commonly used form, the assessment comprises endometrial thickness measurement and description of the pattern (see Chapters 2 and 6). Endometrial

thickness below 7 mm is associated with a low chance of conception [22]; however, pregnancies have been reported with a thickness of 4 mm [23]. A large study of 2896 IVF/intra-cytoplasmic sperm injection (ICSI) cycles by Chen et al., investigating endometrial thickness and pattern on the day of hCG administration, demonstrated that a thin ($\leq$7 mm) and non-triple-layer endometrium was associated with very poor outcomes (clinical pregnancy rate of 14.3 versus 24.4 per cent in women with thin endometrium and a triple-layer appearance; number of patients = 52, $p > 0.05$). In the same study, increasing endometrial thickness was associated with increasing clinical pregnancy rates, with no differences in

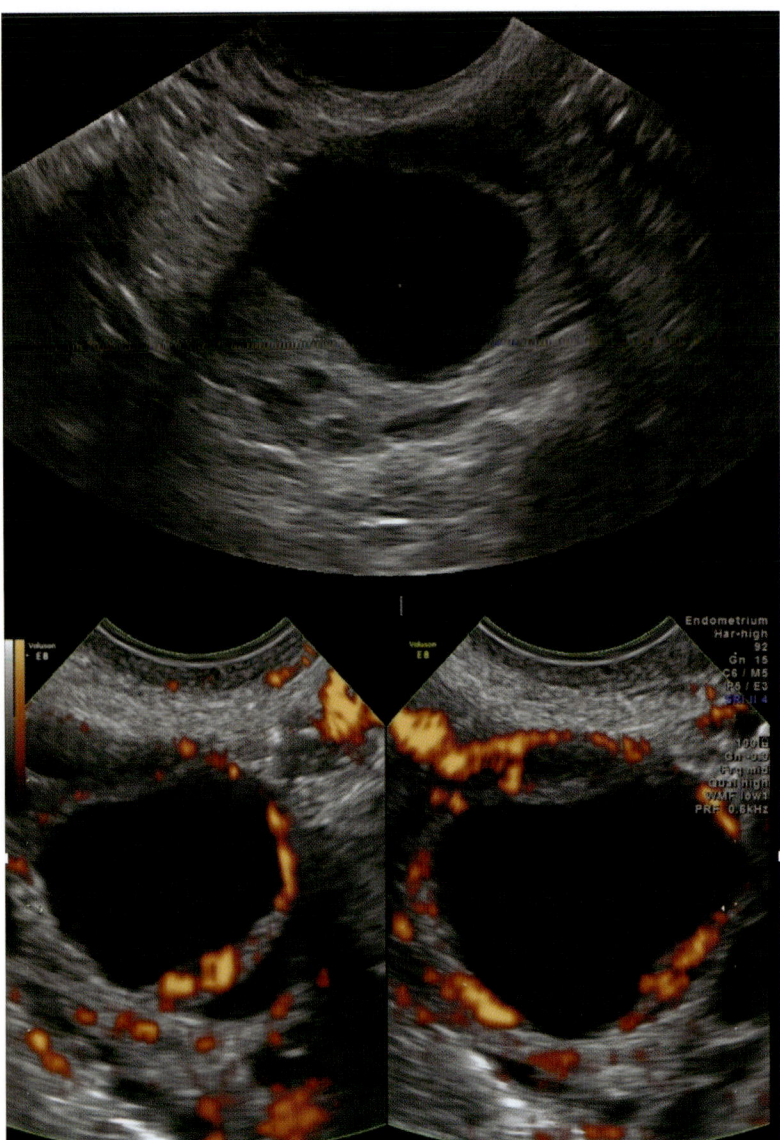

Figure 11.6 Periovulatory follicle with blurred edges and increasing peripheral vascularity.

miscarriage rates. The endometrial pattern did not discriminate between the conception and non-conception cycles; however, miscarriage was much higher in the non-triple-layer appearance of the endometrium (15.6 versus 7.9 per cent; $p < 0.05$) [24]. Similar findings have been reported by other authors [25,26]. It is believed that the premature luteinization of the endometrium, as demonstrated by uniformly hyperechoic appearance with loss of midline echo, may be out of phase with the transferred embryo, and as such, leads to lower implantation rates [27]. In a study by Friedler et al., the authors demonstrated that a homogeneous endometrium on the day of hCG administration has a negative predictive value for conception of 87.5 per cent versus a positive predictive value for conception of 33.1 per cent (specificity 13.7 per cent) for a trilaminar pattern [28].

Studies of endometrial blood flow assessed using 2D colour or power Doppler, or pulse wave Doppler, report discrepant results, with some suggesting low resistance spiral artery waveforms associated with pregnancy [29], and others finding no such correlation [30,31]. The measurement of

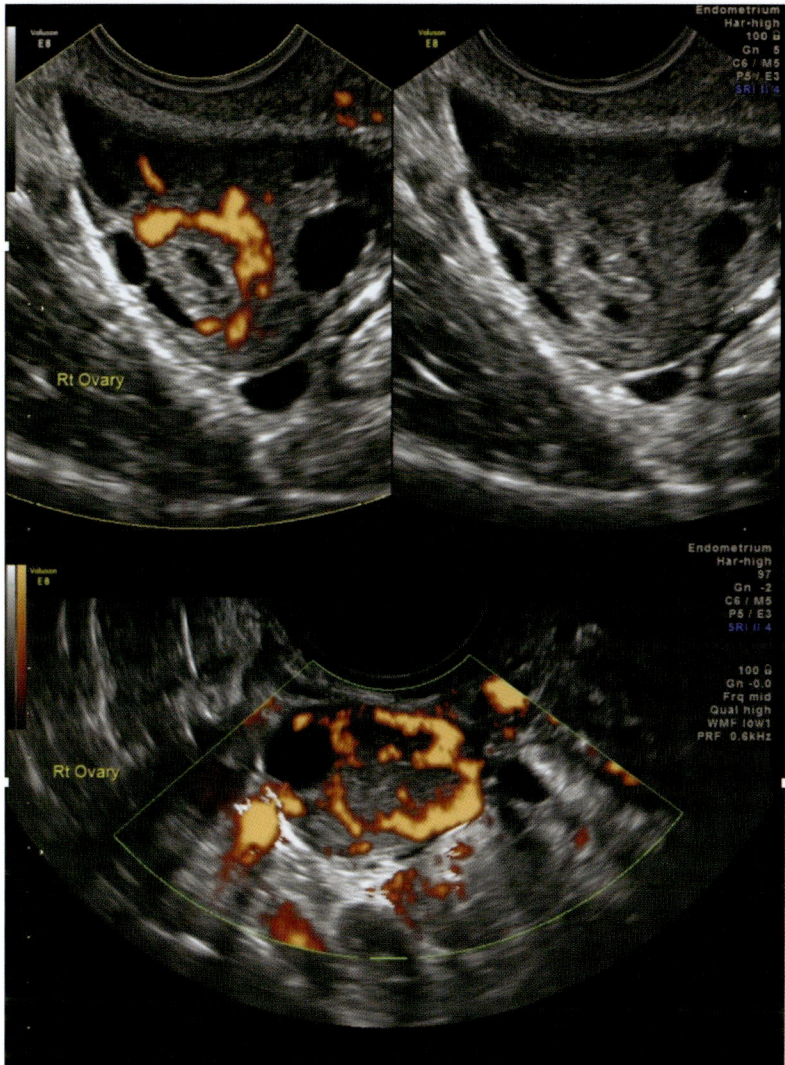

Figure 11.7 Various sonographic appearances of a *corpus luteum*. The single unifying feature is significant vascularity on the periphery, termed the 'ring of fire'.

Doppler indices on endometrial spiral arteries is a difficult and time-consuming process, and is dependent on the distance of the artery from the transducer and the angle of insonation. As such, it is not used in routine clinical practice. Similarly, 3D power Doppler assessment of endometrial and subendometrial vascularity does not clarify the usefulness of this modality as a marker of endometrial receptivity and predictor of ART outcome [32,33]. Finally, endometrial contractions of five or more per minute have been associated with a reduced chance of conception, and can be considered as a potential marker of endometrial receptivity [34,35].

Transvaginal Ultrasound Guided Oocyte Retrieval

Successful oocyte retrieval needs to be fast and precise, aiming to retrieve the maximal number of undamaged oocytes from the ovarian follicles without complications. It is a critical process, as increasing the number of mature oocytes suitable for IVF procedures improves the likelihood of generating good-quality embryos and achieving a successful pregnancy. The evolution and chain of events in the developments in oocyte retrieval techniques (Figure 11.10) have led to increased safety and better pregnancy rates in ART treatment.

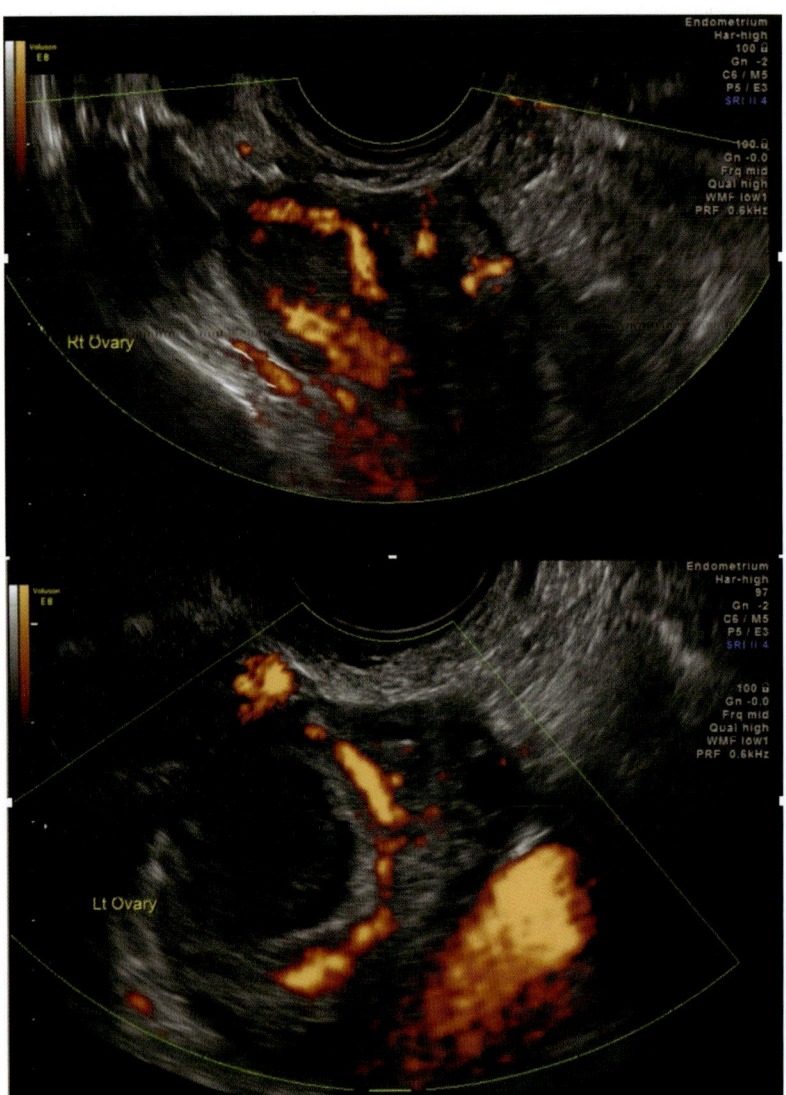

Figure 11.7 (cont.)

Commonly, the final oocyte maturation trigger is administered when ≥3 follicles of ≥17 mm size are documented on ultrasound [36,37]. The trigger can also be given when ≥3 follicles have a diameter of 18 mm [38], or when ≥1 follicle is of ≥18 mm in size and 3 follicles of ≥15 mm [39,40]. Higher pregnancy, implantation and live birth rates were seen in patients when the 17 mm to 10 mm follicle ratio on the day of hCG administration reached 60 per cent and the peak estradiol per oocyte level was within 100–399 pg/ml [41]. Although flexibility in the administration of the oocyte maturation trigger provides convenience for the physician and the patient [42], there is a risk of early progesterone rise causing premature closing of the implantation window [43]. Oocyte retrieval is usually scheduled for 36 hours post-administration of the final oocyte maturation trigger [44], although it could be performed between 32 and 36 hours, with a chance of obtaining mature oocytes reported at 39 hours [45–47].

Appropriate equipment selection, adequate anaesthesia and patient preparation are essential for the procedure to be carried out safely and with optimal results. The transvaginal transducer should be

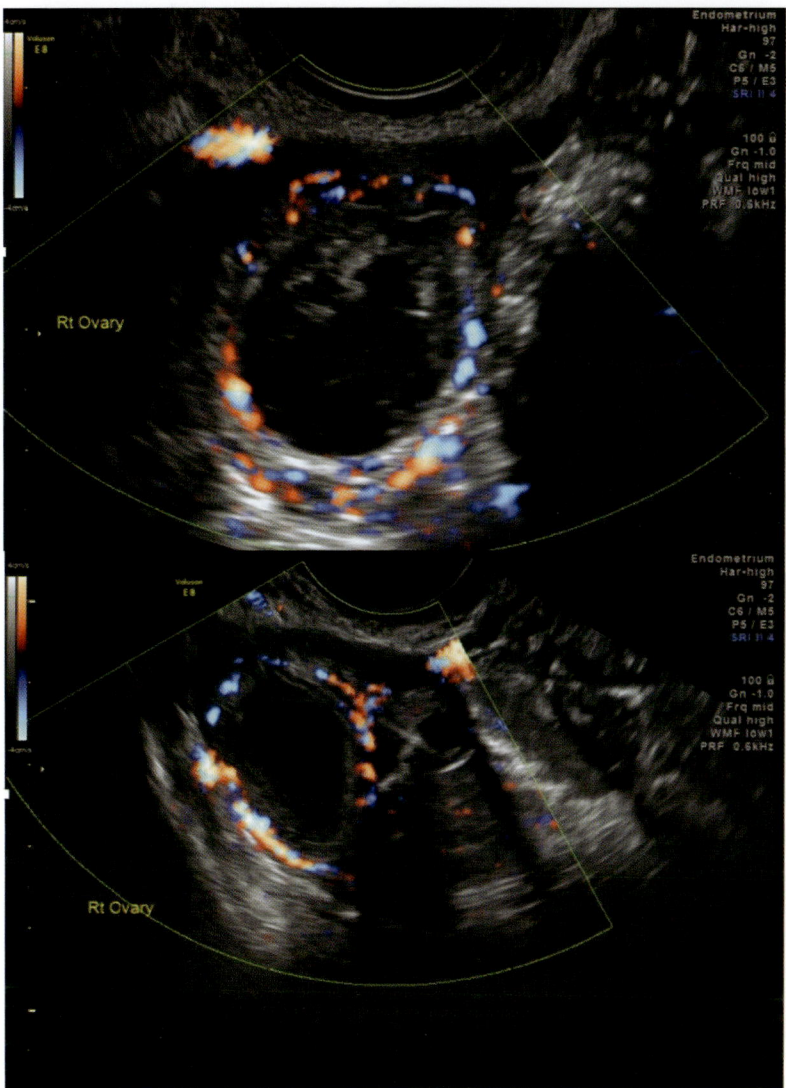

Figure 11.7 (cont.)

covered with a sterile latex-free probe cover with ultrasound gel to assure optimal pelvic organ visualization. A sterile, well-fitting needle guide is attached to the transducer and its patency is tested by passing the oocyte retrieval needle through it before inserting the transducer into the patient. Following introduction of the transducer into the vagina, a scan should be carried out to evaluate the pelvis and the presence of any free fluid, and to assess the ovaries and the uterus (Figure 11.11). At the same time, assessment of the possible entry points is carried out after studying the vaginal wall vascularity by power Doppler and the relationship of the ovary with the neighbouring vessels (Figure 11.12). Rotation of the probe helps to distinguish a uniformly spherical follicle from a vessel that in one plane may be circular but becomes a tubular structure in another plane. Addition of Doppler imaging may also help to differentiate these structures (Figure 11.13); however, Doppler signal may be absent or very weak when the angle between the beam and the blood flow is 90 degrees. When choosing a point of entry of the oocyte collection needle, areas where the bladder (Figure 11.14), bowel, cervix, ureter or other pelvic structures could be inadvertently injured should be avoided. If no obvious point of safe entry can be identified,

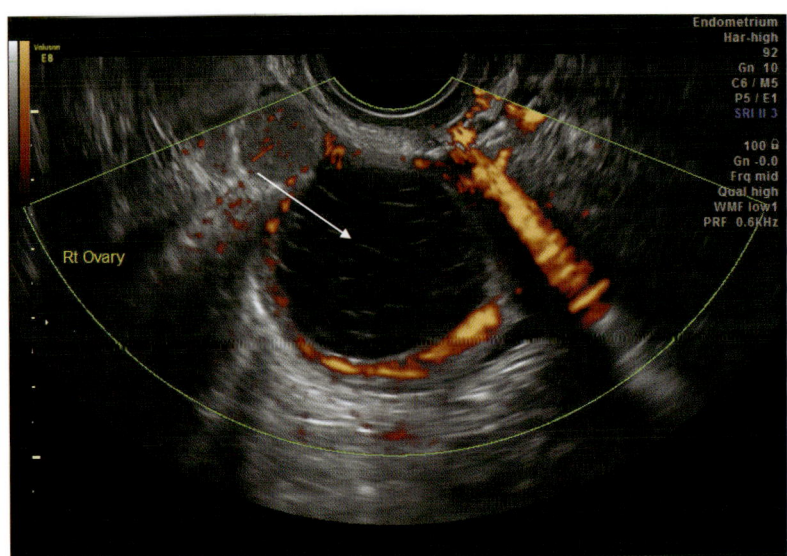

Figure 11.8 Unruptured follicle with haemorrhagic content (spider-web appearance, arrow). The periphery demonstrates significant vascularity indicating luteal transformation.

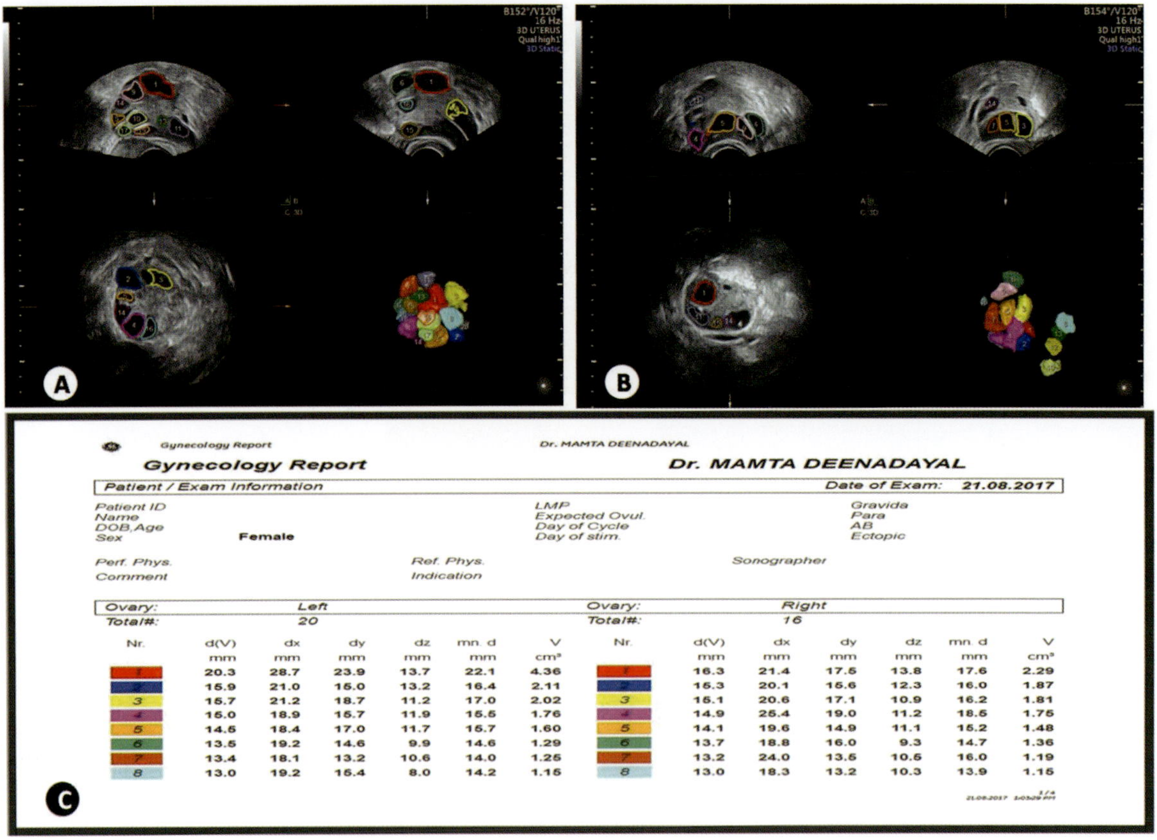

Dr. MAMTA DEENADAYAL

Dr. MAMTA DEENADAYAL

Gynecology Report

Patient / Exam Information		Date of Exam: 21.08.2017
Patient ID	LMP	Gravida
Name	Expected Ovul.	Para
DOB,Age	Day of Cycle	AB
Sex Female	Day of stim.	Ectopic
Perf. Phys.	Ref. Phys.	Sonographer
Comment	Indication	

Ovary:	Left						Ovary:	Right					
Total#:	20						Total#:	16					
Nr.	d(V) mm	dx mm	dy mm	dz mm	mn. d mm	V cm³	Nr.	d(V) mm	dx mm	dy mm	dz mm	mn. d mm	V cm³
1	20.3	28.7	23.9	13.7	22.1	4.36	1	16.3	21.4	17.5	13.8	17.6	2.29
2	15.9	21.0	15.0	13.2	16.4	2.11	2	15.3	20.1	15.6	12.3	16.0	1.87
3	15.7	21.2	18.7	11.2	17.0	2.02	3	15.1	20.6	17.1	10.9	16.2	1.81
4	16.0	18.9	15.7	11.9	15.5	1.76	4	14.9	25.4	19.0	11.2	18.5	1.75
5	14.5	18.4	17.0	11.7	15.7	1.60	5	14.1	19.6	14.9	11.1	15.2	1.48
6	13.5	19.2	14.6	9.9	14.6	1.29	6	13.7	18.8	16.0	9.3	14.7	1.36
7	13.4	18.1	13.2	10.6	14.0	1.25	7	13.2	24.0	13.5	10.5	16.0	1.19
8	13.0	19.2	15.4	8.0	14.2	1.15	8	13.0	18.3	13.2	10.3	15.9	1.15

21.08.2017

Figure 11.9 (a,b) The left and right stimulated ovaries by 3D transvaginal ultrasound (3DTVU) scanning plus SonoAVC software one day before oocyte pickup, showing colour encoded 3D reconstruction of follicles. (c) Detailed SonoAVC report showing measured diameters (dx, dy, dz), automatically calculated mean diameter and volumes, with the colour-coded corresponding follicle.

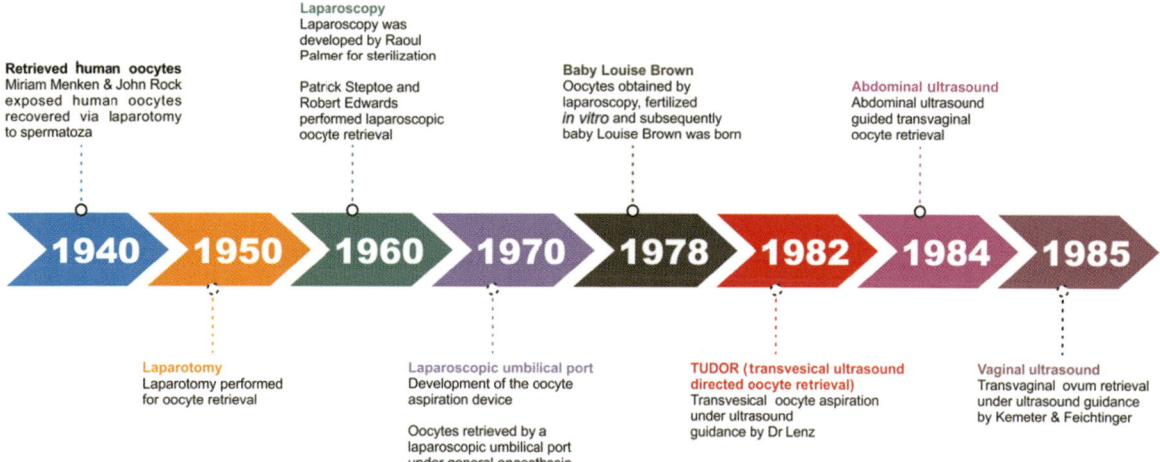

Chain of events in the development of oocyte retrieval techniques

Retrieved human oocytes
Miriam Menken & John Rock exposed human oocytes recovered via laparotomy to spermatozoa

Laparoscopy
Laparoscopy was developed by Raoul Palmer for sterilization

Patrick Steptoe and Robert Edwards performed laparoscopic oocyte retrieval

Baby Louise Brown
Oocytes obtained by laparoscopy, fertilized *in vitro* and subsequently baby Louise Brown was born

Abdominal ultrasound
Abdominal ultrasound guided transvaginal oocyte retrieval

1940 **1950** **1960** **1970** **1978** **1982** **1984** **1985**

Laparotomy
Laparotomy performed for oocyte retrieval

Laparoscopic umbilical port
Development of the oocyte aspiration device

Oocytes retrieved by a laparoscopic umbilical port under general anaesthesia

TUDOR (transvesical ultrasound directed oocyte retrieval)
Transvesical oocyte aspiration under ultrasound guidance by Dr Lenz

Vaginal ultrasound
Transvaginal ovum retrieval under ultrasound guidance by Kemeter & Feichtinger

Figure 11.10 History and evolution of oocyte retrieval techniques.

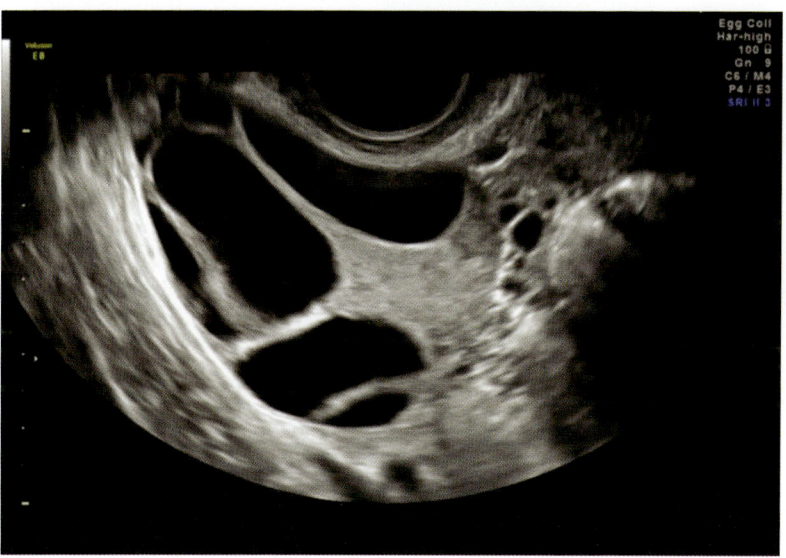

Figure 11.11 Assessment before oocyte collection. Following introduction of the vaginal transducer into the posterior vaginal fornix, both ovaries are visualized in relationship to surrounding structures and the aspiration strategy is planned.

abdominal pressure by the assistant may move structures and create a safe window for passage of the needle (Figure 11.15). When access to the ovary is possible only through the uterus, transuterine puncture is a safe alternative. In this instance, the needle is passed through the myometrium, avoiding the endometrium and uterine vessels [48]. Due to a small increase in miscarriage rates with transuterine oocyte collection, a freeze-all strategy may be applied [49].

Following identification of a safe access point, the ovary should be positioned in the centre of the field of view with the depth and angle of vision set to allow visualization of the entire ovary and parts of the underlying structures. Firm, constant pressure on the probe should be applied throughout the procedure. The needle is then advanced through the vaginal wall and into the follicle, with the needle tip always kept within view in the centre of the follicle (Figure 11.16). Rotating the needle reflects the bevel, allowing

155

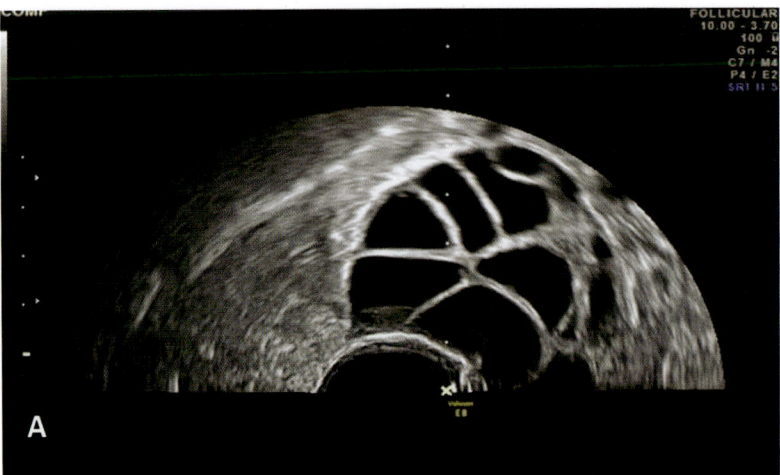

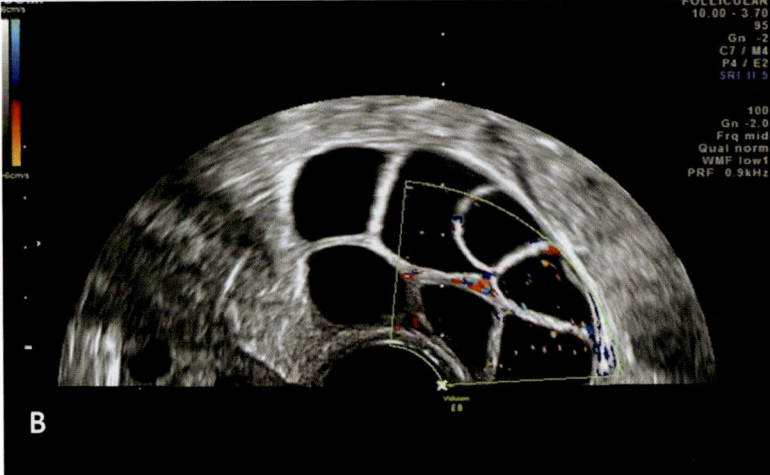

Figure 11.12 After determining the point of entry by greyscale imaging (a), power Doppler imaging (b) is used to evaluate the vascularity at the point of entry.

for better visualization. The aspiration pump should be activated while entering the follicle, with deactivation only when all the possible follicles along the needle line (biopsy guide line) are aspirated, as withdrawing the needle without negative pressure may cause loss of follicular fluid and oocytes. Before moving the probe to focus on the next follicle(s), the needle is withdrawn to the outer edge of the ovary to reduce the risk of ovarian shearing and damage.

Advancement to the next follicle should be carried out systematically, ensuring the needle is in the centre of the follicle and not abutting the follicular wall, as this may impede complete aspiration of the follicular fluid. Rotating the needle assures complete aspiration of the fluid and maximizes the chances of obtaining an oocyte. In the case of large ovaries, aspirating all follicles from a single vaginal puncture may be associated with shearing of the ovarian stroma, resulting

in haemorrhage. In this case, multiple vaginal entries are associated with a higher risk of infection, but lower risk of significant bleeding and injury of pelvic structures [50]. When all follicles have been aspirated, the needle is withdrawn and flushed with the culture medium, followed by a quick scan to assess presence of free fluid in the pouch of Douglas, which might indicate haemorrhage and helps to monitor its progress (Figure 11.17).

In cases of Mullerian agenesis, intra-abdominal adhesions distorting the anatomy, prophylactic ovarian transposition prior to radiotherapy or enlarged uterus displacing the ovaries cephalad, when transvaginal access is not possible, transabdominal ultrasound-guided oocyte retrieval is carried out in preference to laparoscopic procedures, with a combination of transvaginal and transabdominal procedures as an option (Figure 11.18). The same safe

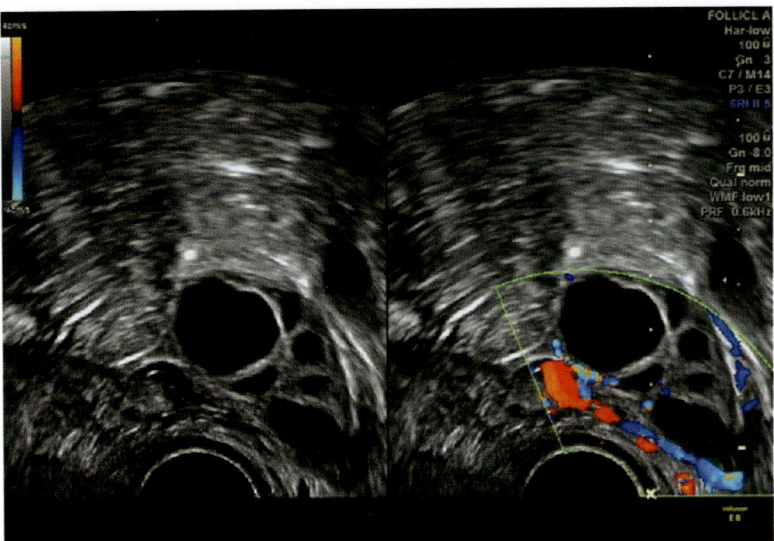

Figure 11.13 Colour Doppler imaging may be used to study the relationship of the vascularity around the ovary to assess the point of entry.

sonographic principles are followed when these procedures are carried out.

Embryo Transfer

Embryo transfer constitutes a crucial step of IVF, in which embryos are replaced into the adequately prepared endometrial cavity. Two ways of carrying out the procedure exist: the clinical touch or the ultrasound-guided technique. The ultrasound-guided method has been associated with significantly improved outcomes of ART compared to the clinical touch technique, and as such is the recommended method of embryo transfer [51]. Transabdominal imaging is used for this procedure, with a moderately filled bladder to aid visualization of the uterus. Too full a bladder causes discomfort and should be discouraged. The endometrial cavity is visualized in the longitudinal section in its entirety, starting with the cervical canal. Speculum blades may obscure the external cervical os at this stage, but introduction of the embryo transfer catheter allows for adjusting the view appropriately (Figure 11.19). Minimal manipulation of the US transducer while introducing the catheter into the endometrial cavity allows for real-time visualization of the catheter tip. Echo-dense catheter tips or air bubbles within the catheter allow for clear visualization on ultrasound scan. Maternal high body mass index (BMI) or axial or retroverted uterus may prevent obtaining adequate views. Emptying the bladder in the latter cases may provide some image quality improvement.

The fluid containing the embryos is secured between two air bubbles, which once injected into the endometrium are evident on ultrasound scan as hyperechoic specks (Figure 11.20). Ultrasound guidance also prevents the tip from reaching the top of the endometrial cavity, which may cause discomfort and may induce endometrial contractions associated with reduced chances of successful treatment outcome [52]. Randomized controlled studies have been carried out in order to assess the most favourable place to deposit the embryos, with no clear conclusions. Higher pregnancy rates were observed by Coroleu et al. when the embryos were replaced 1.5–2 cm away from the fundus [53]. Other studies have called this finding into question, with no difference in pregnancy rates when embryos were replaced in the upper or lower half of the endometrial cavity [54].

Anatomical distortions of the uterus with an acute angle between the cervix and body of the uterus may pose problems with embryo transfer and, as such, contribute to treatment failure. Some authors suggest measuring the angle between the cervix and uterus before embryo transfer and moulding the malleable catheter to match the version. This approach has been associated with higher pregnancy rates and lower rates of difficult or bloody transfers when compared to the blind clinical touch technique [55].

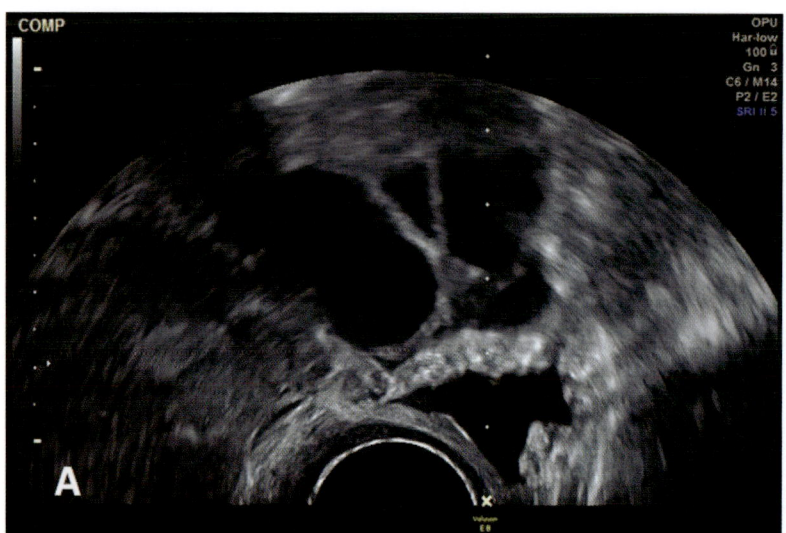

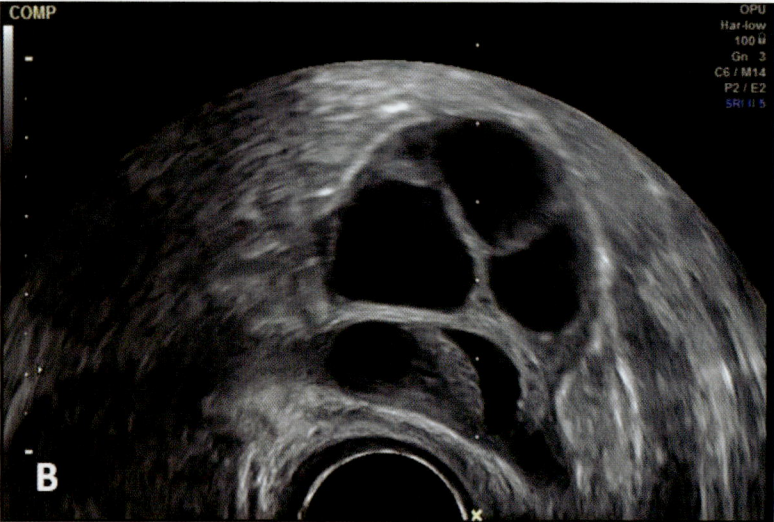

Figure 11.14 (a) The intervening bladder between the vaginal wall and the follicle to be aspirated. On further exploration an area free of the bladder without intervening structure is used as the point of entry (b) (the dotted line indicates the intended tract of the needle – the needle guide).

As a predictor of successful treatment, ultrasound guidance while carrying out embryo transfer may be a poor marker; however, the advantages of the procedure justify its routine use. Direct visualization of the embryos reaching the endometrial cavity provides a strong positive visual cue and reassurance for the couple undergoing the treatment, as well as for the clinician that the embryo transfer was carried out successfully. Incidental findings of endometrial polyps of fluid within the endometrial cavity, which may have arisen since the oocyte retrieval, may lead to a decision to abandon the cycle and freeze embryos in order to maximize chances of conception; similarly, assessment of risk of OHSS just prior to the embryo transfer may prevent the condition from worsening if implantation were to occur. Additionally, scanning during embryo transfer provides a training opportunity for health professionals.

Monitoring of Outcome and Complication

Ultrasound scans are used to monitor the outcome of ART, as well as any possible complications that might have arisen. It is customary to carry out an early viability scan at 6–8 weeks' gestation to ensure the presence of a clinical pregnancy, confirm the number of foetuses and exclude an ectopic gestation. These scans are carried out in a standard fashion, as described in Chapter 14.

Table 11.1 Complications of oocyte retrieval

Common complications
1. Ovarian hyperstimulation syndrome (OHSS)
2. Pain
3. Vaginal bleeding
4. Haemoperitoneum
5. Pelvic infection

Rare complications
Massive retroperitoneal bleeding
Ovarian abscess
Uro-retroperitoneum
Vertebral osteomyelitis
Urethral injury
Ureterovaginal fistula
Bowel injury
Ruptured dermoid
Infected dermoid
Ruptured endometrium
Perforated appendix
Adnexal torsion
Ovarian necrotizing vasculitis

Possible complications directly related to ART include intra-abdominal haemorrhage, infection, OHSS, and others as detailed in Table 11.1. Ovarian hyperstimulation syndrome is a potentially fatal iatrogenic complication of COH related to ovarian enlargement with systemic increase in vascular permeability. The condition can occur following any form of ovarian stimulation, including clomiphene citrate and gonadotrophins, with the latter being responsible for the majority of cases. Spontaneous, unrelated to ovulation induction OHSS has been reported, but is a very rare event [56].

The reported incidence of OHSS is 2–10 per cent of IVF cycles, with the milder forms possibly occurring in up to 23 per cent of cycles [57]. Due to varying classification systems and potential underreporting, the actual prevalence of the condition may be much higher [56]. Ovarian hyperstimulation syndrome can be divided into early and late onset, and mild, moderate, severe and critical. Ultrasound is used to help classify the severity of the condition as an aid, as mainly the clinical picture should lead the investigations and subsequent management. A recent OHSS classification combines the ultrasound findings, clinical signs and symptoms and laboratory investigations [56,58,59]. The resolution of symptoms of OHSS is expected by the sixth week of gestation. Mild OHSS is associated with mild clinical symptoms of abdominal distension,

associated discomfort and nausea. Ultrasound assessment demonstrates mildly enlarged ovaries (<8 cm) with no ascites (Figure 11.21). The critical form is associated with respiratory distress, tense ascites, renal failure and venous thrombo-embolic events. Marked leucocytosis (>25 000/ml), ovarian size >12 cm, hydrothorax and ascites are common features. Table 11.2 contains a description of each of the forms of OHSS, with a focus on ultrasound findings.

Intra-abdominal haemorrhage following oocyte recovery has been reported in 0–0.35 per cent of cycles. This complication is related to direct injury to the ovary, bleeding from the ruptured follicle or injury to pelvic vessels [60]. Pre-existing coagulation disorders, inherited or iatrogenic, increase the risk of these types of complications.

While carrying out oocyte retrieval, careful visualization of the follicle and neighbouring iliac vessels with application of power Doppler (if in doubt as to the nature of the structure) allows for unequivocal identification of follicles and avoidance of puncturing the iliac, ovarian or uterine blood vessels. For monitoring intra-abdominal haemorrhagic complications, abdominal ultrasound should be sufficient to identify free fluid in the abdomen (Figure 11.22); however, organized blood collections or retroperitoneal haematomas might not be immediately visible on transabdominal or transvaginal scans, and may necessitate employment of computed tomography (CT). In contrast to ascites, blood will appear as particulate fluid, with particles moving freely when agitated by gentle pressure on the ultrasound transducer. Pus may have a similar sonographic appearance, but the clinical picture (pyrexia, tachycardia, raised inflammatory markers and stable haemoglobin levels) should suffice to differentiate between haemorrhagic and septic complications on scan.

Visceral injury (mainly bowel), though rare, occurring in 0–1.3 per cent of women following oocyte retrieval procedures [56], may lead to significant morbidity. Ultrasound is rarely employed in these cases as this modality does not lend itself well to direct visualization of bowel injury. Erect chest x-ray may identify free air under the diaphragm and point towards the diagnosis. CT imaging would be the modality of choice for diagnosis and identification of the level of injury.

159

Table 11.2 Leuven University Fertility Centre classification system of OHSS

Grade of OHSS	Symptoms
Mild OHSS	Mild abdominal bloating and pain No weight gain Ovarian size <8 cm
Moderate OHSS	Moderate abdominal pain controlled with rest and simple analgesia Nausea Weight gain up to 1 kg Ultrasound evidence of ascites (deepest pool <3 cm) Ovarian size 8–10 cm
Severe OHSS	Uncontrolled abdominal pain Weight gain >1 kg Clinical ascites (with occasional hydrothorax) Oliguria Haematocrit >45 per cent Ultrasound evidence of significant ascites (deepest pool >3 cm in the upper abdomen; e.g. right upper quadrant) Ovarian size >10 cm
Critical OHSS	Tense ascites or large hydrothorax Haematocrit >55 per cent White cell count >25 000/ml Oligo/anuria Venous-thromboembolic events Adult respiratory distress syndrome

Source: adapted from [56].

Ultrasound of the Testes

Occasionally, ultrasound is used when evaluating the male partner prior to fertility treatment. Irregularities found on clinical examination, suggestion of a hydrocele or varicocele form an indication for sonographic assessment of the testicle.

Supine position is usually used for this procedure, with scrotal support if required. Linear array transducers with scan frequency range 7–10 MHz are used in order to provide optimal views. The testicles should be screened in their entirety, with measurements recorded of all three dimensions. The textures and dimensions are compared between sides. A Valsalva manoeuvre or an upright position is required to assess the venous blood flow characteristics to the testicle [61].

Application of Doppler imaging may differentiate between obstructive and non-obstructive causes of azoospermia, with testicular vasculature usually intact in the former case and absent or significantly reduced in the latter case [62]. When considering surgical sperm retrieval, some authors suggest targeting areas with visible Doppler perfusion, as biopsies from vascular regions were more likely to produce viable spermatozoa [63]. In the case of suspected varicocele, ultrasound reveals multiple, dilated, tortuous tubular structures, mainly located superior and to the side of the testicle. In extremis, dilated vessels may occupy the space posteriorly and inferiorly to the affected testicle. Doppler assessment optimized for low-velocity blood flow demonstrates venous flow pattern with retrograde flow and phasic variation, with best demonstration of these findings during a Valsalva manoeuvre [61]; additionally, decreased blood flow within the testicular artery may be present [62,64].

Conclusion

Ultrasound has become an essential component of ART. It aids in the identification of the cause of infertility, and it is used for monitoring the response to COH and recording the outcomes of treatment. Its use allows for safe oocyte retrieval and provides reassurance to couples when 'seeing' their embryos being safely deposited in the endometrial cavity. No modern IVF unit will be able to carry out any procedures without access to ultrasound, as patients' expectations are high and safety demands its utilization at every step of the COH process.

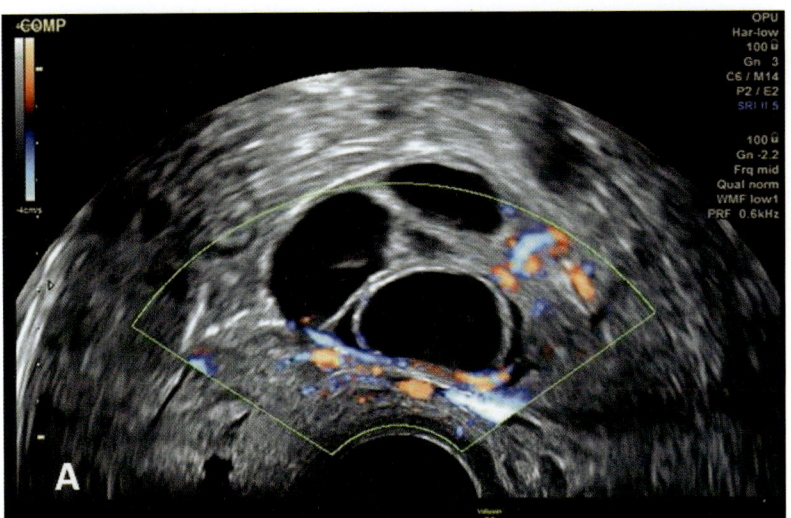

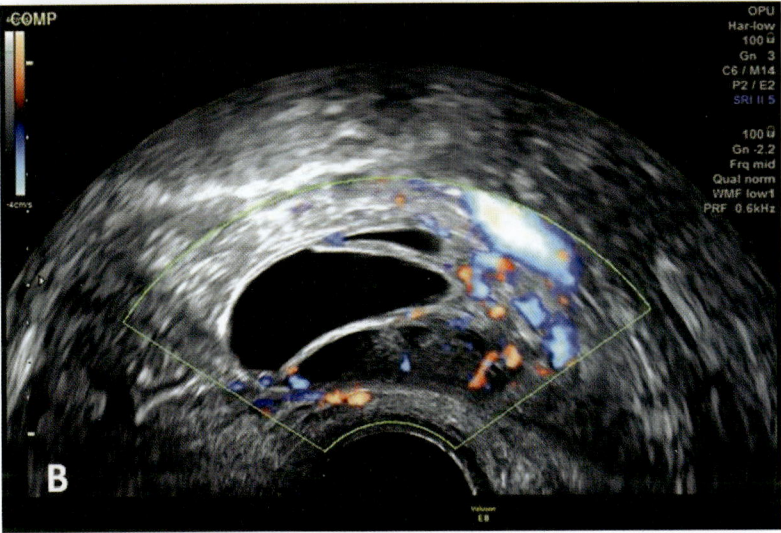

Figure 11.15 (a) Infundibulo-pelvic vessels interposed between the vaginal wall and ovary. (b) After external abdominal manipulation, an area for safe needle entry was achieved.

Tips and Tricks

- For AFC measurement, obtain the best-quality image of the ovary in every plane.
- In order to maximize the reliability of AFC as a predictive marker for ART outcome, aim to carry out the scan between days 2 and 4 of a spontaneous or oral contraceptive menstrual cycle.
- Only include follicles measuring 2–10 mm when assessing AFC.
- Follicle tracking may be carried out live with 2D scanning, measuring the diameters of each follicle, or with 3D scanning used offline. Both methods provide adequate clinical information as to the timing of administration of the final oocyte maturation trigger.

- A good-quality ultrasound machine with a high-frequency vaginal and abdominal transducer, with a needle guide for both, is essential for safe oocyte retrieval.
- Power Doppler helps to identify the vasculature in the pelvis and in combination with rotation of the transducer avoids inadvertent vessel puncture.
- Harmonics (ultrasound machine setting) may be used to improve image quality, especially in cases with hazy ovaries.
- Recording videos of oocyte retrieval or embryo transfer can help to review a particular case in the future and may serve as educational material.
- Abdominal pressure by an assistant may help to mobilize a high ovary into the pelvis and helps to fix it in place for the duration of the oocyte pickup.

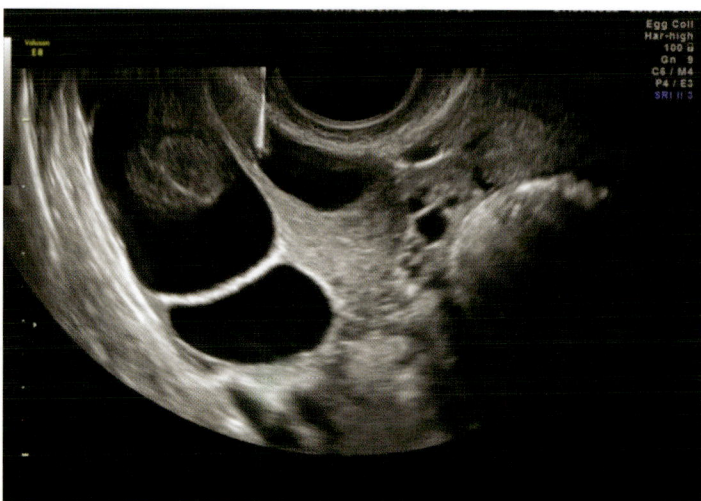

Figure 11.16 The serrated end of the needle is clearly visible within the follicle and must always be maintained in direct view.

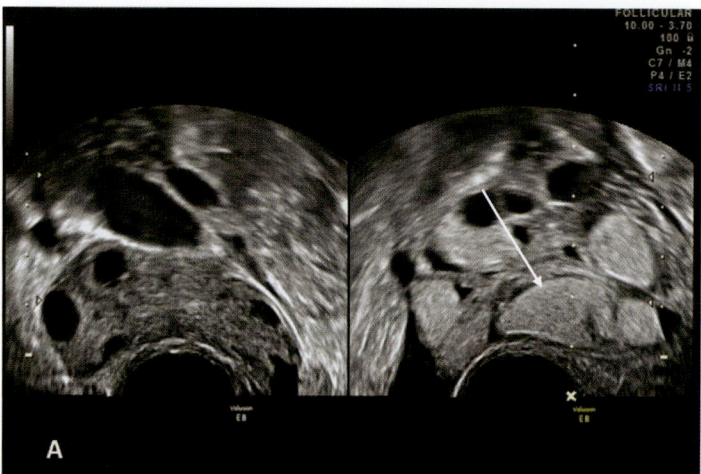

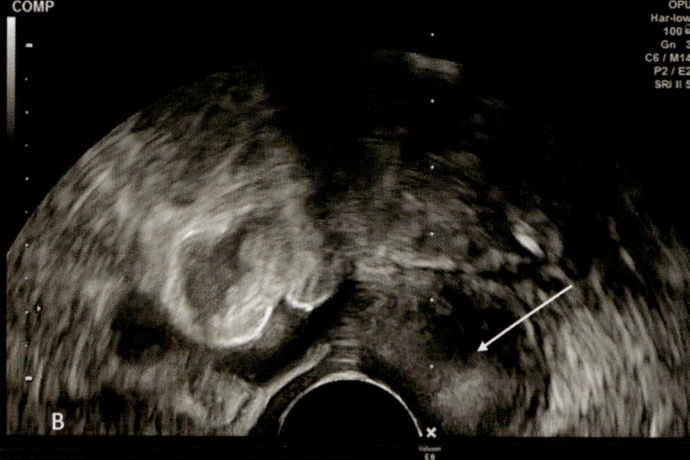

Figure 11.17 (a) Ultrasound image of right and left ovaries immediately post-oocyte retrieval showing intra-follicular haemorrhage (arrow). (b) Post-oocyte collection image showing free fluid in the pouch of Douglas (arrow) which should be measured and recorded.

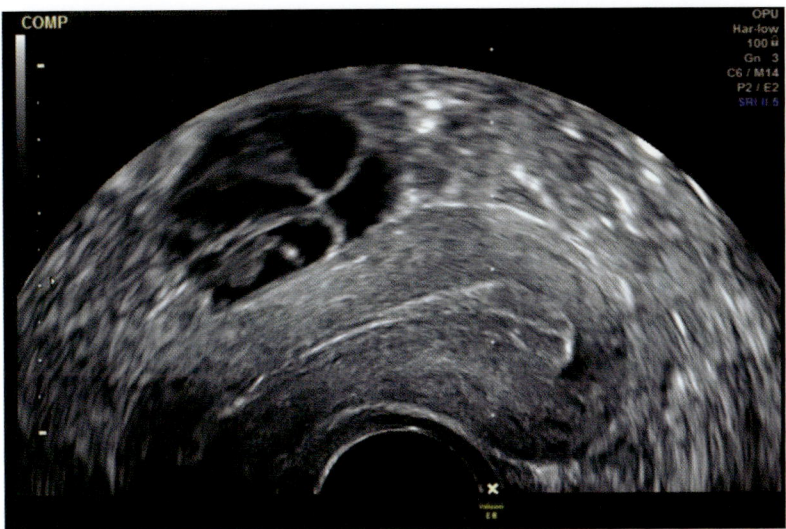

Figure 11.18 Image showing the ovary displaced behind the uterus, inaccessible for transvaginal oocyte retrieval. After transvaginal pickup on one side, transabdominal oocyte collection was performed for this ovary.

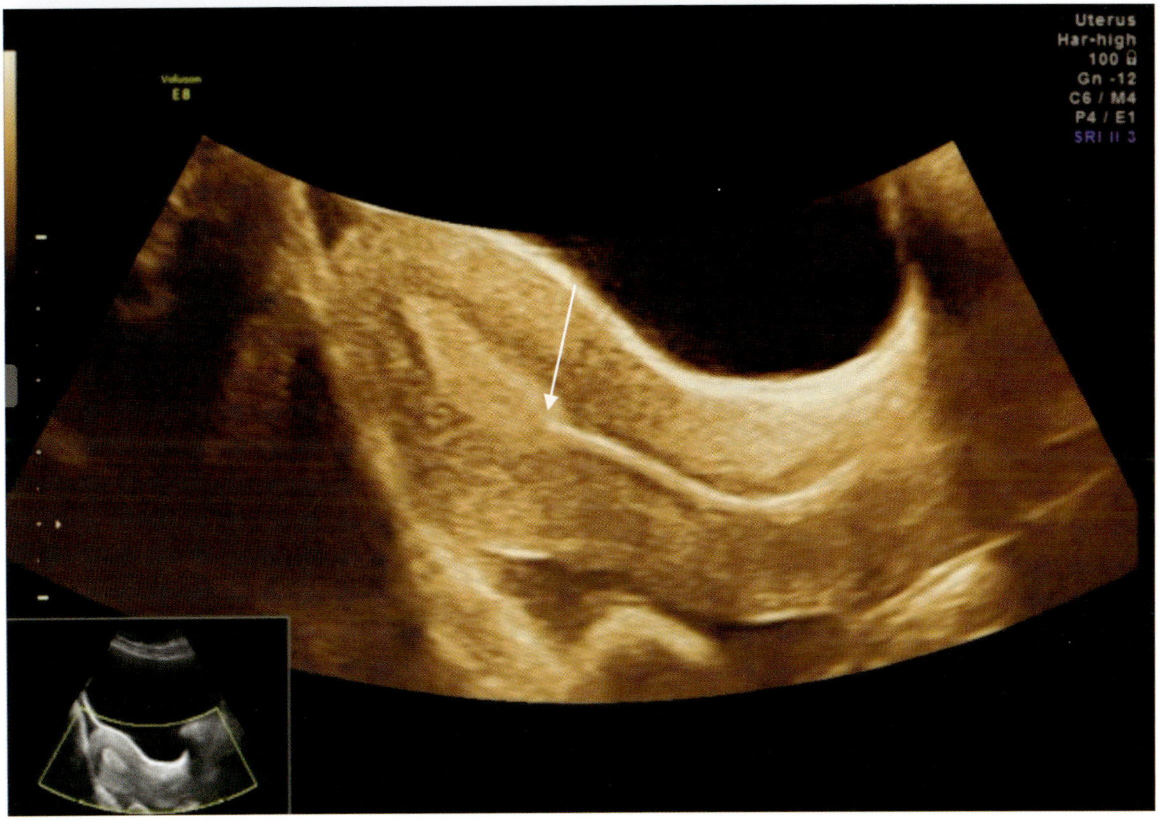

Figure 11.19 Transabdominal US scan at the time of embryo transfer. The uterus is visualized in its entirety in a sagittal section, with the distal end of the embryo transfer catheter (arrow) visible just past the internal os.

- The needle tip must be in constant view throughout the oocyte retrieval process.
- After all the follicles have been aspirated, a scan of the pelvis should be carried out to document any free fluid and check the vaginal vault for bleeding.
- If the transuterine route to access the ovary is the only option, the endometrium should be avoided.

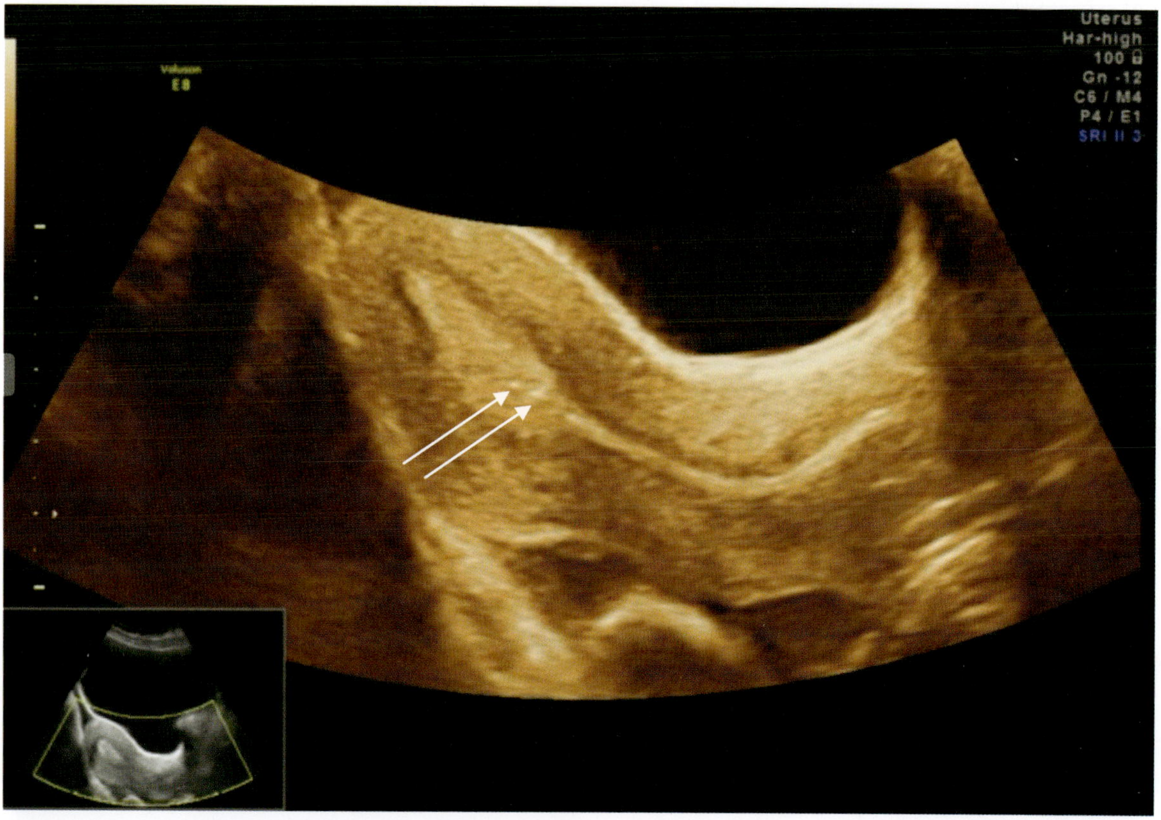

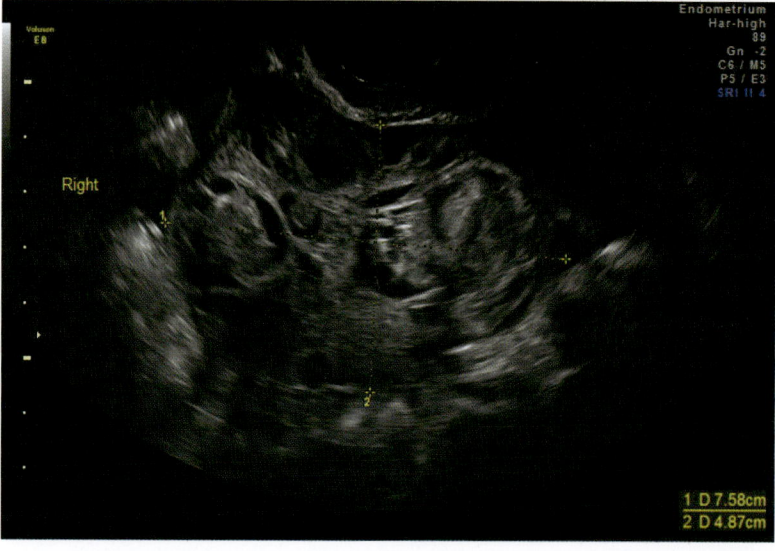

Figure 11.20 Two air bubbles (arrows) indicate a successful embryo replacement.

Figure 11.21 Enlarged ovary post-oocyte collection in a woman who developed mild OHSS. No gross ascites is visible and the largest diameter of the ovary is below 8 cm.

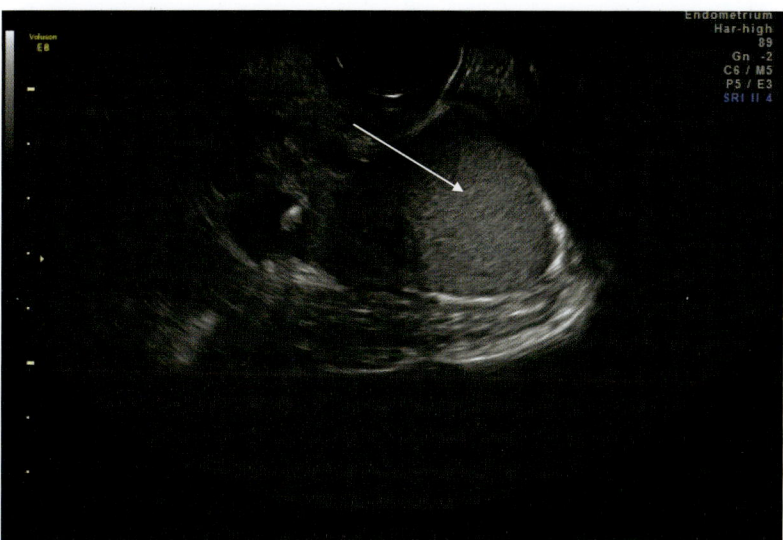

Figure 11.22 Particulate free fluid (arrow) adjacent to the ovary following oocyte collection. This is a haemorrhagic complication of the procedure.

• A moderately filled bladder allows for good visualization of the endometrium at embryo transfer. An empty bladder may improve vision in cases of retroverted and axial uteri.

References

1. Klemetti R, Gissler M, Hemminki E. Comparison of perinatal health of children born from IVF in Finland in the early and late 1990s. *Hum Reprod* 2002;**17**(8):2192–8.

2. Williams C, Sutcliffe A. Infant outcomes of assisted reproduction. *Early Hum Dev* 2009;**85**(11):673–7.

3. Fleming R, Seifer DB, Frattarelli JL, Ruman J. Assessing ovarian response: antral follicle count versus anti-Mullerian hormone. *Reprod Biomed Online* 2015;**31**(4):486–96.

4. Broekmans FJ, de Ziegler D, Howles CM, et al. The antral follicle count: practical recommendations for better standardization. *Fertil Steril* 2010;**94**(3):1044–51.

5. Chang MY, Chiang CH, Chiu TH, Hsieh TT, Soong YK. The antral follicle count predicts the outcome of pregnancy in a controlled ovarian hyperstimulation/intrauterine insemination program. *J Assist Reprod Genet* 1998;**15**(1):12–17.

6. Chang MY, Chiang CH, Hsieh TT, Soong YK, Hsu KH. Use of the antral follicle count to predict the outcome of assisted reproductive technologies. *Fertil Steril* 1998;**69**:505–10.

7. Deb S, Campbell BK, Clewes JS, Pincott-Allen C, Raine-Fenning NJ. Intracycle variation in number of antral follicles stratified by size and in endocrine markers of ovarian reserve in women with normal ovulatory menstrual cycles. *Ultrasound Obstet Gynecol* 2013;**41**(2):216–22.

8. Bauman D. Diagnostic methods in pediatric and adolescent gynecology. *Endocr Dev* 2012;**22**:40–55.

9. Broekmans FJ, Kwee J, Hendriks DJ, Mol BW, Lambalk CB. A systematic review of tests predicting ovarian reserve and IVF outcome. *Hum Reprod Update* 2006;**12**(6):685–718.

10. Broer SL, Mol BW, Hendriks D, Broekmans FJ. The role of antimullerian hormone in prediction of outcome after IVF: comparison with the antral follicle count. *Fertil Steril* 2009;**91**(3):705–14.

11. La Marca A, Sighinolfi G, Radi D, et al. Anti-Mullerian hormone (AMH) as a predictive marker in assisted reproductive technology (ART). *Hum Reprod Update* 2010;**16**(2):113–30.

12. Iliodromiti S, Anderson RA, Nelson SM. Technical and performance characteristics of anti-Mullerian hormone and antral follicle count as biomarkers of ovarian response. *Hum Reprod Update* 2015;**21**(6):698–710.

13. Strandell A, Lindhard A, Waldenstrom U, et al. Hydrosalpinx and IVF outcome: a prospective, randomized multicentre trial in Scandinavia on salpingectomy prior to IVF. *Hum Reprod* 1999;**14**(11):2762–9.

14. Penzias AS, Emmi AM, Dubey AK, et al. Ultrasound prediction of follicle volume: is the mean diameter reflective? *Fertil Steril* 1994;**62**(6):1274–6.

15. Jayaprakasan K, Deb S, Sur S, et al. Ultrasound and its role in assisted reproduction treatment. *Imaging Med* 2010;**2**(2):135–50.

16. Wittmaack FM, Kreger DO, Blasco L, et al. Effect of follicular size on oocyte retrieval, fertilization, cleavage, and embryo quality in in vitro fertilization cycles: a 6-year data collection. *Fertil Steril* 1994;**62**(6):1205–10.

17. Raine-Fenning N. Doppler assessment of uterine artery blood flow for the prediction of pregnancy after assisted reproduction treatment. *Ultrasound Obstet Gynecol* 2008;**31**(4):371–5.

18. Raine-Fenning N, Deb S, Jayaprakasan K, et al. Timing of oocyte maturation and egg collection during controlled ovarian stimulation: a randomized controlled trial evaluating manual and automated measurements of follicle diameter. *Fertil Steril* 2010;**94**(1):184–8.

19. Raine-Fenning N, Jayaprakasan K, Clewes J, et al. SonoAVC: a novel method of automatic volume calculation. *Ultrasound Obstet Gynecol* 2008;**31**(6):691–6.

20. Rodriguez-Fuentes A, Hernandez J, Garcia-Guzman R, et al. Prospective evaluation of automated follicle monitoring in 58 in vitro fertilization cycles: follicular volume as a new indicator of oocyte maturity. *Fertil Steril* 2010;**93**(2):616–20.

21. Shmorgun D, Hughes E, Mohide P, Roberts R. Prospective cohort study of three- versus two-dimensional ultrasound for prediction of oocyte maturity. *Fertil Steril* 2010;**93**(4):1333–7.

22. Oliveira JB, Baruffi RL, Mauri AL, et al. Endometrial ultrasonography as a predictor of pregnancy in an in-vitro fertilization programme after ovarian stimulation and gonadotrophin-releasing hormone and gonadotrophins. *Hum Reprod* 1997;**12**(11):2515–18.

23. Sundstrom P. Establishment of a successful pregnancy following in-vitro fertilization with an endometrial thickness of no more than 4 mm. *Hum Reprod* 1998;**13**(6):1550–2.

24. Chen SL, Wu FR, Luo C, et al. Combined analysis of endometrial thickness and pattern in predicting outcome of in vitro fertilization and embryo transfer: a retrospective cohort study. *Reprod Biol Endocrinol* 2010;**8**:30.

25. Killick SR. Ultrasound and the receptivity of the endometrium. *Reprod Biomed Online* 2007;**15**(1):63–7.

26. Fanchin R, Righini C, Ayoubi JM, et al. New look at endometrial echogenicity: objective computer-assisted measurements predict endometrial receptivity in in vitro fertilization-embryo transfer. *Fertil Steril* 2000;**74**(2):274–81.

27. Bosch E, Valencia I, Escudero E, et al. Premature luteinization during gonadotropin-releasing hormone antagonist cycles and its relationship with in vitro fertilization outcome. *Fertil Steril* 2003;**80**(6):1444–9.

28. Friedler S, Schenker JG, Herman A, Lewin A. The role of ultrasonography in the evaluation of endometrial receptivity following assisted reproductive treatments: a critical review. *Hum Reprod Update* 1996;**2**(4):323–35.

29. Kupesic S, Bekavac I, Bjelos D, Kurjak A. Assessment of endometrial receptivity by transvaginal color Doppler and three-dimensional power Doppler ultrasonography in patients undergoing in vitro fertilization procedures. *J Ultrasound Med* 2001;**20**(2):125–34.

30. Jinno M, Ozaki T, Iwashita M, et al. Measurement of endometrial tissue blood flow: a novel way to assess uterine receptivity for implantation. *Fertil Steril* 2001;**76**(6):1168–74.

31. Zaidi J, Campbell S, Pittrof R, Tan SL. Endometrial thickness, morphology, vascular penetration and velocimetry in predicting implantation in an in vitro fertilization program. *Ultrasound Obstet Gynecol* 1995;**6**(3):191–8.

32. Raine-Fenning NJ, Campbell BK, Kendall NR, Clewes JS, Johnson IR. Endometrial and subendometrial perfusion are impaired in women with unexplained subfertility. *Hum Reprod* 2004;**19**(11):2605–14.

33. Alcazar JL. Three-dimensional ultrasound assessment of endometrial receptivity: a review. *Reprod Biol Endocrinol* 2006;**4**:56.

34. Fanchin R, Righini C, Olivennes F, et al. Uterine contractions at the time of embryo transfer alter pregnancy rates after in-vitro fertilization. *Hum Reprod* 1998;**13**(7):1968–74.

35. Lesny P, Killick SR. The junctional zone of the uterus and its contractions. *BJOG* 2004;**111**(11):1182–9.

36. Borm G, Mannaerts B. Treatment with the gonadotrophin-releasing hormone antagonist ganirelix in women undergoing ovarian stimulation with recombinant follicle stimulating hormone is effective, safe and convenient: results of a controlled, randomized, multicentre trial. The European Orgalutran Study Group. *Hum Reprod* 2000;**15**(7):1490–8.

37. Kolibianakis EM, Albano C, Kahn J, et al. Exposure to high levels of luteinizing hormone and estradiol in the early follicular phase of gonadotropin-releasing hormone antagonist cycles is associated with a reduced chance of pregnancy. *Fertil Steril* 2003;**79**(4):873–80.

38. Garcia-Velasco JA, Isaza V, Vidal C, et al. Human ovarian steroid secretion in vivo: effects of GnRH agonist versus antagonist (cetrorelix). *Hum Reprod* 2001;**16**(12):2533–9.

39. Kolibianakis EM, Albano C, Camus M, et al. Prolongation of the follicular phase in in vitro fertilization results in a lower ongoing pregnancy rate in cycles stimulated with recombinant follicle-stimulating hormone and gonadotropin-releasing hormone antagonists. *Fertil Steril* 2004;**82**(1):102–7.

40. de Jong D, Macklon NS, Fauser BC. A pilot study involving minimal ovarian stimulation for in vitro

fertilization: extending the "follicle-stimulating hormone window" combined with the gonadotropin-releasing hormone antagonist cetrorelix. *Fertil Steril* 2000;**73**(5):1051–4.

41. Hu X, Luo Y, Huang K, et al. New perspectives on criteria for the determination of HCG trigger timing in GnRH antagonist cycles. *Medicine (Baltimore)* 2016;**95**(20):e3691.

42. Chen Y, Zhang Y, Hu M, Liu X, Qi H. Timing of human chorionic gonadotropin (hCG) hormone administration in IVF/ICSI protocols using GnRH agonist or antagonists: a systematic review and meta-analysis. *Gynecol Endocrinol* 2014;**30**(6):431–7.

43. Falagario M, Trerotoli P, Chincoli A, et al. Dynamics of the development of multiple follicles by early versus late hCG administration in ART program. *Gynecol Endocrinol* 2017;**33**(2):105–8.

44. Wang W, Zhang XH, Wang WH, et al. The time interval between hCG priming and oocyte retrieval in ART program: a meta-analysis. *J Assist Reprod Genet* 2011;**28**(10):901–10.

45. Bokal EV, Vrtovec HM, Virant Klun I, Verdenik I. Prolonged HCG action affects angiogenic substances and improves follicular maturation, oocyte quality and fertilization competence in patients with polycystic ovarian syndrome. *Hum Reprod* 2005;**20**(6):1562–8.

46. Andersen AG, Als-Nielsen B, Hornnes PJ, Franch Andersen L. Time interval from human chorionic gonadotrophin (HCG) injection to follicular rupture. *Hum Reprod* 1995;**10**(12):3202–5.

47. Fleming R, Coutts JR. Induction of multiple follicular development for IVF. *Br Med Bull* 1990;**46**(3):596–615.

48. Wisanto A, Braeckmans P, Camus M, et al. Perurethral ultrasound-guided ovum pickup. *J In Vitro Fert Embryo Transf* 1988;**5**(2):107–11.

49. Davis LB, Ginsburg ES. Transmyometrial oocyte retrieval and pregnancy rates. *Fertil Steril* 2004;**81**(2):320–2.

50. Dicker D, Ashkenazi J, Feldberg D, et al. Severe abdominal complications after transvaginal ultrasonographically guided retrieval of oocytes for in vitro fertilization and embryo transfer. *Fertil Steril* 1993;**59**(6):1313–15.

51. Abou-Setta AM, Mansour RT, Al-Inany HG, et al. Among women undergoing embryo transfer, is the probability of pregnancy and live birth improved with ultrasound guidance over clinical touch alone? A systemic review and meta-analysis of prospective randomized trials. *Fertil Steril* 2007;**88**(2):333–41.

52. Matorras R, Urquijo E, Mendoza R, et al. Ultrasound-guided embryo transfer improves pregnancy rates and increases the frequency of easy transfers. *Hum Reprod* 2002;**17**(7):1762–6.

53. Coroleu B, Barri PN, Carreras O, et al. The influence of the depth of embryo replacement into the uterine cavity on implantation rates after IVF: a controlled, ultrasound-guided study. *Hum Reprod* 2002;**17**(2):341–6.

54. Franco JG, Jr., Martins AM, Baruffi RL, et al. Best site for embryo transfer: the upper or lower half of endometrial cavity? *Hum Reprod* 2004;**19**(8):1785–90.

55. Sallam HN, Agameya AF, Rahman AF, Ezzeldin F, Sallam AN. Ultrasound measurement of the uterocervical angle before embryo transfer: a prospective controlled study. *Hum Reprod* 2002;**17**(7):1767–72.

56. Vloeberghs V, Peeraer K, Pexsters A, D'Hooghe T. Ovarian hyperstimulation syndrome and complications of ART. *Best Pract Res Clin Obstet Gynaecol* 2009;**23**(5):691–709.

57. Golan A, Ron-el R, Herman A, et al. Ovarian hyperstimulation syndrome: an update review. *Obstet Gynecol Surv* 1989;**44**(6):430–40.

58. Aboulghar MA and Mansour RT. Ovarian hyperstimulation syndrome: classifications and critical analysis of preventive measures. *Hum Reprod Update* 2003;**9**(3):275–89.

59. Royal College of Obstetricians and Gynaecologists (RCOG). *The Management of Ovarian Hyperstimulation Syndrome.* Green-top Guideline 5. RCOG, 2006; 1–11.

60. Bodri D, Guillen JJ, Polo A, et al. Complications related to ovarian stimulation and oocyte retrieval in 4052 oocyte donor cycles. *Reprod Biomed Online* 2008;**17**(2):237–43.

61. Dogra V, Gottlieb R, Oka M, Rubens D. Sonography of the scrotum. *Radiology* 2003;**227**(1):18–36.

62. Schurich M, Aigner F, Frauscher F, Pallwein L. The role of ultrasound in assessment of male fertility. *Eur J Obstet Gynecol Reprod Biol* 2009; 144(1):S192–8.

63. Foresta C, Garolla A, Bettella A, et al. Doppler ultrasound of the testis in azoospermic subjects as a parameter of testicular function. *Hum Reprod* 1998;**13**(11):3090–3.

64. Tarhan S, Gumus B, Gunduz I, Ayyildiz V, Goktan C. Effect of varicocele on testicular artery blood flow in men: color Doppler investigation. *Scand J Urol Nephrol* 2003;**37**(1):38–42.

167

Operative Ultrasound in Gynaecology

Kanna Jayaprakasan and Uchechukwu N. Ijeneme

Introduction

Ultrasound has been used as a guide during gynaecological operative procedures, in addition to the role in diagnostic testing. In the field of gynaecology, some of the interventions, especially intrauterine procedures, are carried out without imaging guidance or with limited view, and are performed based on clinical skills and experience alone. Operative ultrasound provides concurrent visualization of the structures and contents and, therefore, has the potential to improve efficacy and safety of the operative interventions.

Application of intraoperative ultrasound will depend on a good understanding of the ultrasound features of the normal female pelvic anatomy. The introduction of intraoperative ultrasound in obstetrics and gynaecology is still progressing at a very slow pace, despite some available evidence that it will help to reduce complication rates. Even with endoscopic procedures like hysteroscopy, the perforation rate or trauma is still high – quoted as 1.7 per cent [1]. The use of ultrasound-controlled operative hysteroscopy will help to reduce this known complication of uterine perforation, especially in women with known intrauterine pathologic factors, thereby avoiding the use of unnecessary laparoscopy [2]. This, in turn, has the potential to reduce operating time and cost, and lower potential morbidity. Performing blind intrauterine procedures such as surgical evacuation of the uterus, intrauterine device placement in the presence of uterine abnormalities or complex cases under ultrasound guidance has the benefit of confirmation of procedure completion and reduced risk of injury to the uterus and internal visceral organs. In assisted reproduction treatment (ART), ultrasound has established its indispensable role in egg collection and embryo transfer, as described in Chapter 11. Ultrasound guidance is also used in cases like ovarian cyst aspiration, hydrosalpinx aspiration prior to *in vitro* fertilization embryo transfer (IVF-ET) and aspiration of ascitic fluid resulting from ovarian hyperstimulation syndrome.

Ultrasound-Guided Intrauterine Surgery

Most commonly, abdominal ultrasound is used to guide hysteroscopic and intrauterine procedures. It is best for the patient to have a moderately filled bladder, to have a better view of the uterus and cervix. The abdominal probe is covered with a sterile sheath and is positioned to obtain a longitudinal view of the uterus. Transvaginal and transrectal probes are only used if the abdominal ultrasound view is limited, but this may restrict the vaginal access and manipulation of instruments used for the procedure.

The ultrasound probe is positioned at the start of the procedure to provide a clear delineation of cervical canal, endometrial cavity, myometrial depth and boundaries (Figure 12.1). The bladder, if underfilled, can be filled with sterile normal saline to optimize visualization. Insertion of dilators, if cervical dilation is required, is done under ultrasound guidance to ensure the dilation follows the cervical canal and to minimize the risk of perforation or creation of a false passage. Once the procedure is started, the probe is dynamically manipulated to provide real-time images of the instruments, especially at its distal or operative end, operative site, correct plane of dissection and myometrial thickness/depth.

Resection of Uterine Septum

Uterine septum, resulting from incomplete septal resorption during embryogenesis, is a protrusion of fibromuscular tissue from the fundal region into the uterine cavity, and it can be partial or complete. While most women with uterine septum have normal reproductive function, some may be affected by adverse reproductive outcomes. Although randomized controlled trials on the efficacy and safety of surgical

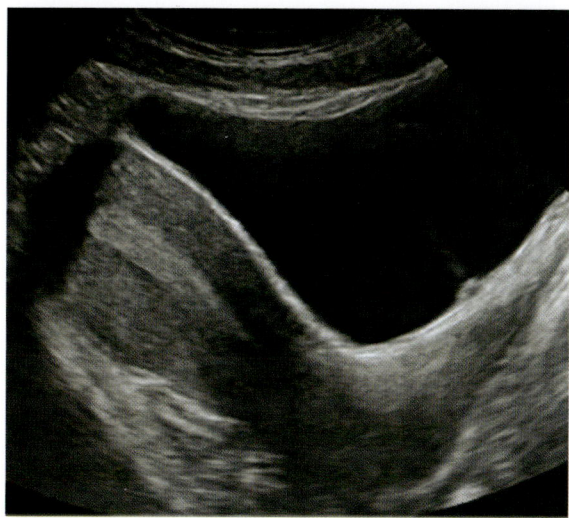

Figure 12.1 Abdominal scan demonstrating the uterus, including the cervix in its longitudinal plane.

treatment of septum to improve reproductive outcomes are lacking, controlled studies have indicated that hysteroscopic septal resection reduces miscarriage rates and increases live birth rates. The National Institute for Health and Care Excellence (NICE) has recommended that the evidence on the efficacy of hysteroscopic metroplasty of a uterine septum for recurrent miscarriage is adequate to support the use of this procedure, provided that normal arrangements are in place for clinical governance, consent and audit [3]. However, for management of septum in primary infertility patients, current evidence on efficacy is inadequate, and this procedure should therefore only be performed with appropriate arrangements for clinical governance [4].

Hysteroscopic septal division is not free of complications, although the procedure is technically less challenging in experienced hands. Some of the complications include incomplete resection of the septum and perforation of the uterus and uterine scarring. During hysteroscopic resection of the uterine septum, it is difficult to perceive the depth despite it being done under direct vision, which provides only an estimate of where the fundus is and may result in either partial/incomplete resection or perforation of the uterus. Partial resection is known to cause recurrent miscarriage [5] and uterine rupture in midtrimester after uterine septal resection has been reported [6]. Pre-operative preparation and measurement of the septal length using 3D ultrasound and

subsequent live scanning during the procedure may improve the outcomes and safety of uterine septal resection. With ultrasound, an accurate measurement of the distances, including the thickness of the fundus just lateral to the base of the septum, may be obtained. Contemporaneous sonographic visualization of the top of the fundus will confirm complete resection of the septum and avoid resecting into the myometrium without the subsequent risk of perforation and scarring. The procedure can be considered complete once both ostia are simultaneously visualized and when the fundal myometrial thickness is 8–10 mm [7]. Ultrasound guidance during the procedure has shown a trend towards lower perforation rates and is less expensive than laparoscopic guidance; therefore it has been suggested as the optimal means of intraoperative guidance during hysteroscopic division of septum or adhesions [8].

Resection of Uterine Fibroids

Submucous fibroids can cause menstrual symptoms and are associated with adverse reproductive outcomes, including subfertility and miscarriage. Hysteroscopic resection of fibroids is the standard treatment for submucous myoma to improve menstrual symptoms and to optimize fertility. While removal of type 0 fibroids (100 per cent intracavitary) may not benefit from ultrasound guidance, removal of type 1 and 2 fibroids (<50 per cent and >50 per cent intramural components) may benefit from ultrasound guidance, as this allows identifying the exact locations of fibroids, the portion of fibroids protruding into the cavity, their intramural extension and myometrial free margin. The common intra-operative and immediate postoperative complications when treating type 1 and 2 fibroids are incomplete removal, perforation and fluid overload. Korkmazer et al. described the technique of ultrasound-guided hysteroscopic resection of submucous fibroids with intramural component using the cutting loop of a monopolar or bipolar resectoscope [9]. The intracavitary component is excised by slicing from the top to basal part and from back to front until reaching the plane of the endometrial surface without causing undesired endometrial ablation. Once the cleavage plane between the fibroid and underlying myometrium with fibroid-free myometrial thickness is identified, the intramural part of the myoma is excised using the cavitation technique by slicing the tissue. Once the procedure is completed, the resectoscope is withdrawn back to the cervix, the uterine cavity is filled with distention media and then the margins of the uterus and fibroid are evaluated sonohysterographically. A prospective multicentre study evaluating 64 women undergoing hysteroscopic resection of type 1 and 2 fibroids under ultrasound guidance reported complete resection with no perforations. The authors concluded that ultrasound-guided hysteroscopy is a safe and effective method for resection of submucous fibroids with an intramural component [9].

Treatment of Intrauterine Adhesions

Intrauterine adhesions result from previous infection or uterine surgeries and manifest as hypomenorrhoea or amenorrhoea, infertility or recurrent miscarriage. Hysteroscopic division of adhesions is the treatment of choice to improve the symptoms. In moderate to severe cases, it is difficult to identify where to enter and which part of the uterine cavity is visualized while doing hysteroscopy. Ultrasound guidance allows the accurate localization of the instruments within the cervical canal and uterine cavity and visualization of myometrial depth (Figure 12.2). Abdominal ultrasound is used to guide the cervical dilation process to ensure the dilator is pushed only along the line of the cervical canal, minimizing the creation of false passage or myometrial or uterine perforation. During the procedure the ultrasonographer is able to provide real-time feedback on the plane of dissection and myometrial thickness. A retrospective cohort review has reported a lower perforation rate and better cost-effectiveness for ultrasound-guided hysteroscopic

adhesiolysis compared to laparoscopic-guided or unguided hysteroscopic procedures [8].

Other Hysteroscopic-Guided Procedures

Ultrasound guidance can be useful in hysteroscopic retrieval of foreign bodies embedded in the myometrium (e.g. bony fragments embedded following therapeutic abortion) when the foreign body is not evident by direct hysteroscopic vision [10]. In cases of haematometra associated with cervical stenosis or following endometrial ablation, concurrent ultrasound can be used to guide cervical dilation and hysteroscopic directed drainage of the uterine content [11]. Where resection of endometrial polyps is not possible using techniques employing direct visualization, ultrasound guidance may be employed in a similar way as when resection of leiomyomas is carried out.

Surgical Management of Miscarriage

The management of miscarriage or termination of pregnancy is one of the commonest gynaecological operations performed within elective and emergency, as well as office and hospital, settings. The procedure can be done either medically or surgically, but even with medical management, surgical intervention may be necessary either to complete a failed procedure or resolve haemorrhagic complications. Surgical management of miscarriage is not without risks, and these include incomplete evacuation and, rarely, perforation of the uterus and the need to return to theatre. All these risks can be potentially minimized by the use of ultrasound during the process of surgical evacuation. Ultrasound can aid in determining cervical orientation and guide the instrument along the cervical canal while dilating the cervix and introducing instruments into the uterine cavity. It helps to evaluate and continually visualize the size and direction of the uterus, position of the gestational sac inside the uterus, insertion and advancement of the instruments and completeness of the procedure.

In the ultrasound-assisted procedure, the orientation of the uterus is confirmed and the location of the product of conception is ascertained. Ultrasound will identify a retroflexed or anteflexed uterus and will help the operator to drop or elevate his or her hand to maintain a straight course to the axis of the uterus, hence avoiding perforation in the anterior or posterior wall of the uterus, which can potentially occur

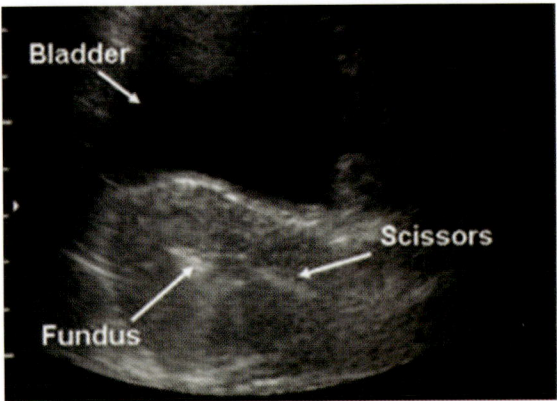

Figure 12.2 Hysteroscopic uterine instrumentation demonstrating the tip of the scissors. Ultrasound guidance allows the accurate localization of the instruments within the uterine cavity and visualization of myometrial depth.

during the blind procedure. Once the procedure is finished, the completeness can be confirmed by ultrasound. The ultrasound-guided procedure has the potential to reduce the risk of adhesion formation as it is performed with minimal trauma, with the instruments (suction and curette) directed towards the product of conception and the procedure is stopped once the empty uterus is demonstrated on the ultrasound scan. In contrast, the blind procedure may be associated with overzealous curettage in order to ensure completeness of the procedure, leading to subsequent damage of the endometrium. Controlled studies have reported that ultrasound-guided surgical management of miscarriage has the advantage of reduced blood loss and operating time, and less chance of retained products of conception when compared to the conventional blind procedure [12].

Caesarean Scar Ectopic Pregnancy

Caesarean scar pregnancy (CSP) is a rare type of ectopic pregnancy in which the gestational sac is implanted in the scar caused by a previous Caesarean section (Figure 12.3). While two types of CSP – type 1 (endogenic) and type 2 (exogenic) – are described, the management approach is the same. Type 1 CSP is where implantation occurs on the scar and the gestational sac grows towards the cervico-isthmic or uterine cavity with the potential to reach a viable gestational age, but with the risk of massive bleeding from the implantation site. Type 2 CSP occurs when the gestational sac is deeply embedded in the scar and the surrounding myometrium and grows towards the bladder. In exogenic types, a layer of myometrium may be seen between the gestational sac and the bladder at an earlier stage; this becomes thin and eventually disappears, with bulging of the gestational sac through the gap as the pregnancy progresses, thus carrying a greater risk of earlier rupture. In two-thirds of cases the thickness of the scar may be less than 5 mm [13].

While most women present with slight vaginal bleeding and mild abdominal discomfort, some may present with acute pain and profuse vaginal bleeding. Incidental diagnosis is sometimes made in asymptomatic women on routine early pregnancy scanning. Haemodynamic instability and collapse in a suspected Caesarean scar pregnancy strongly indicates rupture with intra-abdominal bleeding. Given the potential for serious life-threatening complications, accurate and reliable diagnosis and appropriate management are crucial.

Transvaginal ultrasound is the primary diagnostic modality, with supplementation by transabdominal imaging, if required. Key to the diagnosis of CSP is

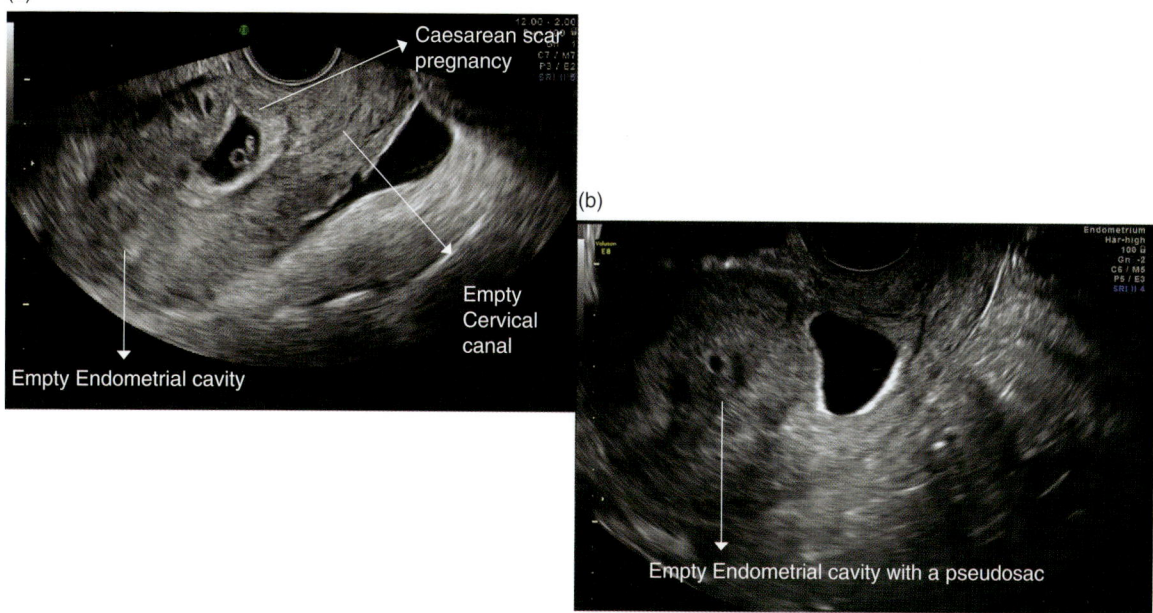

(a)

Caesarean scar pregnancy

Empty Cervical canal

Empty Endometrial cavity

(b)

Empty Endometrial cavity with a pseudosac

Figure 12.3 Caesarian scar pregnancy. TV scan showing a pregnancy sac (with foetal pole and yolk sac) attached to Caesarean scar. Oval gestational sac in the lower uterine segmant (a). Triangular gestational sac with a pseudosac in the endometrial cavity (b).

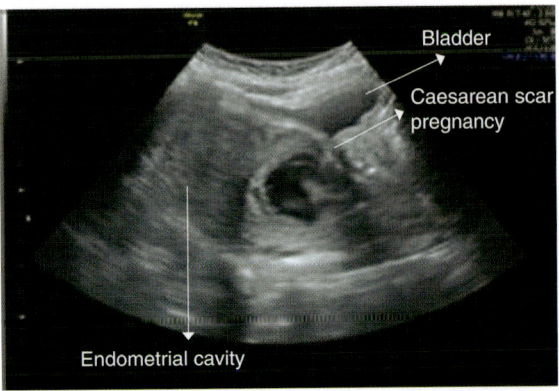

Figure 12.4 Caesarean scar pregnancy on abdominal scan. Note the thin myometrium between the pregnancy sac and bladder.

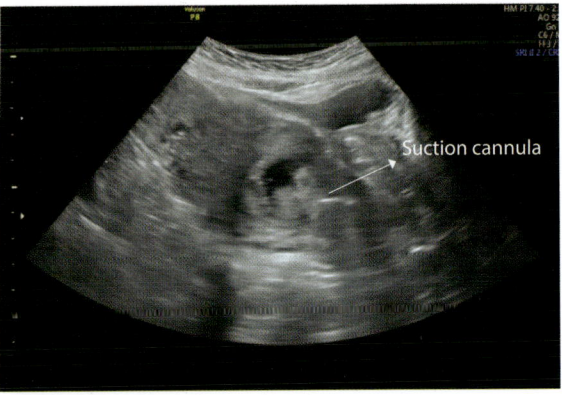

Figure 12.5 Evacuation of Caesarean scar pregnancy under ultrasound guidance.

a high index of suspicion followed by an ultrasound assessment demonstrating characteristic features.

Ultrasound *diagnostic criteria* for diagnosing CSP are:

- empty uterine cavity;
- empty cervical canal;
- gestational sac or solid mass of trophoblast located anteriorly at the level of the internal os embedded at the site of the previous lower uterine segment Caesarean section scar;
- a triangular/round or oval-shaped gestational sac that fills the niche of the scar;
- a thin or absent myometrial layer between the gestational sac and the bladder;
- discontinuity in the anterior wall of the uterus adjacent to the gestational sac;
- yolk sac, embryo and cardiac activity may or may not be present;
- evidence of prominent trophoblastic/placental circulation on colour flow Doppler examination;
- negative 'sliding organ' sign (gentle pressure with the transvaginal probe at the level of the internal os may slide the gestational sac against the endocervical canal seen in inevitable miscarriage, with tissues loosely seen in the isthmal or cervical area; this is absent in CSP as the pregnancy sac is attached to the isthmal region).

Medical and surgical interventions, with or without additional haemostatic measures, should be considered in women with first-trimester CSP. While there are various medical and surgical options available, there is insufficient evidence to recommend any one specific intervention over another for CSP.

However, the current literature supports a surgical rather than medical approach as the most effective option. Dilation of cervix and evacuation under ultrasound guidance is suitable for symptomatic CSP and endogenic CSP with myometrial thickness of at least 2 mm. Various techniques to reduce the bleeding during and after the procedure have been reported. Cervical cerclage applied prior to surgical evacuation and tied after the procedure is an effective method of reducing bleeding following evacuation. Other haemostatic techniques include the use of an intrauterine Foley catheter inserted intra-/post-operatively and pre-operative uterine artery embolization [13].

Abdominal ultrasound is done to obtain a sagittal view of the uterus, cervix and CSP in one plane if possible (Figure 12.4). In our unit, we give 800 mcg of misoprostol rectally in theatre immediately before starting the procedure. A cervical cerclage using a Merseline tape is inserted, but not tied at this stage. Dilation of the cervix under ultrasound guidance is done so that the suction cannula can be inserted with ease. Suction evacuation of the decidua from the uterine cavity (to ensure the uterine cavity is emptied to reduce the risk of post-procedure bleeding) and then CSP is done under ultrasound guidance (Figure 12.5). It is important to suction the CSP using a high suction pressure as quickly as possible as the blood loss is maximal during the procedure. Real-time ultrasound is utilized to ensure CSP tissue is completely removed. Once the procedure is completed, the Merseline tape (cervical cerclage suture) is tied. The suture is then removed 2–4 days later in the outpatient setting. Follow-up is recommended a week after the

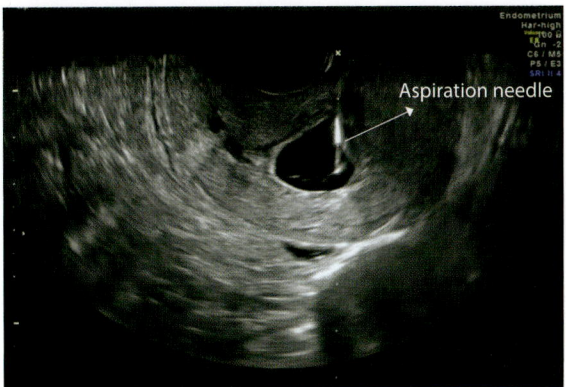

Figure 12.6 Caesarean scar ectopic. Aspiration of gestational sac and injection of methotrexate directly into the sac under TV ultrasound guidance.

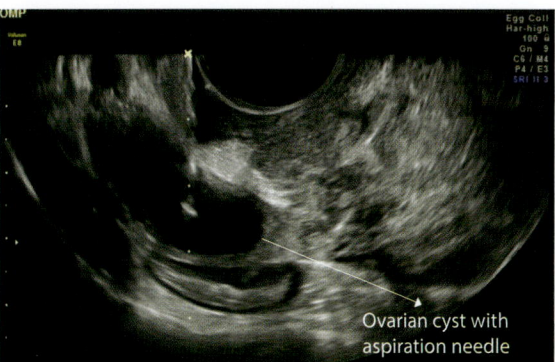

Figure 12.7 Ovarian cyst aspiration under TV ultrasound guidance.

procedure to ensure complete resolution of the ectopic pregnancy with either serum hCG estimation or urine pregnancy test, with or without ultrasound. Long-term follow-up beyond 1–2 weeks is rarely needed.

Medical management of CSP includes local or systemic injection of methotrexate, although long-term follow-up is required. Gestational sac aspiration with the administration of methotrexate into the sac is the preferred approach for exogenic CSP with thin myometrial tissue between the gestational sac and bladder. This approach alone, or combined with systemic administration of methotrexate, appears to have a better success rate and requires fewer additional interventions. In this effective technique, the gestational sac is aspirated and methotrexate injected into it under ultrasound guidance. While transabdominal and transvaginal injection approaches are both feasible, the transvaginal approach is recommended as it has the advantage of being anatomically closer to the target lesion and so helps to avoid visceral injury. This procedure is like 'transvaginal egg collection' done as part of IVF, with a biopsy guide attached to the vaginal ultrasound probe. The 16–18 Fr needle is inserted through the vagina and into the gestational sac (Figure 12.6). The time required for complete resolution of the ectopic mass correlates with the initial sac size and hCG levels. The dose of the methotrexate, pre-procedure evaluation, counselling and follow-up are similar to that for systemic methotrexate injection for ectopic pregnancy management.

Ovarian Cyst and Hydrosalpinx Aspiration

Ovarian Cyst Aspiration

Ovarian cysts, especially functional, if present before starting ovarian stimulation during IVF are not desired as they may interfere with stimulation response and IVF outcome [14]. Ovarian cysts can be aspirated transvaginally under ultrasound guidance (Figure 12.7). The procedure is similar to 'transvaginal oocyte collection' and is a relatively easy procedure in experienced hands. The transvaginal probe is used with the biopsy guide attached. A routine egg collection needle – a 16–18 gauge long needle with Teflon tubing – is used. The tubing is attached to the aspiration (suction) pump. When all the fluid is aspirated and the cyst is empty, the needle is removed. A scan is done to rule out any bleed or fluid collection in the pelvis. Usually, postoperative pain is very mild, but if required analgesics may be given. Aspirated fluid, especially if there is uncertainty as to the nature of the cyst, is sent to pathology for cytological evaluation. As the refilling and recurrence risk is high after aspiration, it is best to start the ovarian stimulation soon after ovarian cyst aspiration.

Hydrosalpinx Aspiration

Available evidence suggests that hydrosalpinx has a negative impact on IVF outcome [15]. This may be due to the toxic effect of tubal fluid on the implanting embryo or from a direct mechanical flushing effect. Salpingectomy or tubal ligation/clipping has been recommended to improve IVF outcome in those affected with hydrosalpinx. In patients who have had complex abdominal surgery, where

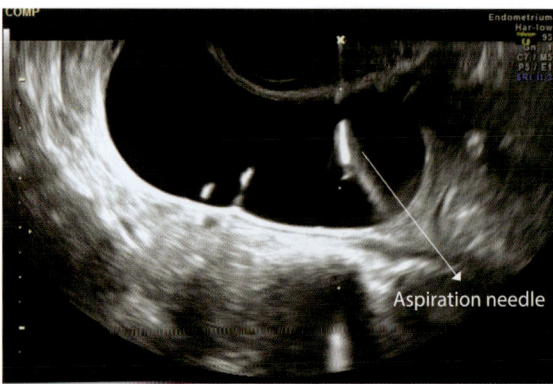

Figure 12.8 Hydrosalpinx aspiration under TV ultrasound guidance.

laparoscopy poses significantly increased surgical risks or if hydrosalpinx is seen during the ovarian stimulation stage of IVF treatment, ultrasound-guided transvaginal aspiration of hydrosalpinx has been suggested as a treatment option to improve embryo implantation and IVF outcome [16] (Figure 12.8). As the potential for re-accumulation of the tubal fluid exists, aspiration of the hydrosalpinx could be considered as an intermediate measure, until definitive treatment in the form of clipping or surgical resection can be safely carried out. The procedure is again similar to that of 'transvaginal oocyte collection'. Perioperative antibiotics are generally given because of the risk of infection.

Conclusion

Due to the ability of ultrasound to provide direct visualization of pelvic structures, contents, planes and operating instruments, ultrasound guidance improves the safety and efficacy of various gynaecological procedures discussed in this chapter. Ultrasound should be used in our operating theatres more often to guide various intrauterine procedures in order to reduce the intra-operative risks and complications, including uterine perforations and visceral injury. The use of ultrasound necessitates an additional assistant experienced in ultrasound in the theatre, but regular use of ultrasound improves the training opportunities of the trainees and clinicians.

Tips and Tricks

- While abdominal ultrasound is commonly used, transrectal or transvaginal ultrasound could also be used to guide operative procedures.

- A moderately filled bladder during an abdominal ultrasound-guided procedure helps to provide a better view of the uterus and cervix.
- The uterus and cervix are displayed in the sagittal plane during the procedure.
- Ultrasound guidance allows the accurate localization of the instruments within the cervical canal and uterine cavity and visualization of myometrial depth.
- Always keep in view the distal end of the instrument used (e.g. dilator, hysteroscope, scissors or resectoscope). The probe is dynamically moved (rotational/angling) to keep the distal tip of the instrument within view.

References

1. Royal College of Obstetricians and Gynaecologists (RCOG). *Best Practice in Out Patient Hysteroscopy.* Green-top Guideline 59. RCOG, 2011.

2. Shalev E, Shimoni Y, Peleg, D. Ultrasound controlled operative hysteroscopy. *J Am Coll Surg* 1994;**179**(1):70–1.

3. NICE. Hysteroscopic metroplasty of a uterine septum for recurrent miscarriage. Available at: www.nice.org.uk/guidance/ipg510, 2014.

4. NICE. Hysteroscopic metroplasty of a uterine septum for primary infertility. Available at: www.guidance.nice.org.uk/ipg509, 2015.

5. Kormanyos Z, Molnar BG, Pal A. Removal of a residual portion of a uterine septum in women of advanced reproductive age: obstetric outcome: *Hum Reprod* 2006;**21**(4):1047–51.

6. Satiroglu MH, Gozukucuk M, Cetinkaya SE, et al. Uterine rupture at the 29th week of subsequent pregnancy after hysteroscopic resection of uterine septum. *Fertil Steril* 2009;**91**(3):934e1.

7. Fedele L, Bianchi S, Marchini M, et al. Residual uterine septum of less than 1 cm after hysteroscopic metroplasty does not impair reproductive outcome. *Hum Reprod* 1996;**11**(4):727–9.

8. Kresowik J, Syrop C, Van Voorhis B, Ryan G. Ultrasound is the optimal choice for guidance in difficult hysteroscopy. *Ultrasound Obstet Gynecol* 2012;**39**:715–18.

9. Korkmazer E, Tekin B, Solak N. Ultrasound guidance during hysteroscopic myomectomy in G1 and G2 submucous myomas: for a safer one step surgery. *Eur J Obstet Gynecol Reprod Biol* 2016;**203**:108–11.

10. Wu MH, Hsu CC, Lin YS. Three-dimensional ultrasound and hysteroscopy in the evaluation of intrauterine retained fetal bones. *J Clin Ultrasound* 1997;**25**(2):93–5.

11. Kohlenberg CF, Pardey J, Ellwood DA. Transabdominal ultrasound as an aid to advanced hysteroscopic surgery. *Aust N Z J Obstet Gynaecol* 1994;**34**(4):462–4.

12. Abbas, AM, Ali MK, Abdel-Reheem M, et al. Surgical evacuation of first trimester missed miscarriage with & without use of transabdominal ultrasound: a randomized clinical trial. *J Gynecol Neonatal Biol* 2016;**2**(1):1–4.

13. Jayaram P, Okunoye G, Konje J. Caesarean scar ectopic pregnancy: diagnostic challenges and management options. *Obstet Gynaecol* 2017;**19**:13–20.

14. Qublan HS, Amarin Z, Tahat YA, Smadi AZ, Kilani M, et al. Ovarian cyst formation following GnRH agonist administration in IVF cycles: incidence and impact. *Hum Reprod* 2006;**21**(3):640–4.

15. Strandell A, Lindhard A, Waldenstrom U, et al. Hydrosalpinx and IVF outcome: a prospective randomized multicentre trial in Scandinavia on salpingectomy prior to IVF. *Hum Reprod* 1999;**14**:2762–9.

16. Hammadieh N, Coomarasamy A, Bolarinde O, et al. Ultrasound-guided hydrosalpinx aspiration during oocyte collection improves pregnancy outcome in IVF: a randomized controlled trial. *Hum Reprod* 2008;**23**:1113–17.

Sonographic Assessment of Complications Related to Assisted Reproductive Techniques

Miriam Baumgarten and Lukasz Polanski

Introduction

Assisted reproductive techniques (ARTs) are the only hope for biologically own progeny for couples that fail to conceive naturally. In the developed world, up to 4.0 per cent of all children born are the result of assisted conception, be it *in vitro* fertilization (IVF) or intracytoplasmic sperm injection (ICSI) [1,2]. The treatment-associated interventions, though well established, are not without complications to which the couples are often oblivious, as the hope of having a child may diminish one of the most significant and basic human instincts of self-preservation.

Complications in ART may arise at any stage of the process, starting at ovulation induction and concluding with obstetric complications of an achieved pregnancy. Due to under-reporting or the benign nature of some of the complications, the actual prevalence is most likely underestimated. Complication rates vary from 0.02 to 23 per cent for infectious complications and miscarriage, respectively [3,4]. When discussing the complications of ART, separation into procedure-related and pregnancy-related complications should be made, with procedure-related complications including ovarian torsion, bleeding and infection following transvaginal ultrasound-guided oocyte retrieval (TVOR) with associated co-morbidities, and ovarian hyperstimulation syndrome (OHSS). When a pregnancy is achieved, it might be in the form of an ectopic pregnancy, heterotopic pregnancy or multiple pregnancy, or it might end in a miscarriage. There is evidence to suggest that ART pregnancies that progress past the first trimester are at an increased risk of congenital anomalies, preterm birth, low birth weight, gestational diabetes and pre-eclampsia [5,6]. The exact cause of the increase in the adverse outcomes can be sought in the technology or underlying maternal factors [7].

In this chapter we cover the sonographic aspects of the procedure and pregnancy-related complications of ART.

Ovarian Hyperstimulation Syndrome

Ovarian hyperstimulation syndrome is a potentially fatal condition related to ovarian enlargement with systemic increase in vascular permeability. It may occur following any form of ovarian stimulation, including clomiphene citrate and gonadotrophins, with the latter being responsible for the majority of cases. Spontaneous – unrelated to ovulation induction – OHSS has been reported but is a rare event [8].

Varying classification systems and potential underreporting allow for an estimate of overall incidence approximating 2–10 per cent of IVF cycles [8], with the severe form complicating 0.1–2 per cent of all IVF cycles and a mild form occurring in up to 23 per cent of IVF cycles [9]. The reported mortality rate related directly to OHSS or indirectly (due to complications) is estimated to be between 1 in 400,000 and 1 in 500,000 ovarian stimulation cycles [10].

The main pathogenic changes leading to clinical manifestations of the condition are shifts in fluid from the intravascular to the extravascular compartment. The release of vascular endothelial growth factor (VEGF) from the stimulated and punctured follicles and associated activation of the renin-angiotensin system (RAS) is the pathway responsible for the increase in global vascular permeability [8]. The exact mechanism of this process is still under debate, with various factors such as oestrogens, progestogens, interleukins, angiogenins, endothelins, prostaglandins, histamine, prolactin and kinins thought to play a role [11]. The described molecular changes lead to clinical findings of relative hypovolaemia, hypotension, tachycardia, haemoconcentration with increasing haematocrit, renal hypoperfusion with associated renal failure, and acute respiratory failure. Increased vascular permeability leads to the development of albumin-rich ascites and pleural effusions causing abdominal discomfort and distension, as well as respiratory distress. Pericardial effusions can be present in the more severe forms of the

Table 13.1 Leuven University Fertility Centre classification system of OHSS

Grade of OHSS	Symptoms	Management
Mild OHSS	Mild abdominal bloating and pain No weight gain Ovarian size <8 cm	Conservative, outpatient based If symptoms deteriorate, advice is to seek medical help
Moderate OHSS	Moderate abdominal pain controlled with rest and simple analgesia Nausea Weight gain up to 1 kg Ultrasound evidence of ascites (deepest pool <3 cm) Ovarian size 8–10 cm	Conservative, outpatient based
Severe OHSS	Uncontrolled abdominal pain Weight gain >1 kg Clinical ascites (with occasional hydrothorax) Oliguria Haematocrit >45 per cent Ultrasound evidence of significant ascites (deepest pool >3 cm) Ovarian size >10 cm	Hospital based
Critical OHSS	Tense ascites or large hydrothorax Haematocrit >55 per cent White cell count >25,000/ml Oligo/anuria Venous-thromboembolic events Adult respiratory distress syndrome	Admission to critical care unit

Source: adapted from [8].

syndrome [12]. Gastrointestinal symptoms (diarrhoea and vomiting) and liver function derangements are attributed to an increase in intra-abdominal pressure, which may lead to compression of the low-pressure abdominal vessels supplying intra-abdominal organs (liver, intestines) [13]. Haemoconcentration and hyperoestrogenaemia lead to an altered thrombotic state which can cause a severe venous thrombotic event (VTE), and if undiagnosed and untreated significantly contributes to mortality.

Clinically, OHSS can have an early or late onset, be mild, moderate, severe or critical [14]. The most often quoted, older classification of OHSS was based on ultrasound findings of ovarian enlargement and ascites [9]. A newer classification combines ultrasound findings, clinical signs and symptoms and laboratory investigations [8,15,16]. The detailed description of each clinical form is shown in Table 13.1. The resolution of OHSS symptoms is expected by the sixth week of gestation.

Ultrasound assessment should be performed via the abdominal and transvaginal route when assessing women with suspected OHSS. This approach allows visualization of the pelvic organs, often-enlarged ovaries that have moved out of the pelvis, and the upper abdomen with quantification of ascites.

Ovarian size >12 cm may preclude complete ovarian assessment due to ultrasound attenuation, and bleeding into the ovarian follicles may be missed. In such cases, clinical judgement or computed tomography (CT) in the absence of pregnancy may be carried out.

Following oocyte collection, the ovaries change their appearance dramatically. There is a significant enlargement, with the follicles refilling with fluid and blood. The vascularity significantly increases and multiple *corpora lutea* are formed. These range in size and appearance, with some being filled with clear fluid, some appearing solid and some having a mixed content of blood, blood clot and clear fluid (Figure 13.1). Greyscale ultrasound shows these to be isoechoic with the ovarian stroma. The dominant feature is the presence of strong peripheral Doppler signal signifying rapid neo-angiogenesis.

The abdominal scan should be performed first, with the vaginal scan to follow. In the assessment, the standard description of the pelvic organs should be undertaken as described in Chapter 2. Special focus should be placed on assessment of any points of tenderness, the presence of large haemorrhagic cysts within the enlarged ovaries (signifying bleeding into the ovaries), absence of vascularity within one or both

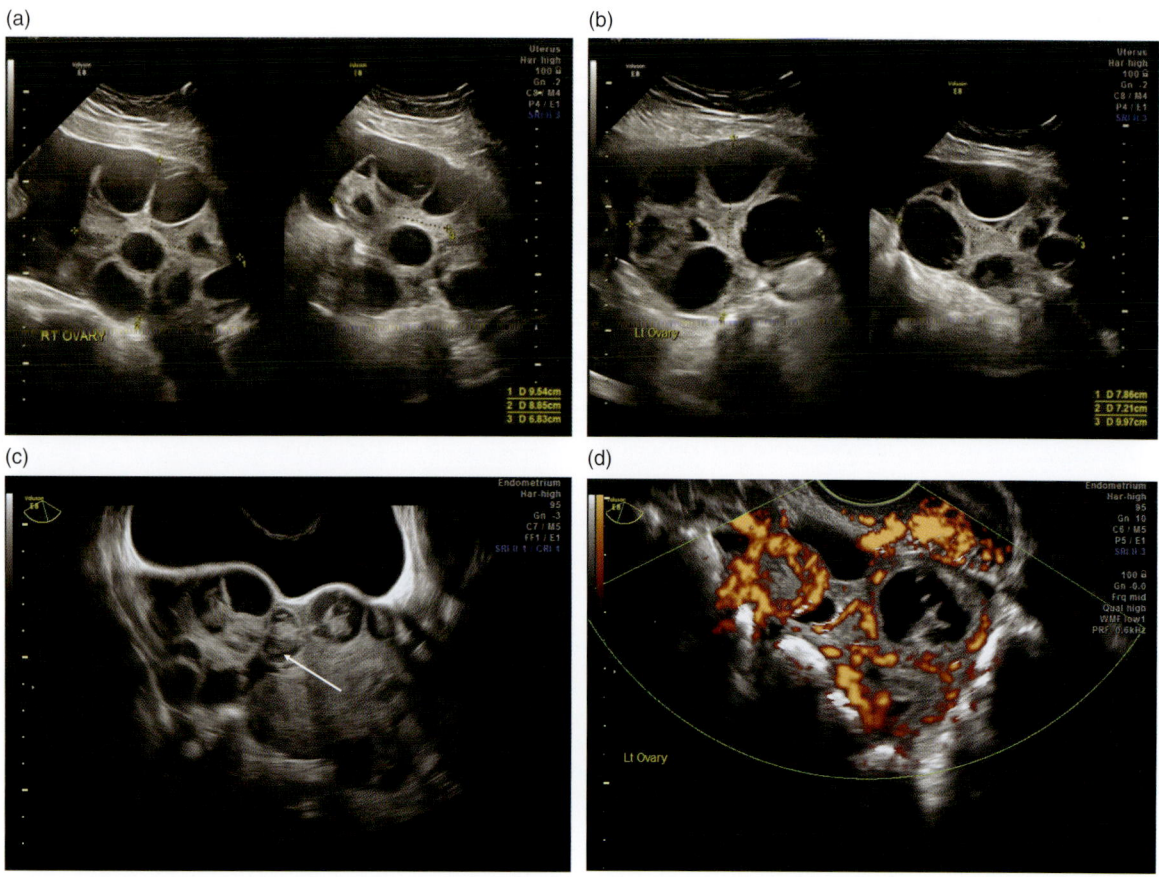

Figure 13.1 (a,b) Transabdominal ultrasound scan of moderately enlarged ovaries following ART with post-oocyte collection follicles of varying size. (c) Transvaginal ultrasound scan of bilaterally enlarged ovaries following ART. Both ovaries are displaced superiorly above the uterus and meet in the midline ('kissing ovaries'). Some of the follicles contain blood clots (arrow). (d) Transvaginal ultrasound scan of post-oocyte retrieval ovary with significantly increased vascularity as demonstrated by power Doppler modality.

ovaries, the deepest vertical pool of fluid in the pouch of Douglas and pouch of Morrison (upper abdomen), presence of intra-abdominal blood clots, and appearance of the fluid (clear or particulate, with the latter representing blood or pus) (Figure 13.2).

According to the Royal College of Obstetricians and Gynaecologists (RCOG), clinical assessment of women with mild to moderate OHSS should include body weight recording, abdominal girth measurement and pelvic ultrasound, and should be carried out every 2–3 days in order to determine deterioration of condition [16]. In more severe cases, with tense ascites causing severe discomfort or impeding respiration, ultrasound-guided paracentesis should be considered [17,18]. Similarly, women with inadequate urine output, despite appropriate rehydration, and ascites could benefit from decreased intra-abdominal pressure, as this might improve renal circulation and restore urine production [19]. Gradual drainage of ascites and the use of pigtail catheters should be encouraged to prevent cardiovascular collapse due to rapid fluid shifts [20].

Oocyte Retrieval-Related Complications

Transvaginal ultrasound-guided oocyte retrieval is currently the procedure of choice for oocyte collection in most IVF centres worldwide [21]. Though the procedure is safe overall, associated risks exist, such as bleeding, intra-abdominal sepsis and injury to pelvic organs.

Bleeding

Visible vaginal bleeding can be limited by minimizing the number of vaginal punctures, which are the

(a) (b)

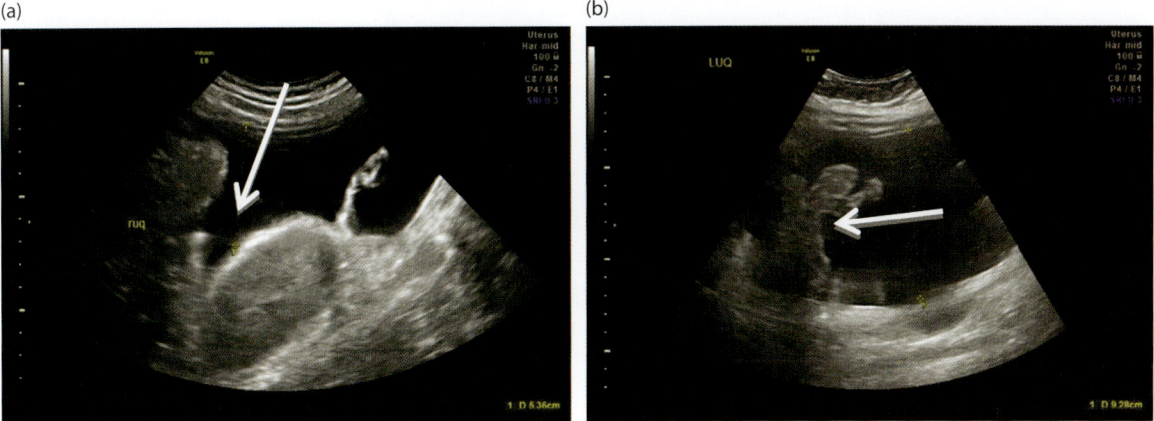

Figure 13.2 Transabdominal scan of the right upper quadrant demonstrating the liver and right kidney (a). In cases of severe OHSS, free fluid can be seen in the pouch of Morrison (arrow). The left upper quadrant can also be filled with free fluid in severe cases of OHSS (b). Note free-floating loops of bowel (arrow).

most common form of haemorrhagic complications, occurring in 0.5–8.6 per cent of oocyte retrievals, with significant vaginal bleeding exceeding >100 ml reported to occur in 0.8 per cent of cases [22]. Occult haemorrhage into the ovary or peritoneal cavity is a more severe complication, with an incidence of 0–0.35 per cent. This complication is related to direct injury to the ovary, bleeding from the ruptured follicle or injury to large pelvic vessels [23]. Coagulation disorders, inherited or iatrogenic, increase the risk of haemorrhagic complications.

Careful visualization of the follicle and neighbouring iliac vessels and application of power Doppler if there is doubt as to the nature of the structure allows for unequivocal identification of follicles and avoidance of puncturing the neighbouring blood vessels. A more detailed description of oocyte collection can be found in Chapter 12.

In the event of an uncomplicated TVOR, the expected blood loss should not exceed 250 ml, with a haematocrit drop of approximately 5 per cent. Larger visible loss, unexpectedly low haemoglobin values following TVOR, or symptomatic hypovolaemia should warrant further investigations [24]. Abdominal and transvaginal ultrasound scan should be performed and should suffice to identify and quantify presence of free fluid in the abdomen (Figure 13.2). Organized blood collections localized above the pelvic brim, retroperitoneal and broad ligament haematomas might not be immediately visible and

may necessitate employment of other imaging modalities such as computed tomography (CT).

As in the case of OHSS, thorough and systematic assessment of the pelvis and abdomen should be undertaken, with abdominal scan carried out first. The appearance of the ovaries should be described, with identification and size quantification of haemorrhagic cysts – fresh with liquid blood, as well as old where blood has organized to produce a blood clot (Figure 13.3).

The amount of fluid in the pelvis and abdomen should be commented on, with the presence of fluid in the upper abdomen in the space between the liver and right kidney (pouch of Morrison) signifying bleeding in excess of 400 ml [25]. Particulate fluid with moving particles when pressure is applied signifies bleeding. If the bleeding stops, organized, mixed echogenicity or avascular mass could be seen in the pouch of Douglas or surrounding the ovary or uterus (Figure 13.4). When pressure is applied on the transducer, the mass may not move, or move with the organ it is attached to (the ovary). The timing of investigation, as well as the number of oocytes retrieved, should be taken into account when scanning a patient presenting with abdominal distension and pain, as OHSS might have developed rather than intra-abdominal haemorrhage, or these two complications might co-exist.

Visceral Injury

Injury to the bowel, bladder or ureters is a very uncommon complication, with injury to the bowel

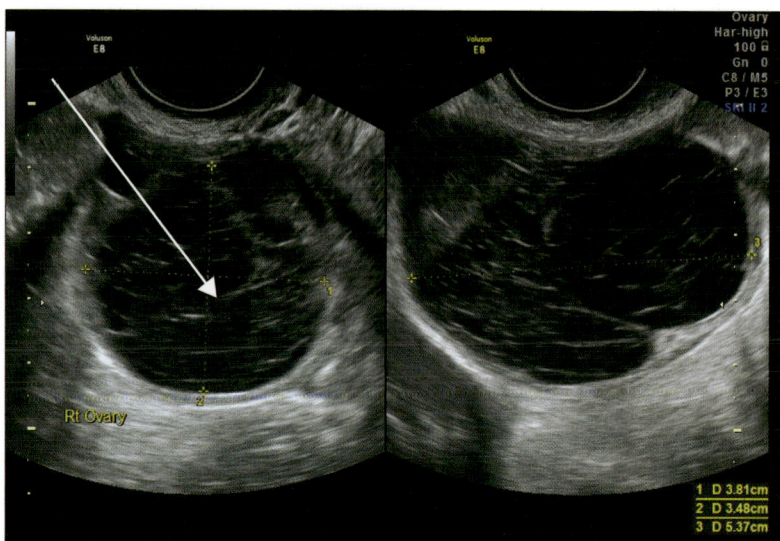

Figure 13.3 Haemorrhagic follicular cyst following TVOR. Note the extensive fibrin deposits within the cysts (arrow) and lack of Doppler signal within the cyst.

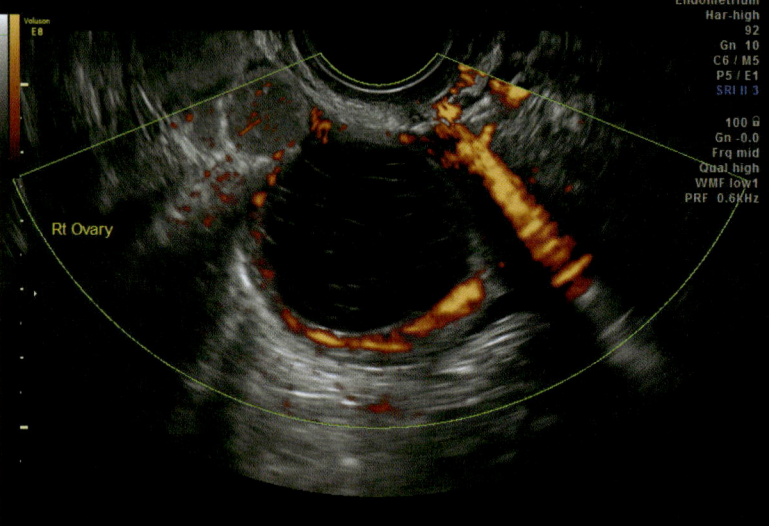

possibly being more common; however, most cases resolve spontaneously with no clinical manifestations [26]. Two case reports of repeated perforations of the appendix following TVOR have been described [27,28]. Urinary retention, haematuria or loin pain should raise the suspicion of bladder [29] or ureteric [26,30] injury, respectively.

Ultrasound imaging in cases of visceral injury is of limited value, with contrast CT providing superior images of the kidneys, their collection system, as well as the ureter throughout its entire length, and possible collections attributable to bowel injury. Erect chest x-ray may be considered to exclude bowel injury, with free air under the diaphragm confirming presence of the complication.

Infection

Pelvic infection or infected pelvic collection (abscess) is a serious complication of TVOR occurring in 0–1.3 per cent of women following TVOR [8], with possible mechanisms related to bowel injury, reactivation of quiescent pelvic inflammatory disease or introduction of pathogens from the vagina [31]. Treatment should be prompt in accordance with national sepsis guidelines. In this complication, ultrasound scan may be considered as well as CT

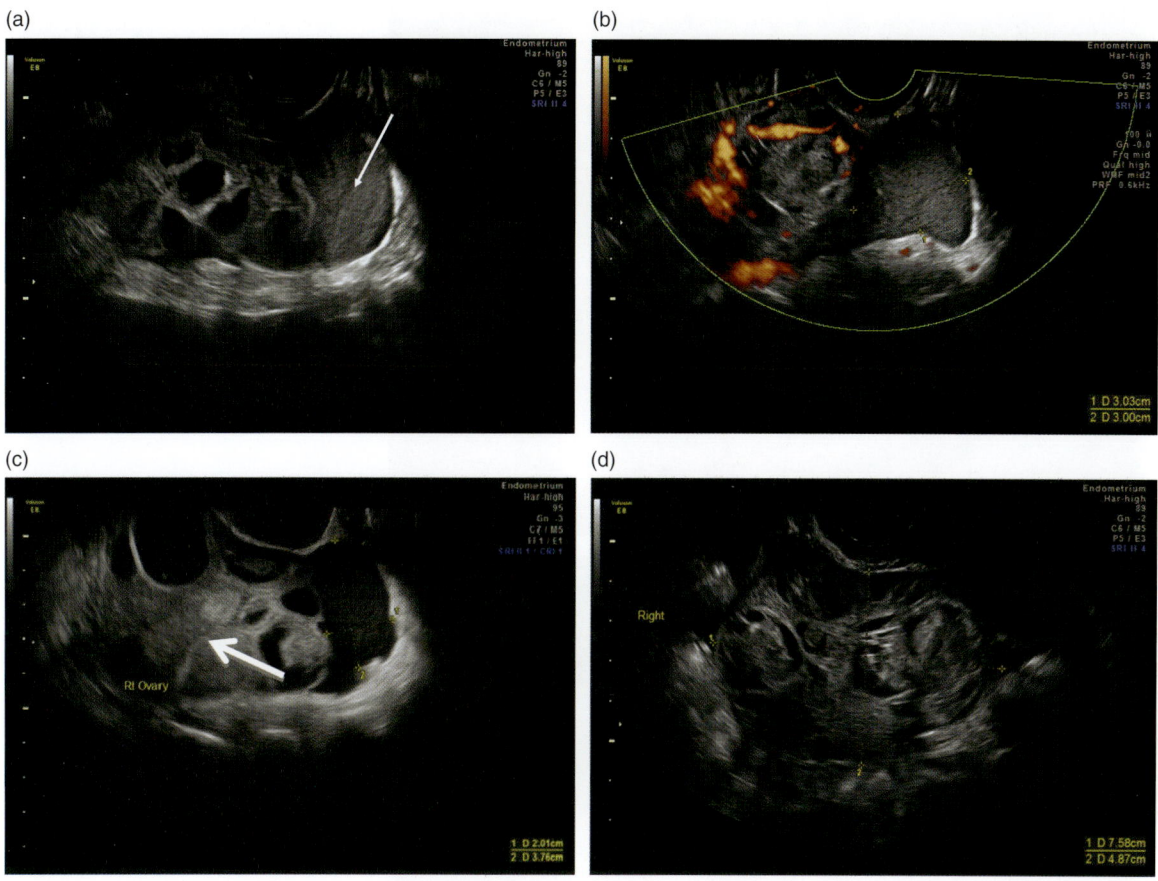

Figure 13.4 (a,b) Fresh bleeding into the pouch of Douglas immediately following TVOR. Note the particulate appearance of the fluid (arrow). Live scanning would reveal movement of the particles. (c) Hypoechoic fluid in the pouch of Douglas representing 'old' bleeding (examination performed two days after TVOR). The ovary is enlarged (arrow). (d) Enlarged right ovary with mixed content within the aspirated follicles. Appearance at embryo transfer (day 5).

imaging. Due to limitations of ultrasound in assessment of bowel or deeper pelvic or abdominal structures, CT is superior but exposes the woman to significant doses of ionizing radiation, which is not desired after the embryo has been replaced. Pelvic and abdominal ultrasound is an easy, safe and accessible modality in such cases and might yield relevant additional information.

In the case of a pelvic collection, particulate free fluid will be visible in the pouch of Douglas. Tenderness on scanning will be an additional diagnostic feature. Pyosalpinx will have the appearance of a tortuous, tubular lesion with hemi-septations, thick wall and mixed echogenicity content. When Doppler signal is applied, significant vascularity will be present within the tube wall. Tubo-ovarian abscess will take the form of a mixed echogenic mass

with abundant Doppler signal; accompanying particulate free fluid in the pouch of Douglas may be an additional finding.

Other Complications

Torsion of the enlarged ovary is a rare but serious complication of ART, with a reported incidence of 0.08–0.2 per cent of women undergoing ovarian hyperstimulation [8,23,28,32]. Ultrasound findings in this case include blurred ovarian margins and enlargement of the ovary with absent Doppler signal. These signify stromal oedema and absence or a decrease in blood flow, respectively. A vortex pattern of blood flow in the region of the ovarian pedicle can be another helpful sign to diagnose adnexal torsion. It is, however, possible to retain arterial blood flow in the early stages of torsion due to the higher perfusion

181

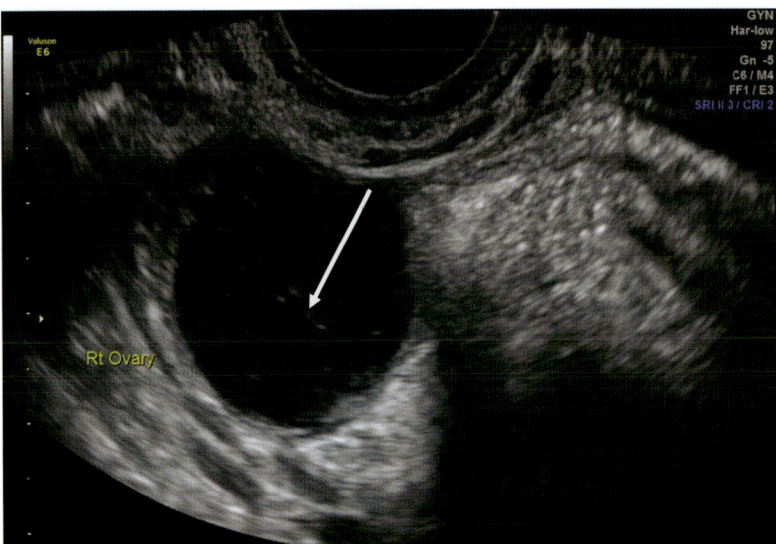

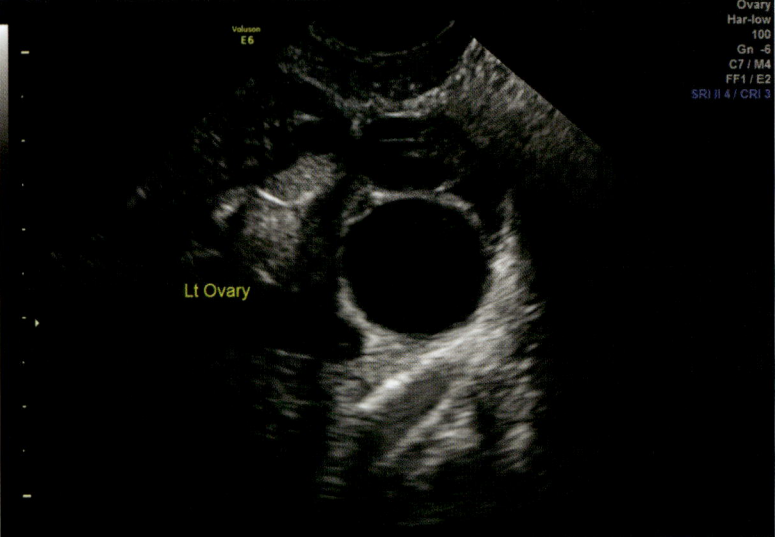

Figure 13.5 Appearance of the ovaries eight weeks after oocyte collection. Note the enlarged ovaries with evidence of haemorrhage into the larger follicle on the right ovary as demonstrated by fine fibrin deposits (arrow).

pressure and thicker arterial walls. As the process progresses, these may also become occluded, with complete absence of vascularity; thus diagnosis of ovarian torsion should be made on clinical grounds where sudden onset of pain in the presence of ovarian cyst or enlarged ovaries co-exist [8,33].

Pregnancy-Related Complications

The most favourable outcome of ART is a live birth; however, other outcomes may be encountered, with ectopic and heterotopic pregnancies, miscarriages and multiple pregnancies posing significant health risks to patients. The sonographic assessment of pregnancies conceived using ART does not differ from spontaneous conceptions. Some differences exist and need to be taken into consideration when performing ultrasound assessments. These include increased ovarian size and the presence of multiple ovarian cysts of varying appearance and the presence of free fluid in the pouch of Douglas. Depending on the number of follicles present in the ovary and the number of oocytes retrieved, the ovaries might still appear enlarged at the 6–8-week scan (Figure 13.5). Development of OHSS might prolong this period considerably; however, all changes would be expected to return to normal by the 20-week anomaly scan.

Further detailed description of sonographic assessment of early pregnancy complications is given in Chapter 14.

> **Tips and Tricks**
>
> - Systematic assessment is crucial with transabdominal and transvaginal approaches to scanning.
> - Anatomy is altered due to enlarged ovaries following oocyte collection.
> - Free fluid is likely to be present following oocyte collection – assess the appearance and quantity.
> - Two complications might co-exist – OHSS and intra-abdominal bleeding; maintain clinical suspicion at all times.
> - Colour or power Doppler modality may be useful when aiming to exclude ovarian torsion, but torsion may still have happened when blood is still flowing!

References

1. Klemetti R, Gissler M, Hemminki E. Comparison of perinatal health of children born from IVF in Finland in the early and late 1990s. *Hum Reprod* 2002;**17**:2192–8.

2. Williams C, Sutcliffe A. Infant outcomes of assisted reproduction. *Early Hum Dev* 2009;**85**:673–7.

3. Ferraretti A, Goossens V, Kupka M, et al. Assisted reproductive technology in Europe, 2009: results generated from European registers by ESHRE. *Hum Reprod* 2013;**28**:2318–31.

4. Klemetti R, Sevon T, Gissler M, Hemminki E. Complications of IVF and ovulation induction. *Hum Reprod* 2005;**20**:3293–300.

5. Isaksson R, Gissler M, Tiitinen A. Obstetric outcome among women with unexplained infertility after IVF: a matched case-control study. *Hum Reprod* 2002;**17**:1755–61.

6. Talaulikar VS, Arulkumaran S. Reproductive outcomes after assisted conception. *Obstet Gynecol Surv* 2012;**67**:566–83.

7. Talaulikar VS, Arulkumaran S. Maternal perinatal and long-term outcomes after assisted reproductive techniques (ART): implications for clinical practice. *Eur J Obstet Gynecol Reprod Biol* 2013;**170**:13–19.

8. Vloeberghs V, Peeraer K, Pexsters A, D'Hooghe T. Ovarian hyperstimulation syndrome and complications of ART. *Best Prac Res Clin Obstet Gynaecol* 2009;**23**:691–709.

9. Golan A, Ron-el R, Herman A, et al. Ovarian hyperstimulation syndrome: an update review. *Obstet Gynecol Surv* 1989;**44**:430–40.

10. Brinsden PR, Wada I, Tan SL, Balen A, Jacobs HS. Diagnosis, prevention and management of ovarian hyperstimulation syndrome. *Br J Obstet Gynaecol* 1995;**102**:767–72.

11. Soares SR, Gomez R, Simon C, Garcia-Velasco JA, Pellicer A. Targeting the vascular endothelial growth factor system to prevent ovarian hyperstimulation syndrome. *Hum Reprod Update* 2008;**14**:321–33.

12. European Society of Human Reproduction (ESHRE). *Special Interest Group (SIG) Guidelines on Ovarian Hyperstimulation Syndrome (OHSS)*. ESHRE, 2005.

13. Vlahos NF, Gregoriou O. Prevention and management of ovarian hyperstimulation syndrome. *Ann NY Acad Sci* 2006;**1092**:247–64.

14. Mathur RS, Akande AV, Keay SD, Hunt LP, Jenkins JM. Distinction between early and late ovarian hyperstimulation syndrome. *Fertil Steril* 2000;**73**:901–7.

15. Aboulghar MA, Mansour RT. Ovarian hyperstimulation syndrome: classifications and critical analysis of preventive measures. *Hum Reprod Update* 2003;**9**:275–89.

16. Royal College of Obstetricians and Gynaecologists (RCOG). *The Management of Ovarian Hyperstimulation Syndrome*. Green-top Guideline 5. RCOG, 2006.

17. Maslovitz S, Jaffa A, Eytan O, et al. Renal blood flow alteration after paracentesis in women with ovarian hyperstimulation. *Obstet Gynecol* 2004;**104**:321–6.

18. Levin I, Almog B, Avni A, et al. Effect of paracentesis of ascitic fluids on urinary output and blood indices in patients with severe ovarian hyperstimulation syndrome. *Fertil Steril* 2002;**77**:986–8.

19. Meldrum DR, Moore FA, Moore EE, et al. Prospective characterization and selective management of the abdominal compartment syndrome. *Am J Surg.* 1997;**174**:667–72.

20. Abuzeid MI, Nassar Z, Massaad Z, et al. Pigtail catheter for the treatment of ascites associated with ovarian hyperstimulation syndrome. *Hum Reprod* 2003;**18**:370–3.

21. Wikland M, Enk L, Hamberger L. Transvesical and transvaginal approaches for the aspiration of follicles by use of ultrasound. *Ann NY Acad Sci* 1985;**442**:182–94.

22. Bennett SJ, Waterstone JJ, Cheng WC, Parsons J. Complications of transvaginal ultrasound-directed follicle aspiration: a review of 2670 consecutive procedures. *J Assist Reprod Genet* 1993;**10**:72–7.

23. Bodri D, Guillen JJ, Polo A, et al. Complications related to ovarian stimulation and oocyte retrieval in 4052

oocyte donor cycles. *Reprod Biomed Online* 2008;**17**:237–43.

24. Dessole S, Rubattu G, Ambrosini G, et al. Blood loss following noncomplicated transvaginal oocyte retrieval for in vitro fertilization. *Fertil Steril* 2001;**76**:205–6.

25. Branney SW, Wolfe RE, Moore EE, et al. Quantitative sensitivity of ultrasound in detecting free intraperitoneal fluid. *J Trauma* 1995;**39**:375–80.

26. Ludwig AK, Glawatz M, Griesinger G, Diedrich K, Ludwig M. Perioperative and post-operative complications of transvaginal ultrasound-guided oocyte retrieval: prospective study of >1000 oocyte retrievals. *Hum Reprod* 2006;**21**:3235–40.

27. Akman MA, Katz E, Damewood MD, Ramzy AI, Garcia JE. Perforated appendicitis and ectopic pregnancy following in-vitro fertilization. *Hum Reprod* 1995;**10**:3325–6.

28. Roest J, Mous HV, Zeilmaker GH, Verhoeff A. The incidence of major clinical complications in a Dutch transport IVF programme. *Hum Reprod Update* 1996;**2**:345–53.

29. Sauer MV. Defining the incidence of serious complications experienced by oocyte donors: a review of 1000 cases. *Am J Obstet Gynecol* 2001;**184**:277–8.

30. Fugita OE, Kavoussi L. Laparoscopic ureteral reimplantation for ureteral lesion secondary to transvaginal ultrasonography for oocyte retrieval. *Urology* 2001;**58**:281.

31. Sharpe K, Karovitch AJ, Claman P, Suh KN. Transvaginal oocyte retrieval for in vitro fertilization complicated by ovarian abscess during pregnancy. *Fertil Steril* 2006;**86**:219e11–e13.

32. Serour GI, Aboulghar M, Mansour R, et al. Complications of medically assisted conception in 3,500 cycles. *Fertil Steril* 1998;**70**:638–42.

33. Fleischer AC, Brader KR. Sonographic depiction of ovarian vascularity and flow: current improvements and future applications. *J Ultrasound Med* 2001;**20**:241–50.

Sonographic Assessment of Early Pregnancy

Anita Jeyaraj

Introduction

Transvaginal ultrasound scan (TVS) is the recommended method for assessing pregnancies in the first trimester [1]. Transabdominal scanning can be performed if women are reluctant to have a TVS, but the limitations of this method over TVS should be explained. Examination with TVS provides a detailed evaluation of the endometrial cavity and ovaries, but the high-frequency transducer that allows improved near-field resolution compared with transabdominal examinations suffers from limited sound penetration (far-field imaging) [2,3]. The vaginal probe, due to its proximity to the uterus, allows excellent views of the uterus and pelvis in order to view and measure the gestational sac and any embryonic structures, which are small in the first trimester.

The main purpose of the early pregnancy scan is to locate the pregnancy, assess the viability and gestational age and establish the number of pregnancies. It is important to consider maternal anatomy also, as this may aid determining between an intrauterine pregnancy and an ectopic pregnancy [1,3]. This assessment can be achieved using four key movements [3], though sliding and panning is restricted when performing a vaginal scan (Table 14.1).

While scanning techniques are described in Chapter 1, this is further discussed here. When beginning to scan, it can be difficult to correlate the movement of the probe with the organs you wish to image. An ordinary pear may serve as an excellent example (Figure 14.1). If you hold the pear in the palm of your hand, with the narrower end pointing towards the wrist, you have in your hand a representation of the uterus, with the broader part of the pear representing the fundus and the narrower end, the cervix.

When you insert the probe into the vagina, the first view you are trying to obtain is in the sagittal view (Figures 14.1 and 14.2). Hopefully you can see the similarity. If we were to continue to slice the pear evenly, as a loaf of sliced bread, we would create a 3D representation of the ultrasound 'slices' that our imaging produces. Similarly, if we slice a pear across its widest circumference and continue to slice evenly like sliced bread (Figure 14.3), we create a representation of the uterus in transverse views (Figure 14.4).

An intrauterine pregnancy will be visualized within the endometrium eccentric to the midline, which is the bright white horizontal line in Figure 14.4.

Systematic Approach

When beginning to scan, it is important to develop a systematic approach in order not to miss any pathology. It is easy to get distracted by an embryo, which catches the operator's attention, and then easily forget to confirm the location of the pregnancy.

Once the sagittal section of the uterus has been obtained, the next step is to scan through the uterus from side to side. Without causing too much discomfort to the patient, it is possible to build an image of the uterus and confirm the location of the gestational sac (Figures 14.5 and 14.6). It is helpful to see the fundus and cervix in the same plane as the sac, as this will help avoid missing an interstitial pregnancy, which will be seen laterally to the midline. Rotate the probe anticlockwise by 90 degrees to move from the longitudinal to transverse view.

Once the surveillance in the longitudinal plane is completed, move the probe back to the midline of the patient, and rotate the probe anticlockwise 90 degrees and tilt the probe upwards and downwards in a gentle motion to view the uterus in transverse. An image of the largest cross-section of the uterus, which features the endometrium and the outline of the uterus, will be almost oval in shape (Figure 14.4). By tilting the probe upwards, the fundus will come into view in an anteverted uterus, and by moving the probe down the cervix will come into view. In

Table 14.1 Movements possible while scanning early pregnancy using the transvaginal approach

The transducer should be moved gently and slowly:

Sliding refers to moving the transducer along the length of the vagina.

Rotating is to move the transducer 90 degrees along its long axis (from the usual position with the groove at the 12 o'clock to 9 o'clock position).

Rocking or tilting of the transducer is a motion made along the long axis of the probe with the transducer array held stationary.

Panning is moving the entire transducer in one plane (horizontal or transverse).

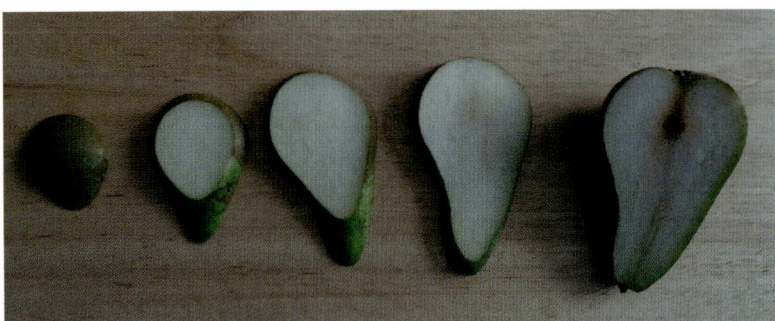

Figure 14.1 Longitudinal views through the pear, as an analogy to scanning through the uterus in a sagittal section.

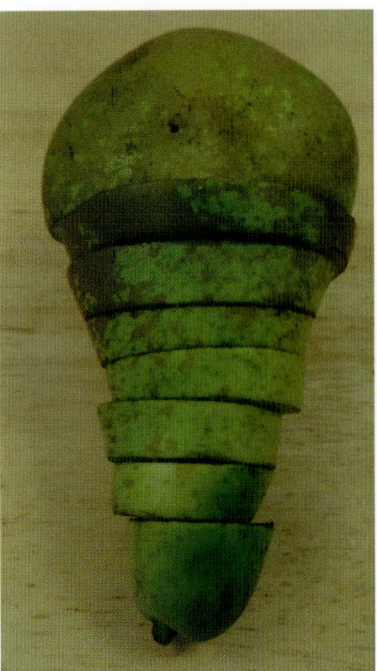
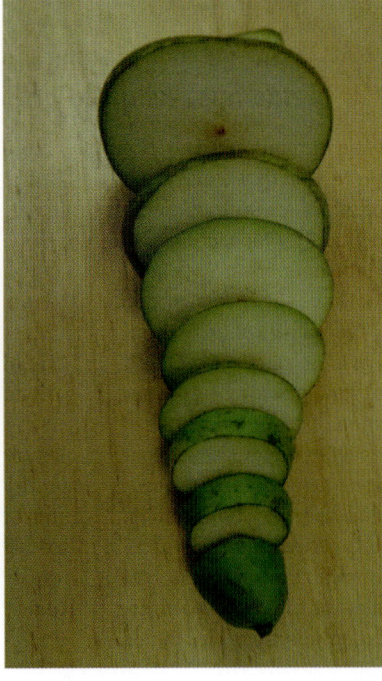

Figure 14.2 Ultrasound longitudinal section of the uterus (mimicking with longitudinal section through the pear).

a retroverted uterus the reverse is true: moving upwards will bring the cervix into view and angling the probe downwards will bring the fundus into view. If the uterus is very anteflexed or retroflexed it may be difficult to complete the scan in this plane due to the limited space in the vagina.

When measuring the gestational sac, the same principles should be followed as for measuring any cystic structure. The sac should be measured in three orthogonal planes: at the maximum longitudinal diameter, the maximum anterior–posterior diameter and the maximum transverse diameter in transverse view.

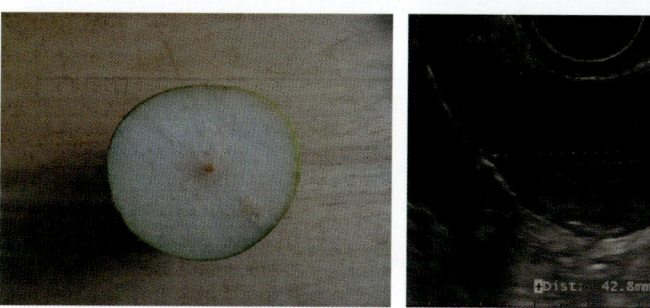

Figure 14.3 Transverse sections through the pear.

Figure 14.4 Ultrasound of transverse section of the uterus (mimicking with transverse section through the pear).

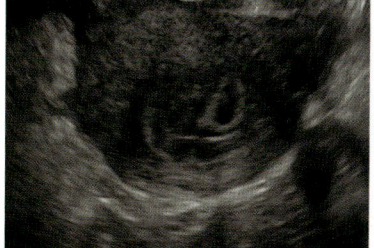
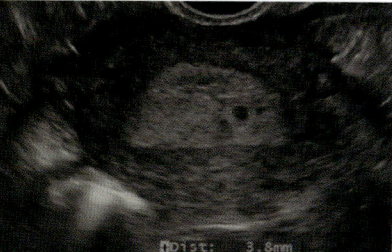

Figure 14.5 Intrauterine pregnancy.

Structures Seen in Normal Intrauterine Pregnancy

The gestational sac is the first definitive sign of an intrauterine pregnancy, which can be seen as early as the fourth week, but generally is clearer from the fifth. Before such structures are visible, the endometrium is thickened and has a hyperechoic appearance due to exposure to progesterone. The gestation sac is filled with clear fluid and therefore does not reflect

187

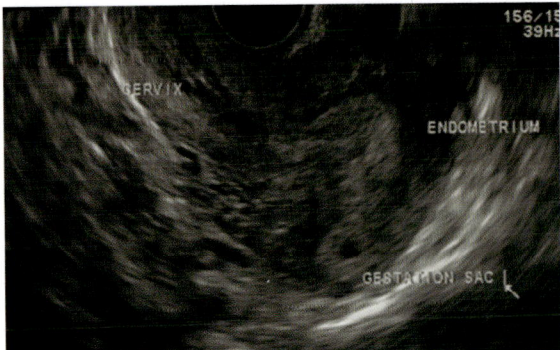

Figure 14.6 Laterally placed gestational sac.

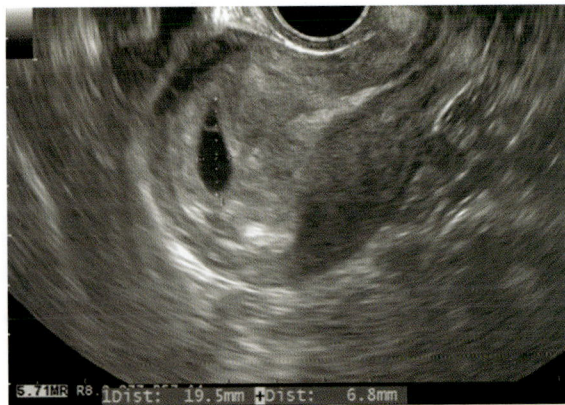

Figure 14.7 Intrauterine gestational sac – note the bright echogenic ring eccentric to the midline of endometrium.

ultrasound. As such, it is described as *anechoic*, which refers to the black appearance on ultrasound of the inside of the gestational sac. This actually consists of two fluid-filled compartments – the inner amniotic cavity and the outer chorionic cavity. The outer edge of the gestational sac, by contrast, is bright and *echogenic* and therefore *hyperechoic* in relation to the fluid within. This ring corresponds to the invading chorionic villi. Depending on length of a woman's cycle, sometimes the sac cannot be visualized until after the fifth week. Due to uncertainty as to the conception dates in cases of recently stopping hormonal contraception, breast feeding and irregular cycle length, visualization of the gestation sac may not correspond with the patient's dates. This should be considered when diagnosing pregnancies of unknown location and intrauterine pregnancies of uncertain viability, as well as ectopic pregnancies.

The bright echogenic rim eccentric to the midline is the distinguishing feature of a true gestational sac (Figure 14.7) versus a 'pseudo sac' (Figure 14.8). It should be noted that a failing intrauterine pregnancy may also have a thinner wall than a normal gestational sac. A word or two should be mentioned about the 'pseudo sac' within the context of ectopic pregnancy diagnosis. This is not a sac *per se* as it has no wall, but a small collection of non-clotted blood within the cavity. It can be differentiated from a normal gestational sac by the lack of a double echogenic ring around its anechoic contents. A normal gestational sac will also appear regular and circular in the longitudinal section, whereas the pseudo sac has a thin, not markedly as echogenic and more elongated appearance as it follows the shape of the uterine cavity (Figure 14.8) [3–5]. In a woman with a

bicornuate uterus, a small amount of bleeding may be present in the empty hemi-uterus, which may also create a pseudo sac appearance. As with any skill requiring pattern recognition, the more normal gestational sacs one sees, the more likely one is to recognize when an anechoic structure within the cavity does not look entirely normal. Decreasing the gain on the machine (making the image darker) may help to highlight the decidual reaction surrounding a normal gestation sac, a feature that will be absent in a pseudo sac.

By contrast to the black, circular appearance of the gestational sac, the yolk sac is seen as a bright echogenic 'ring'-like structure within the gestation sac and may be visualized from around five weeks' gestation. The foetal pole will appear adjacent to this from around six weeks (Figures 14.9 and 14.10). The foetal pole is hypoechoic compared to the yolk sac. Cardiac activity should be detectable once the crown–rump length (CRL) of the embryo measures 7 mm, though it can be, and most of the time is, detected much earlier, when the CRL measures 3 mm. Cardiac activity at this early gestation appears as a small echogenic equals sign (=), where the lines move together and apart in a pulsating manner.

It is worth bearing in mind that dates from the last menstrual period may be unreliable even when the woman reports a regular cycle, as an unusually early or late ovulation may occur. With the introduction of over-the-counter pregnancy dating tests and use of phone apps, there can often be confusion about dates and what these mean in correlation to what the scan reveals. Therefore, although it is important to have an idea of what we should expect to see on a scan based

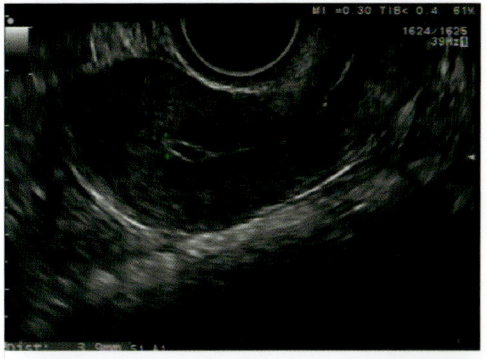

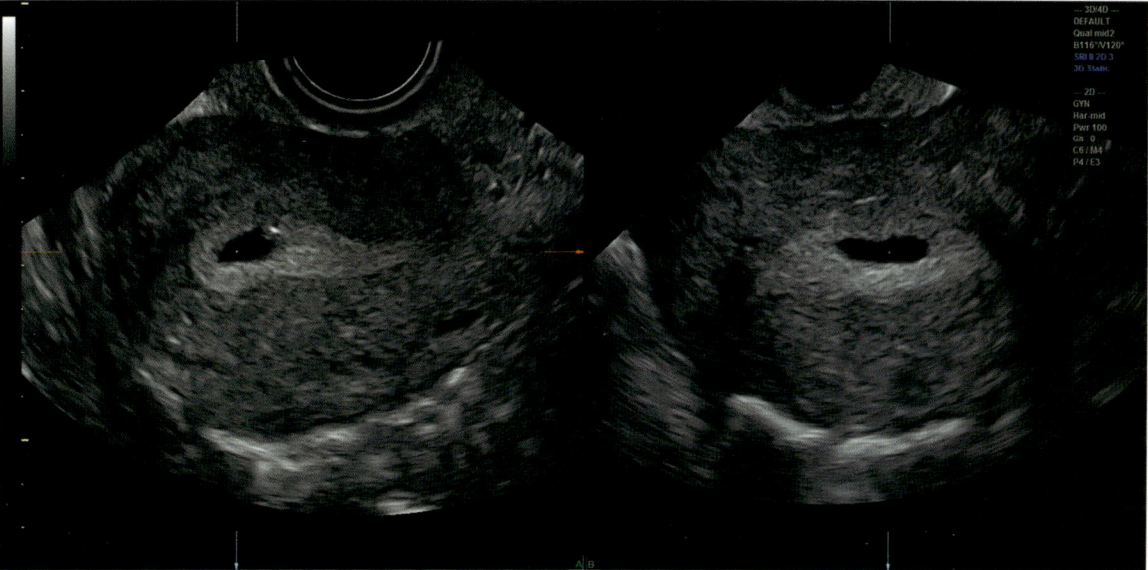

Figure 14.8 Pseudo sac – note the collection of non-clotted blood in the endometrial cavity with irregular outlines and no decidual reaction.

on this information, consideration should be given when interpreting our scan findings.

The gestational sac may occasionally implant in the lower part of the endometrial cavity and result in a normal pregnancy. It is necessary in these cases to differentiate a low implantation from a miscarriage in progress, a Caesarean scar ectopic pregnancy (Figure 14.11) or a cervical ectopic pregnancy. In the case of women who have had a previous Caesarean section, it is important to check that the gestational sac or trophoblastic tissue has not implanted into the scar itself. This is detailed later in this chapter.

The discriminatory hCG level refers to the level at which a gestational sac should be visible in a normal single intrauterine pregnancy in a normal uterus. This has traditionally been 1500 IU/L for a transvaginal scan and 6000 IU/L on transabdominal scan [6], but with the advent of high-resolution ultrasound machines the current discriminatory hCG level is much lower. Therefore, under no circumstances should scanning be delayed in the event that the hCG level is below an arbitrary cutoff of 1500 IU/L, as ectopic pregnancies do occur and rupture below this level. The presence of fibroids and the anatomy of the uterus will affect the ability to visualize an early pregnancy. The yolk sac can be seen when the mean sac diameter (MSD) of the gestational sac is between 5 and 12 mm. Its function is to transport nutrition to the embryo, haematopoiesis and storage of primordial germ cells [2].

Measuring the Crown–Rump Length

To illustrate the measuring of the embryo (or foetus after 10/40 gestation), an analogy can be made

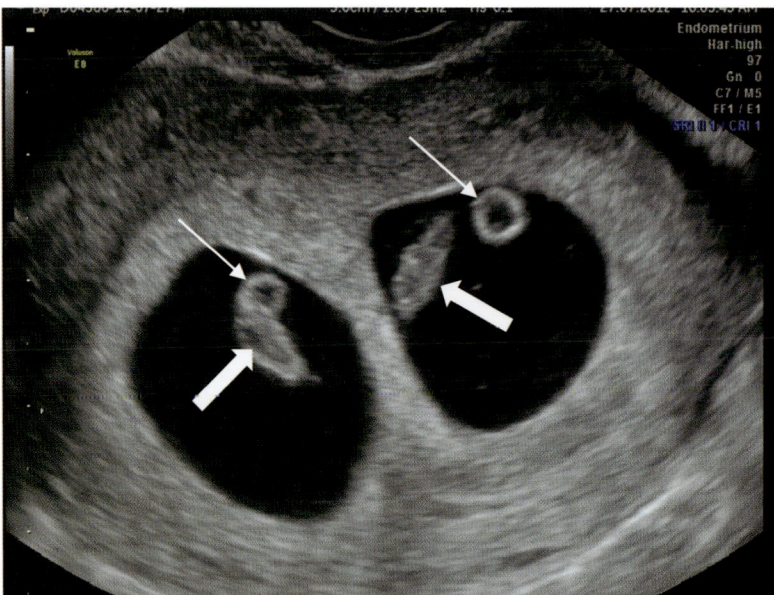

Figure 14.9 Twin gestational sac with yolk sacs (thin arrows) and foetal poles inside (thick arrows).

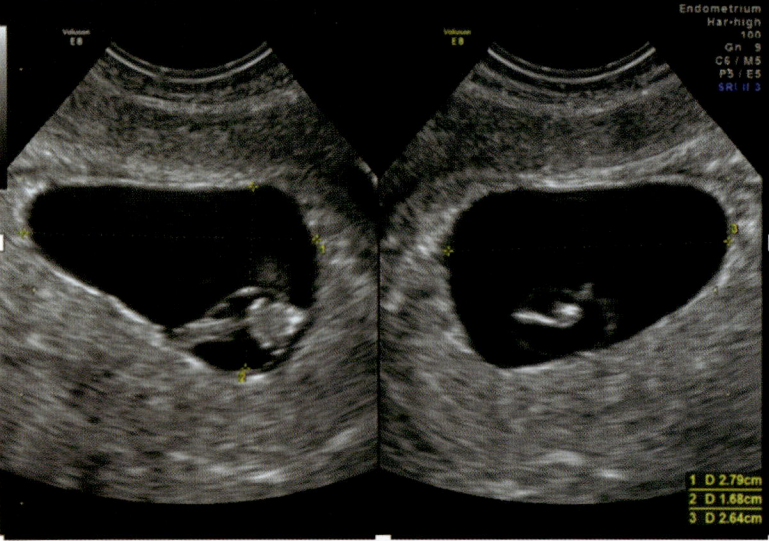

Figure 14.10 Intrauterine pregnancy: gestational sac (callipers) measurements. The gestational sac should be measured in three planes: longitudinal, anterior–posterior and transverse, always from the inner trophoblastic edge.

between a jelly baby (a humanoid-shaped sweet) and an embryo seen on scan. Holding the jelly baby longitudinally between one finger and the thumb and gently squeezing it to create a small curvature approximates a seven-week embryo complete with forebrain, heart bulge and rump. The white lines demonstrate how the measurement of the CRL can differ depending on the plane in which the embryo is viewed and thus the placement of the callipers (Figure 14.12). During a real scan in the very early gestation, these measurements differ only slightly, with no major

impact on the actual due date (Figure 14.13). The crown and the rump are difficult to visualize at the early stages of pregnancy, so always obtain the longest measurement.

Figures 14.12 and 14.13 demonstrate the difference between sagittal and coronal views and how the coronal measurement of CRL may differ from the sagittal one. When the embryo only measures a few millimetres, a millimetre not measured can affect the dating of the pregnancy (Figures 14.14 and 14.15). However, with a TVS and often due to foetal position,

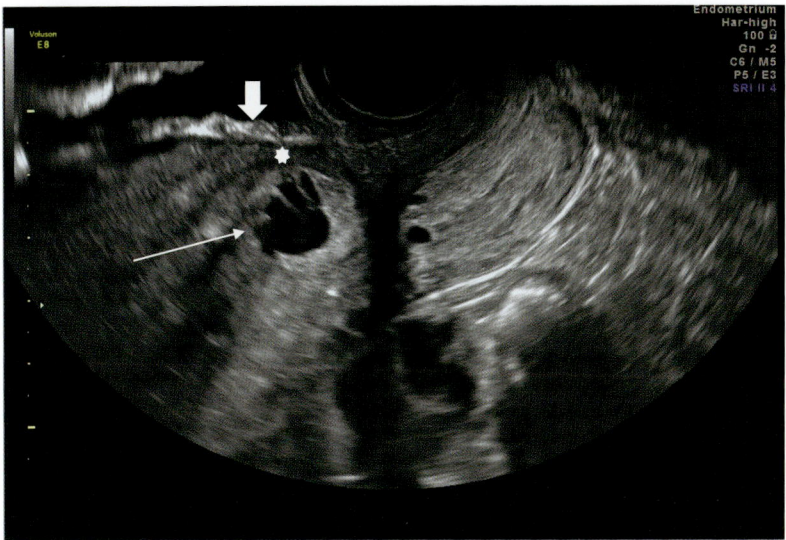

Figure 14.11 Caesarean scar pregnancy with empty uterine cavity and gestational sac at the Caesarean scar site (arrow). Notice the proximity of the gestational sac to the bladder and thin layer of myometrium (star) between the sac and the brighter hyperechoic (thick arrow) posterior bladder wall. The uterine fundus has also been displaced posteriorly due to the sac site (and has not been included in this image).

(a)

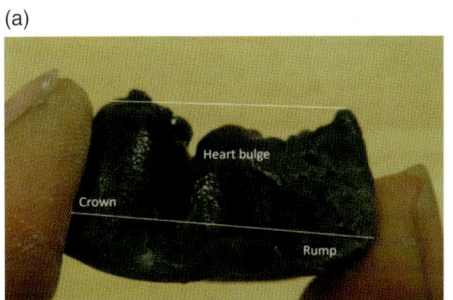

(b)

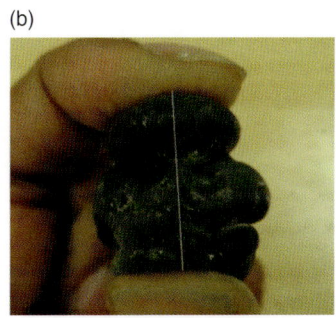

Figure 14.12 Sagittal view of a jelly baby (a) and a coronal view (b).

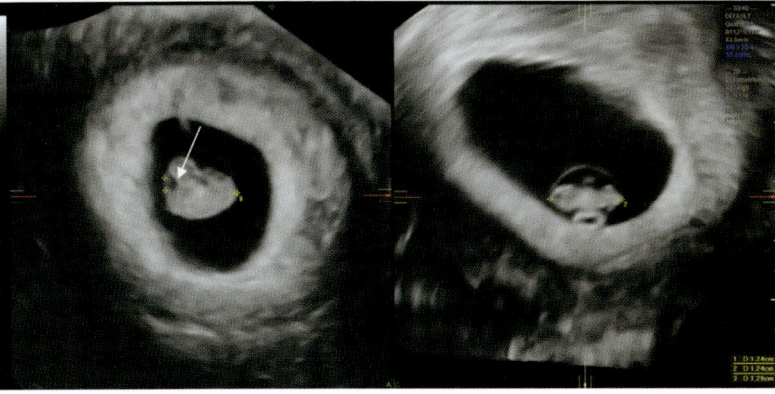

Figure 14.13 Sagittal and coronal view of a seven-week foetus. Measurements 1 and 2 are identical as they are measuring the same distance in two planes (sagittal on the left and coronal on the right); however, the more accurate CRL is represented by measurement 3 as this starts at the top of the crown. The difference in measurement is negligible, however. The crown is characterized by the telencephalon (hypoechoic area marked with an arrow). The images are enhanced by volume contrast imaging (VCI).

it may not be possible to obtain a true sagittal section of the foetus to measure a 'true' CRL, hence a coronal plane may be all that is available. In this case a rescan in 7–14 days may be offered to more accurately date the pregnancy. As foetal structures are very small at this stage of pregnancy, only small movements of the transducer and mainly rotation along the long axis are necessary to produce an acceptable image of the foetus on scan and allow for accurate measurement. This is especially important when confirming miscarriage (see details in the subsequent sections). At 12 weeks' gestation, foetuses, much like the children they may

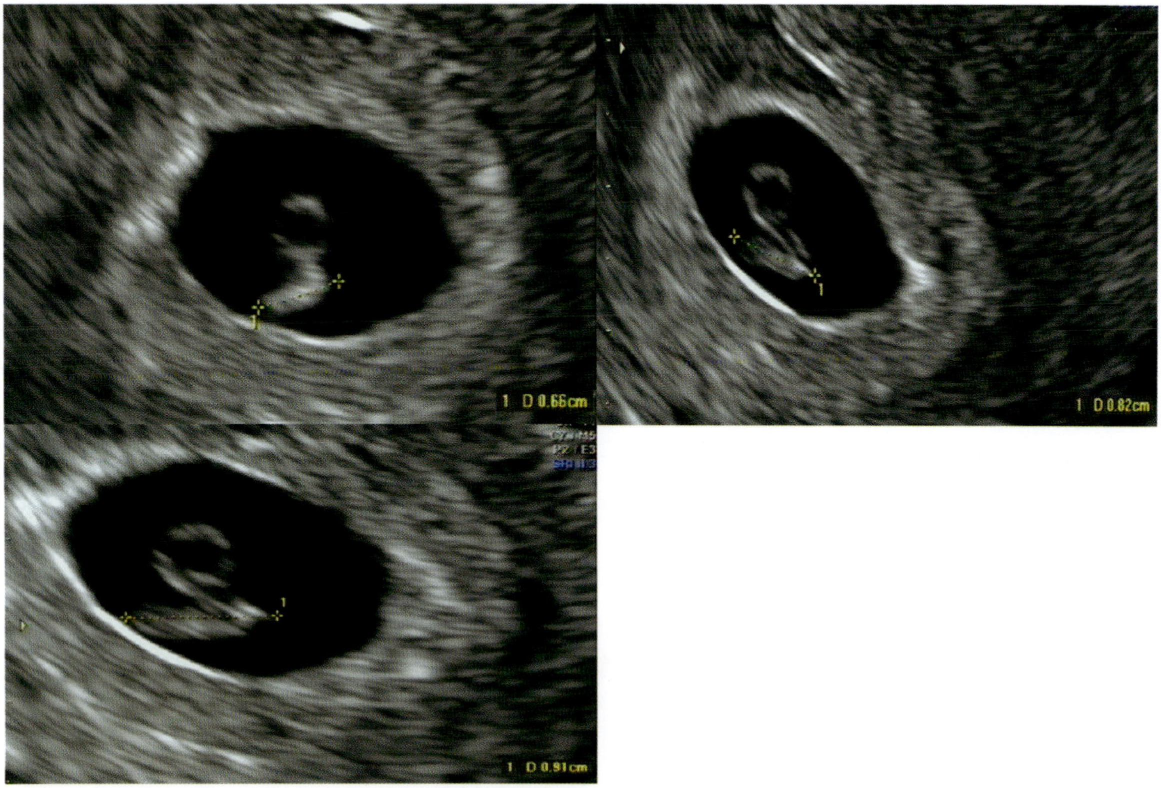

Figure 14.14 Images taken during a single scan. Different calliper placements may alter the measurement of the CRL and affect dating of the pregnancy. Different planes obtained during the scanning may also add to the discrepancy.

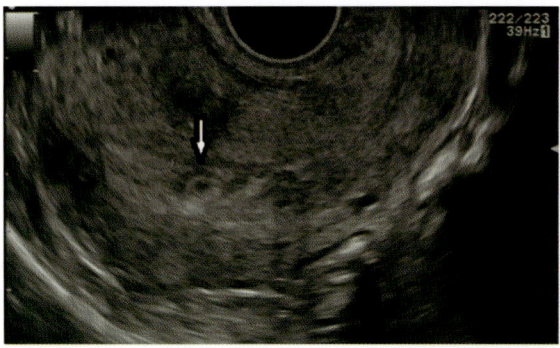

Figure 14.15 Four-plus weeks' gestation. Within an anteverted and anteflexed uterus a small gestation sac is visible (arrow). Note the brighter area surrounding it (decidual reaction). The endometrium is also thickened (callipers).

or try an abdominal scan once it has been confirmed that the pregnancy is intrauterine.

Dating of the pregnancy can be performed by using the inbuilt CRL reference charts (i.e. Hadlock or Chitty charts) on the scanning machine, or after the examination using a database software, where reports can also be written and stored. Figure 14.14 demonstrates the possible differences in measurements depending on the starting points and the obtained planes. The nuchal translucency (NT) scan may be booked based on the early pregnancy scan, so that the CRL on the actual day of the NT screening will be within the acceptable range of 45–84 mm, assuming a 1 mm per day elongation of the CRL. Changes in sonographic appearance of pregnancy and its development are demonstrated in Figures 14.15–14.23.

Multiple Pregnancies

Due to the increased perinatal morbidity and mortality of twin or higher-order pregnancies, it is important to

become, are not always well behaved and their position may inhibit measurement of a true CRL. Options are to wait for a foetus to move, ask the patient to change position (i.e. lift the pelvis up and down, tilt),

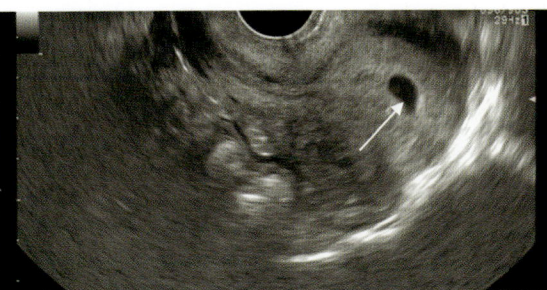

Figure 14.16 Five weeks' gestation. A small anechoic regular gestational sac (arrow) can be seen eccentric to the midline (pale grey line running over the top of the sac in this retroverted uterus). A yolk sac can also be seen within the sac from 5 + 2 weeks' gestation, or when the mean sac diameter of the gestational sac is >12 mm.

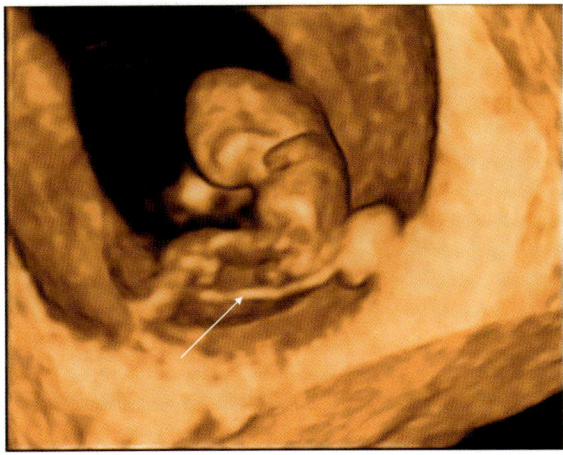

Figure 14.18 Seven weeks' gestation – 3D reconstruction. The embryo is now clearly recognizable and is separated from the yolk sac by the vitelline duct (arrow).

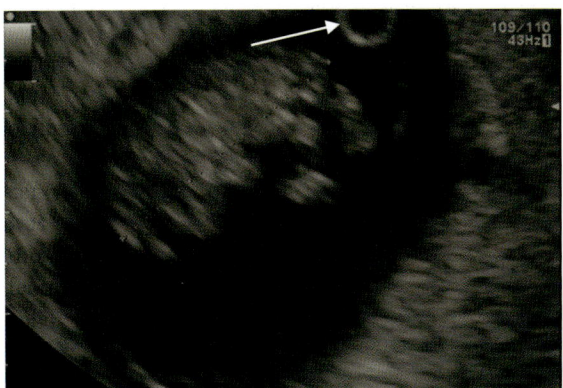

Figure 14.20 Nine weeks' gestation. The limb buds have started to lengthen, the left leg can be seen below the yolk sac (arrow).

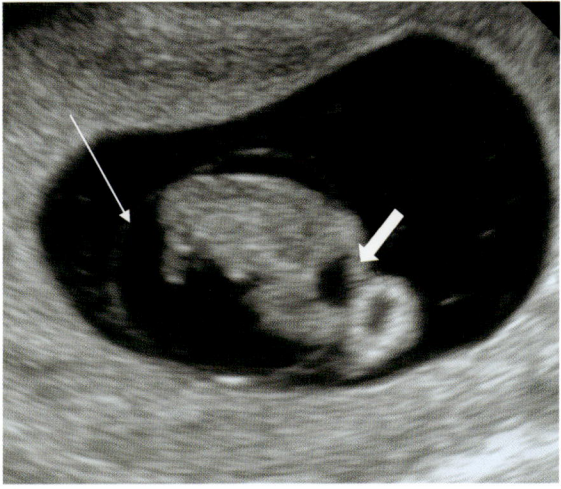

Figure 14.17 Six weeks' gestation. The distinct features of a foetus are seen. The rhombencephalon is the hypoechoic area within the foetal head (arrow). Amnion is clearly seen (thin arrow) and note the yolk sac close to the foetal head. This may produce errors in gestational age estimation if mistaken for the rhombencephalon.

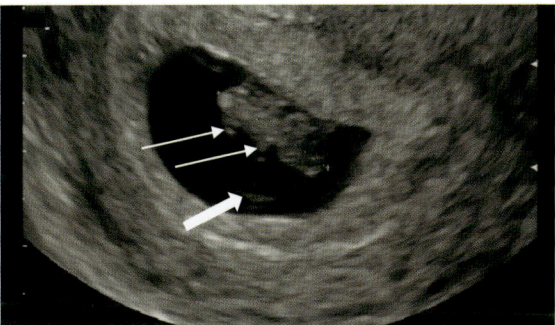

Figure 14.19 Eight weeks' gestation. The embryo's features are more distinguishable and limb buds start to appear (coronal section). The arm and leg buds (thin arrows) can be seen in the image protruding from the body of the embryo. Embryonic movements can also be detected on scan. The amniotic sac can be seen surrounding the embryo (thick arrow). The forebrain, midbrain, hindbrain and skull can be detected [5].

determine chorionicity and amnionicity as early as possible [3–5]. Monochorionic diamniotic (MCDA) twin pregnancies have a 25 per cent chance of developing twin-to-twin transfusion syndrome (TTTS), associated with a very high mortality of one or both twins. Monochorionic monoamniotic (MCMA) twins have high rates of cord accidents due to cord entanglement and polyhydramnios leading to premature delivery. There is also an increase in foetal structural defects and intrauterine growth restriction (IUGR) in monozygotic pregnancies [3–5].

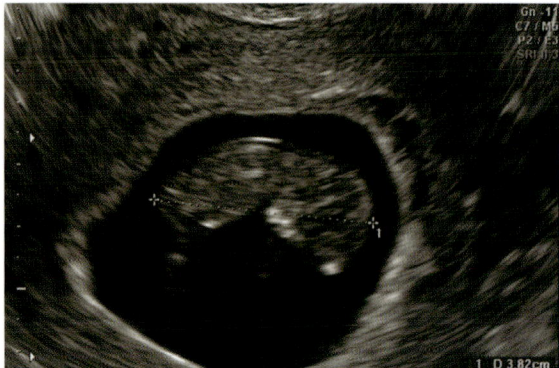

Figure 14.21 Ten weeks' gestation. Further lengthening of limbs. Hands and feet are visible. Yolk sac starts to disappear [3,5]. Physiological herniation of the gut into the cord may be demonstrable at this stage. The bowel content should return into the abdominal cavity by the 12th week of pregnancy.

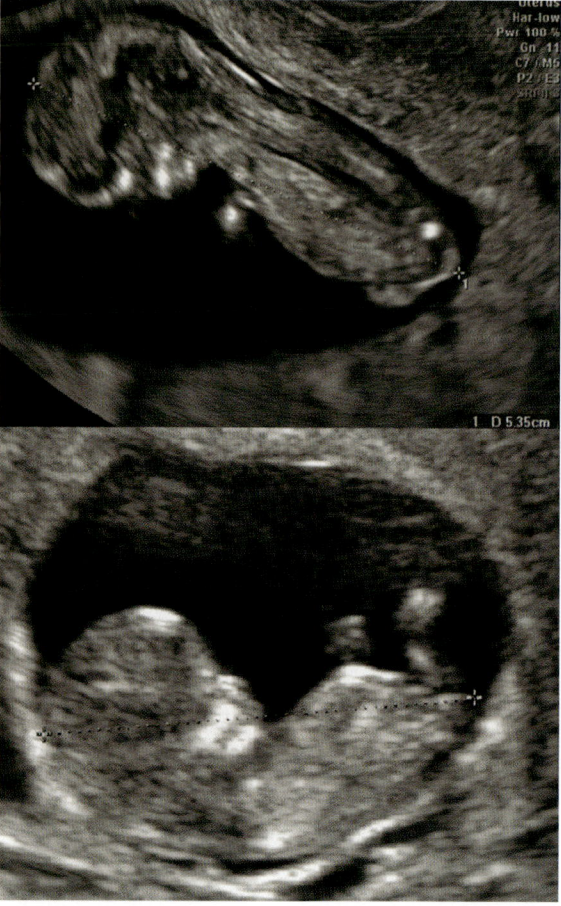

Figure 14.22 Eleven to twelve weeks' gestation. The foetus in this plane is a familiar image seen at many scans. The facial features are more distinguishable and the foetus can often be seen stretching and moving within the amniotic fluid.

The number of gestational sacs can be determined between the fifth and sixth week. By adopting a systematic approach of scanning through the uterus in both longitudinal and transverse planes, the cavity can be fully explored to ensure undercounting of gestational sacs has not occurred. Repeating the scan between weeks 9 and 12 may be worthwhile. The presence and number of amniotic sacs can be identified as early as the seventh week. The lambda (λ) or 'twin peak' sign refers to a wedge shape of the chorions between the two gestation sacs and is characteristic of a dichorionic diamniotic (DCDA) twin pregnancy (Figure 14.24). A 'T sign' occurs when only amnions are fused together and occurs in MCDA twin pregnancies (Figure 14.25). These signs are much easier to visualize in the first trimester than later in the pregnancy. By 20 weeks, about 10 per cent of dichorionic pregnancies will not have a lambda sign [5]. In the absence of amnions, the presence of two foetuses within one gestation sac indicates an MCMA multiple pregnancy (Figure 14.26). Higher-order multiple pregnancies are described in a similar manner (i.e. singleton pregnancy and DCDA/MCDA/MCMA twin pregnancy; monochorionic triamniotic triplet pregnancy) (Figure 14.27). The standard method for labelling twins is to identify them by the proximity of the gestational sac to the cervix. Twin 1 is located nearest the cervix and Twin 2 is furthest away (Triplet 1, 2 and 3, etc.). In a monoamniotic sac twins may only be distinguishable if they have different growth rates or one twin has a structural abnormality.

Occasionally, a bleeding (subchorionic haematoma) may occur and mimic a second (or third) gestation sac. Depending on when the bleeding occurred in relation to the scan, the haematoma may have a variable appearance, from isoechoic, to mixed to hyperechoic, but always conforming to the shape of the other gestation sac(s) and the endometrial cavity. Measurement should be carried out in three orthogonal planes and the relationship to the gestation sac and internal cervical os should be documented (Figure 14.28).

Tips and Tricks

- Make sure it is a genuine multiple pregnancy – a single gestational sac may appear as two in the transverse section of a sub-septated uterus.

(a)

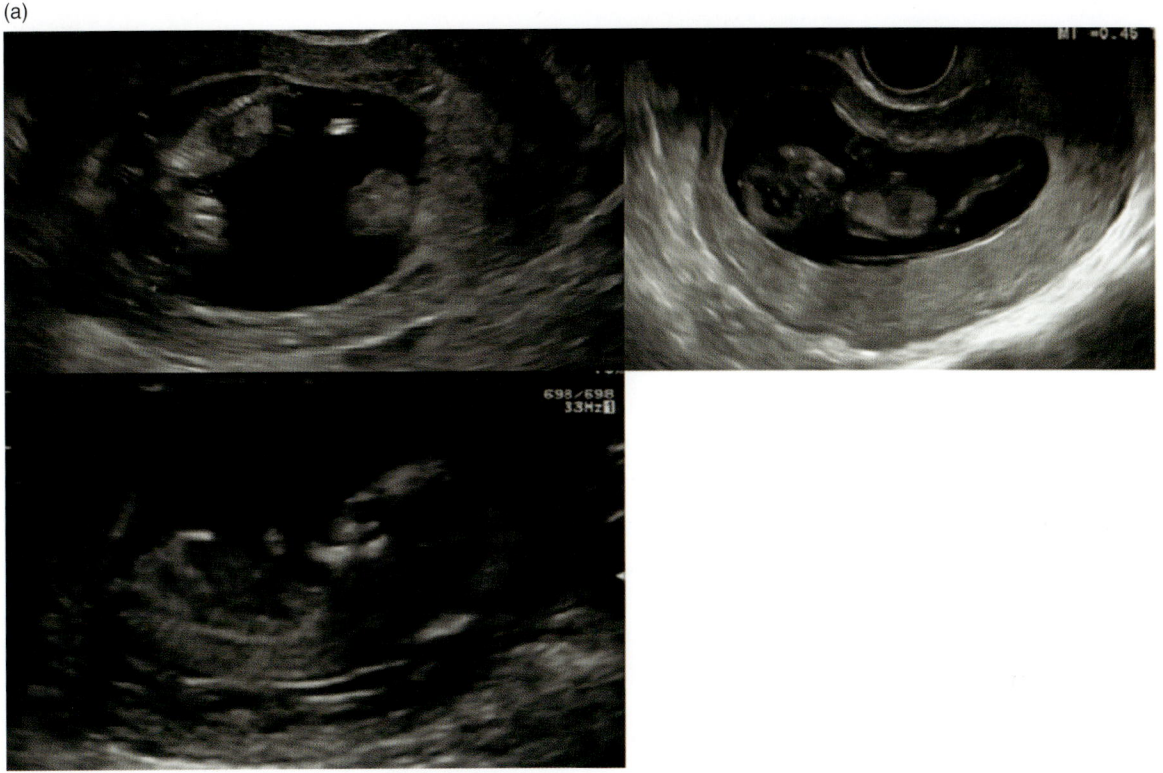

Figure 14.23 At around 12+ weeks. Eye sockets are visible, stomach and bladder can be identified. The two images in (b) represent a 3D rendering of a 12-week foetus with well-formed limbs.

- Visualize both/all embryos on the screen at the same time.
- Other possibilities to rule out are: a haematoma; a lateral artefact that produces the appearance of two sacs in the transverse plane.

Ectopic Pregnancy

The site of an ectopic pregnancy will affect its appearance on scan. Ninety-five per cent of ectopic pregnancies are tubal and are associated with a small, round, inhomogeneous mass in the adnexa, separate to the ovary (blob sign). The other classic description is that of a hyperechoic ring, referred to as the 'bagel' sign (Figure 14.29). These features can be seen in 50–60 per cent of cases, in addition to an empty endometrial cavity. If rupture has occurred, haemoperitoneum may be present in the pelvis, or haemorrhage may be present around the trophoblastic tissue (Figure 14.30). Other sites for an ectopic pregnancy include: interstitial (1–6 per cent), Caesarean section scar (<1 per cent),

ovary (<1 per cent), cervical (<1 per cent), intramural (<1 per cent) and abdominal (<1 per cent) [7].

Increasingly, ectopic pregnancies are being identified on ultrasound at earlier gestation due to better-quality scanning machines, increasing the management options for these patients. Identifying the exact location and type of ectopic is imperative in order that appropriate management can be offered. Confirming that a gestational sac is implanted laterally as opposed to being an interstitial ectopic will prevent unnecessary administration of methotrexate for a healthy intrauterine pregnancy. The interstitial portion of the tubes can be identified in Figure 14.31, which shows a transverse section of the uterus with the endometrium extending from the lateral aspect of the cavity through the myometrium [1]. Three-dimensional ultrasound allows for definitive diagnosis of interstitial ectopic pregnancies and should be considered as the gold standard diagnostic tool.

(b)

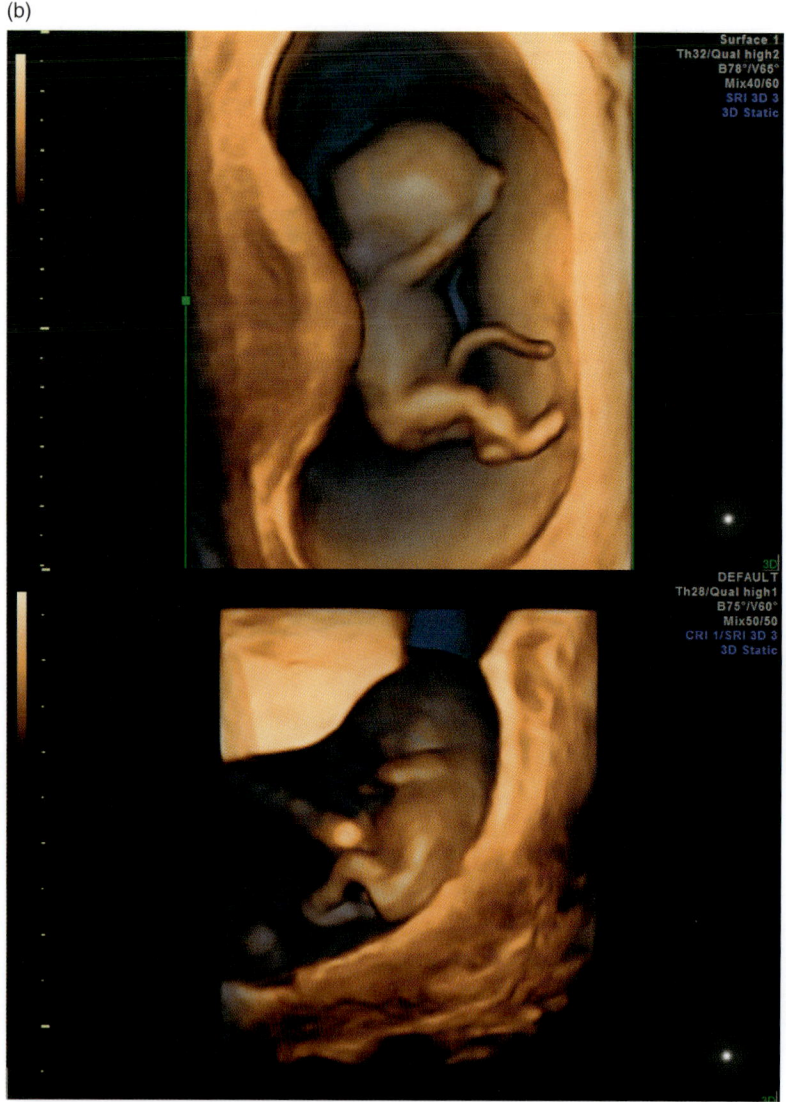

Figure 14.23 (cont.)

Tips and Tricks

- Use the gain to assess the fluid and determine the echogenicity; be aware that increasing the gain can make anechoic fluid appear echogenic.

In order to exclude an ectopic pregnancy located within the interstitial part of the tube, the rudimentary horn or the cervix, the uterus must be examined in the longitudinal section. Identification of the gestation sac along the line leading from the cervical canal, through the endometrial cavity to the pregnancy, confirms its intrauterine (endometrial cavity) location. Inability to visualize a gestation sac in the sagittal view of the uterus may indicate a high lateral implantation of a gestation sac or an interstitial ectopic pregnancy. In order to differentiate one from the other, a second opinion should be sought or, if available and expertise exists, 3D ultrasound scan should be utilized. High-implanting lateral gestation sacs on repeat scan (at least seven days apart) should be visible in the sagittal section of the uterus. In the transverse plane, a normal gestation sac will be positioned medially to the interstitial part of the tubes (Figure 14.32). The endo-myometrial junction

(a)

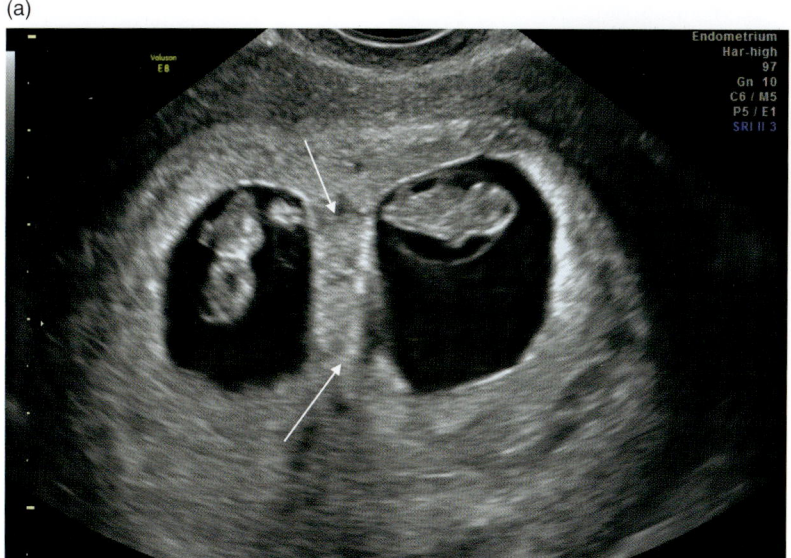

Figure 14.24 Dichorionic diamniotic twin gestation: the lambda sign is clearly seen in the two images in (a) and (b) (arrows). (b) A 3D reconstruction of a DCDA twin pregnancy. (c) At 18 weeks + 5 days' gestation, the lambda sign is not apparent with the chorion in the dividing membrane almost absent (arrow).

(b)

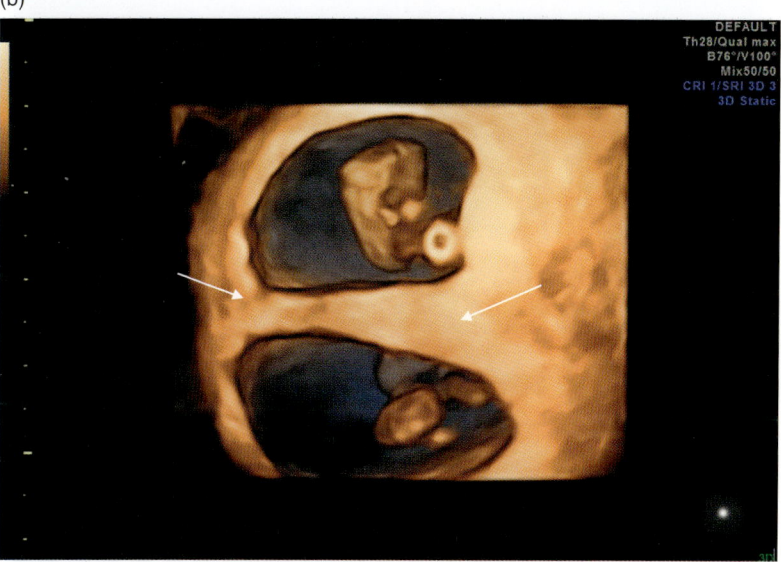

(c)

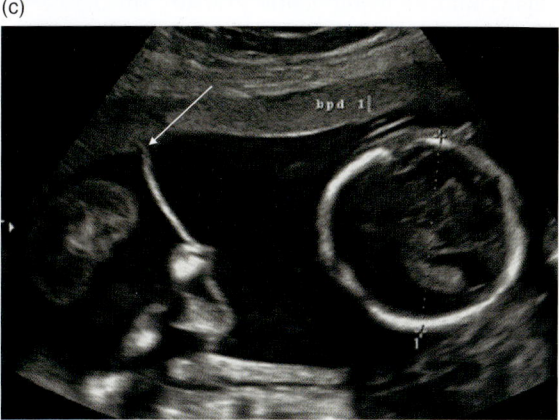

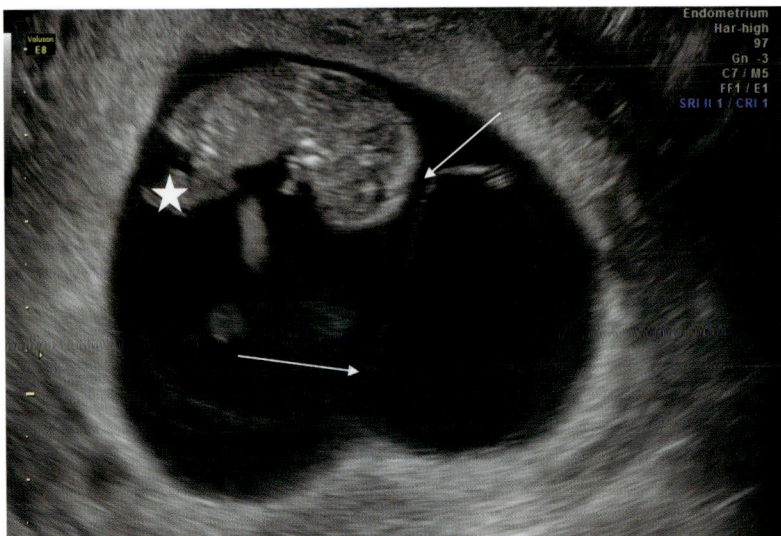

Figure 14.25 Monochorionic diamniotic pregnancy. The fusing amniotic sacs can be seen as a thin white line (T sign; arrow). Due to foetal position, only one twin is visible. Note the physiological hernia (star).

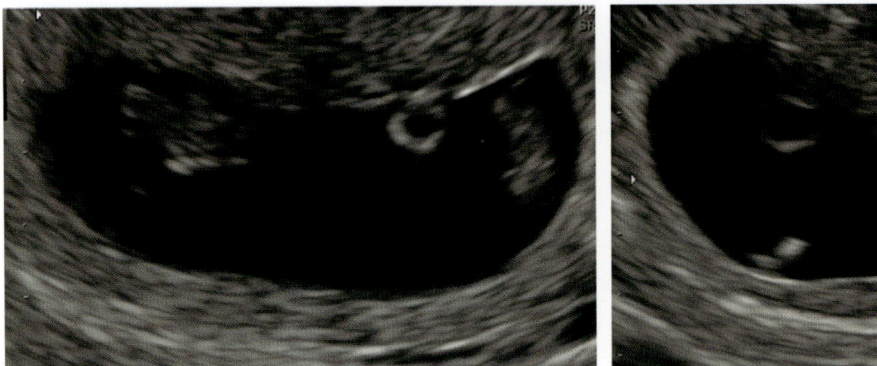

Figure 14.26 Monochorionic monoamniotic pregnancy. Note the presence of foetuses and yolk sacs within a single gestation scan with no visible separate amniotic cavities.

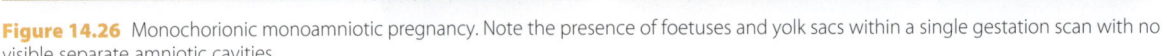

should extend around the gestational sac in contrast to interstitial pregnancies, where only a thin layer of myometrium surrounds the gestational sac (Figure 14.33); 3D ultrasound helps in confirming the diagnosis (Figure 14.34).

If the gestation sac is located low in the cavity or within the cervix, a detailed assessment of these structures needs to be carried out in order to exclude a cervical (Figures 14.35 and 14.36) and Caesarean section scar implantation (Figure 14.37). In a normal pregnancy, the gestational sac should be located above the level of the internal cervical os. If the sac is below the internal os, the practitioner needs to differentiate between the cervical phase of a miscarriage, and cervical and Caesarean

section scar pregnancy. Sliding the probe in the vagina and applying gentle pressure on the cervix may cause the sac to slide along the cervical canal in a miscarriage ('sliding organ' sign positive). Absence of the sliding sign indicates that the gestation sac is attached to the surrounding structures. Colour Doppler may be useful in identifying trophoblastic invasion in the cervix (Figure 14.36) present in a cervical ectopic.

The incidence of heterotopic pregnancy (Figure 14.38) is usually estimated at 1 in 30 000 pregnancies in natural conception, though the actual occurrence may be as high as 1 in 7500 [7]; with the advent of IVF, however, the incidence is increasing.

(a)

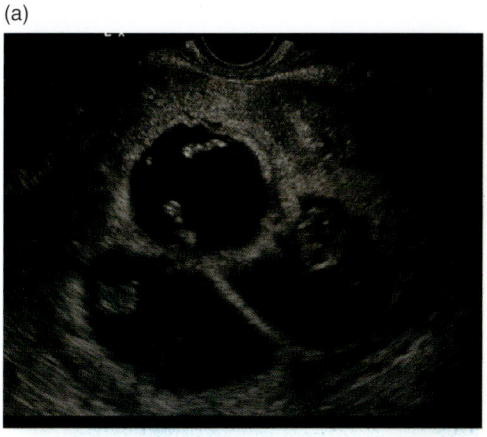

Figure 14.27 Triplet pregnancy. (a) Trichorionic triplet pregnancy. (b) Triplet pregnancy with a singleton and a monochorionic and diamniotic twin. Note the 'lambda' sign (thick arrow) separating the two gestation sacs. The 'T sign' has not yet formed, but two distinct amniotic sacs can be noted (thin arrows).

(b)

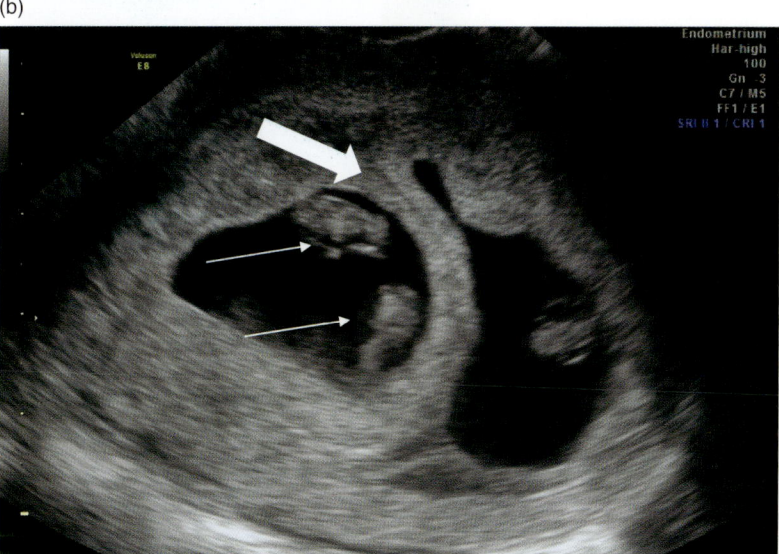

Tip and Tricks

- Once a gestational sac has been identified, its location in relation to the uterus should be confirmed as an ectopic or intrauterine pregnancy.

Diagnosing Miscarriage

Intrauterine Pregnancy of Uncertain Viability

In order to prevent the unnecessary termination of an ongoing pregnancy, it is imperative that the diagnosis of a missed miscarriage is made accurately and patients are aware of the limitations of the predictive value of ultrasound. Despite the anxiety patients may endure waiting up to two weeks for a diagnosis to be made, being certain of the viability of the pregnancy prior to instigating management is imperative [7–9].

If the mean sac diameter (MSD) of the gestational sac measures less than 25 mm and an embryo cannot be visualized, a repeat scan is necessary to confirm an early intrauterine pregnancy or whether a diagnosis of missed miscarriage can be made. In the case of the former, an embryo with foetal heartbeat (FH) can be seen at the scan 7–14 days later. While patients will be anxious about the wait, the longer the time between scans, the more definitive a scan result will be. For example, scanning someone a week after the initial scan may reveal an embryo of <7 mm but with no FH, in which case another scan would be recommended to confirm the viability of the pregnancy [7–9].

(a)

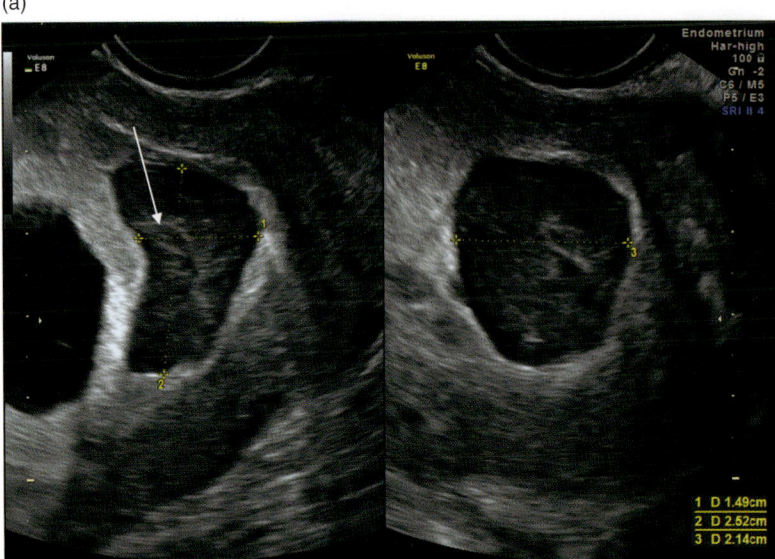

(b)

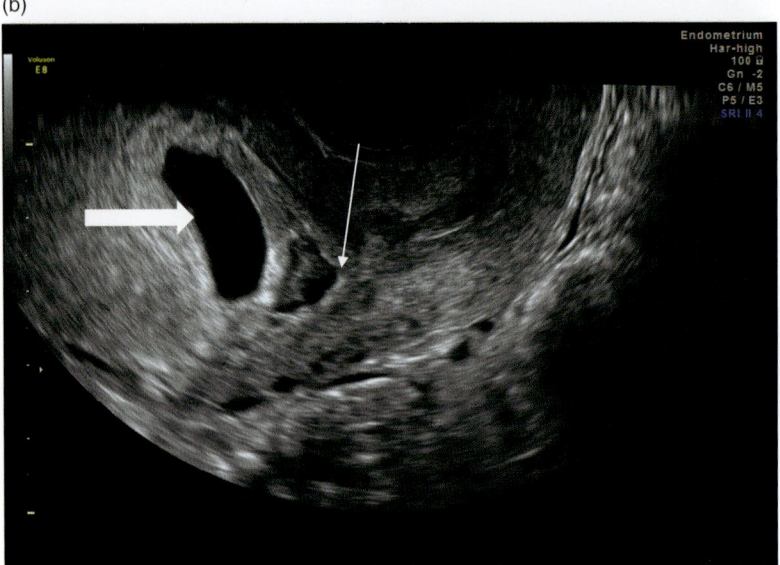

Figure 14.28 Subchorionic haematoma. (a) The measurements are carried out in three orthogonal planes (callipers). The content of the haematoma is beginning to organize and fibrin strands are becoming apparent (thin arrow). (b) In a sagittal section of the uterus, the haematoma is just above the internal cervical os (thin arrow) and below the gestation sac (thick arrow). (c) 'Chorionic bumps' – small haematomas (thin arrows) causing irregularities of the internal wall of the gestation sac – are often a poor prognostic factor. The yolk sac (thick arrow) is seen above the bump.

When a gestational sac and an embryo have been seen at the initial scan, but no FH has been detected and the CRL of the embryo is 7 mm or less, a transvaginal scan should also be repeated in 7–14 days to re-assess for foetal cardiac activity [9]. A pathway for management of such cases may be found in Figure 14.39.

Miscarriage

Due to the high prevalence of miscarriage in the first trimester, women attending the early pregnancy unit (EPU) will often be doing so due to experiencing vaginal bleeding and/or pain, or may be highly anxious due to their previous history of pregnancy loss. While most miscarriages will be due to chromosomal

(c)

Figure 14.28 (cont.)

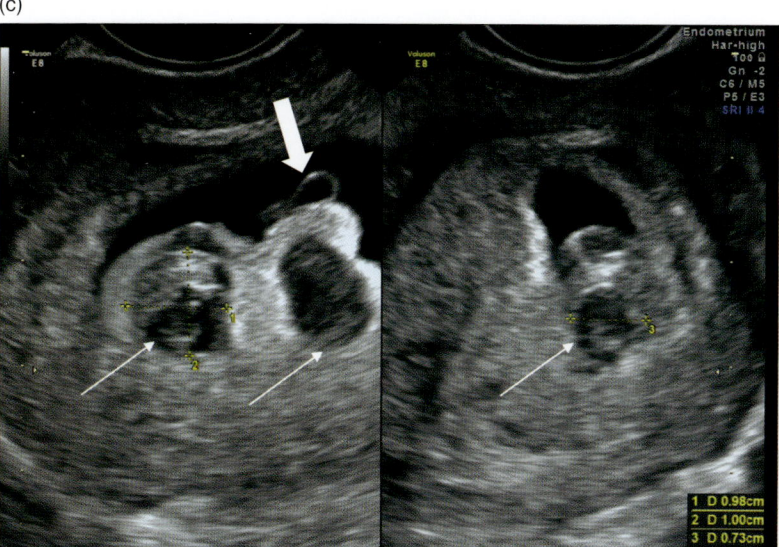

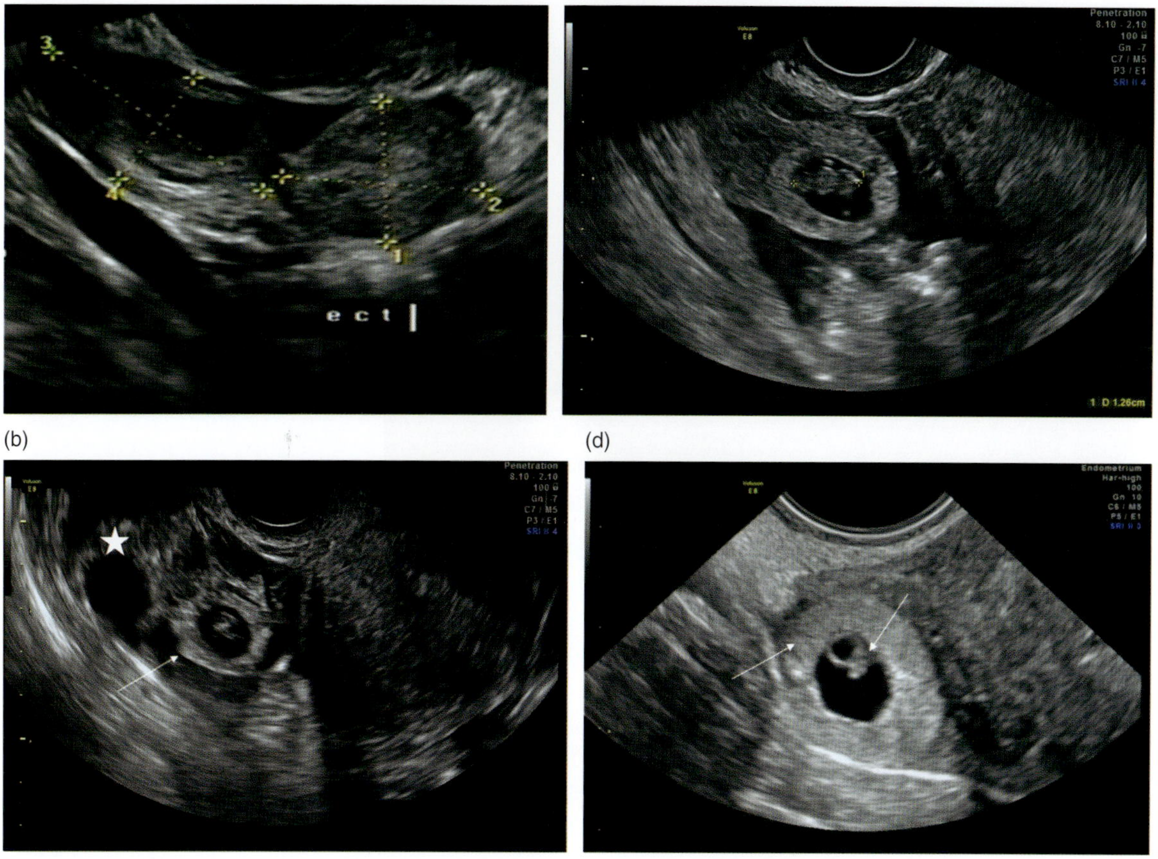

(a)

(c)

(b)

(d)

Figure 14.29 Tubal ectopic pregnancy. (a) Round, inhomogeneous mass ('blob sign'; callipers 1 and 2 adjacent to the ovary) and hyperechoic ring around the gestational sac ('bagel sign'; arrow). (b) Seen separate to the ovary (star). (c) An advanced tubal ectopic pregnancy with a CRL of 12.6 mm (callipers) and foetal heart beat present. The bagel sign is evident. (d) Proximal tubal ectopic pregnancy. Note the very bright placental tissue and the foetus with a yolk sac (arrow) within the ectopic gestation sac.

(a)

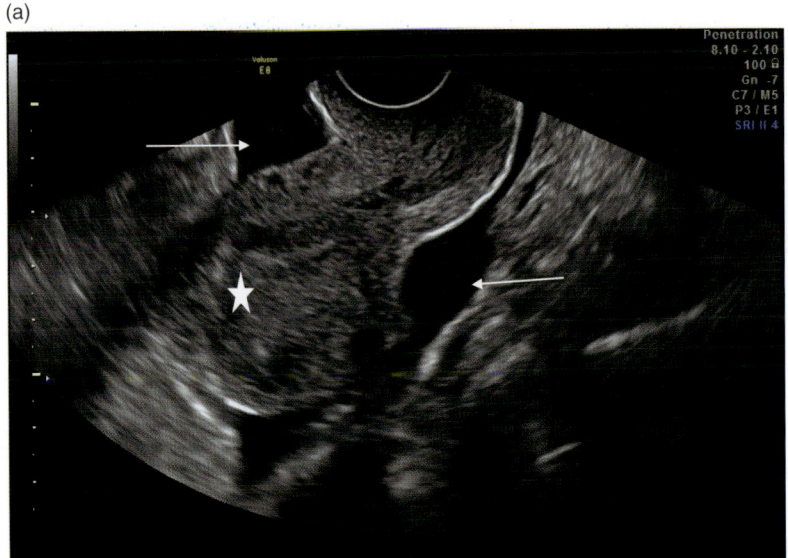

(b)

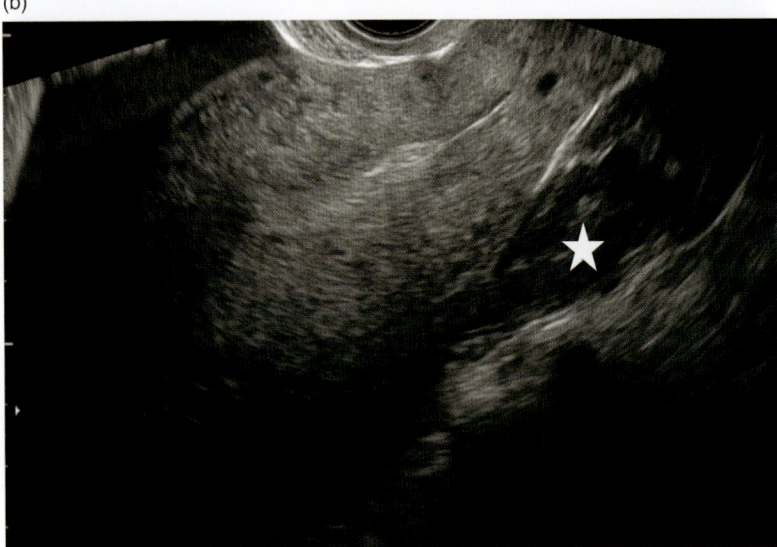

Figure 14.30 Ruptured ectopic pregnancy presenting with haemoperitoneum. (a) The endometrium is thickened and no intrauterine pregnancy is seen (star). Hypoechoic fluid may be seen in the pouch of Douglas and anteriorly (arrows). Careful inspection of the fluid (especially in the uterovesical fold) demonstrates small speckles (particles) and is highly suggestive of blood (in this context). In (b) an organized collection (blood clot) is seen within the pouch of Douglas (star).

abnormality, the loss of a pregnancy, even in the early weeks, may be of great significance to the patient and her partner. It is therefore important to deliver scan findings in a clear and sensitive manner and be aware that patients may receive the news in very different ways. This is especially important when discussing the intrauterine pregnancy of uncertain viability (IUPUV) diagnosis, when often an interval scan is necessary before a diagnosis can be made. Managing the expectations of patients is paramount, especially if there is a possibility that the pregnancy may miscarry before the next appointment. The possibility of heavy bleeding and pain should be explained to patients where appropriate. In the case of assisted fertility patients, treatment

dates should be taken into consideration rather than delaying the diagnosis of miscarriage.

A miscarriage can be diagnosed when any one of the following criteria has been met:

1. Foetal cardiac activity cannot be detected with a CRL of >7 mm.
2. A gestational sac has an MSD >25 mm with no CRL.
3. An interval scan has been performed confirming a miscarriage following an initial scan diagnosis of IUPUV.

Sonographic appearances of miscarriages at different gestations are presented in Figures 14.40 and 14.41.

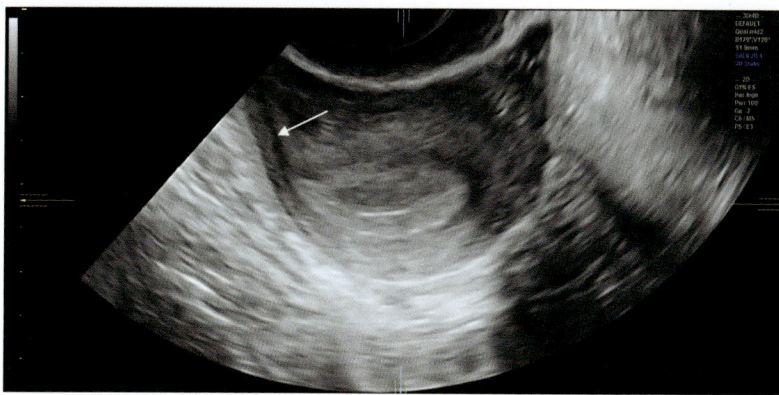

Figure 14.31 Interstitial portion of the right fallopian tube (arrow). It is rarely possible to include both on the same image due to anatomical differences. The image has been enhanced with volume contrast imaging (VCI) to allow for better tissue contrast.

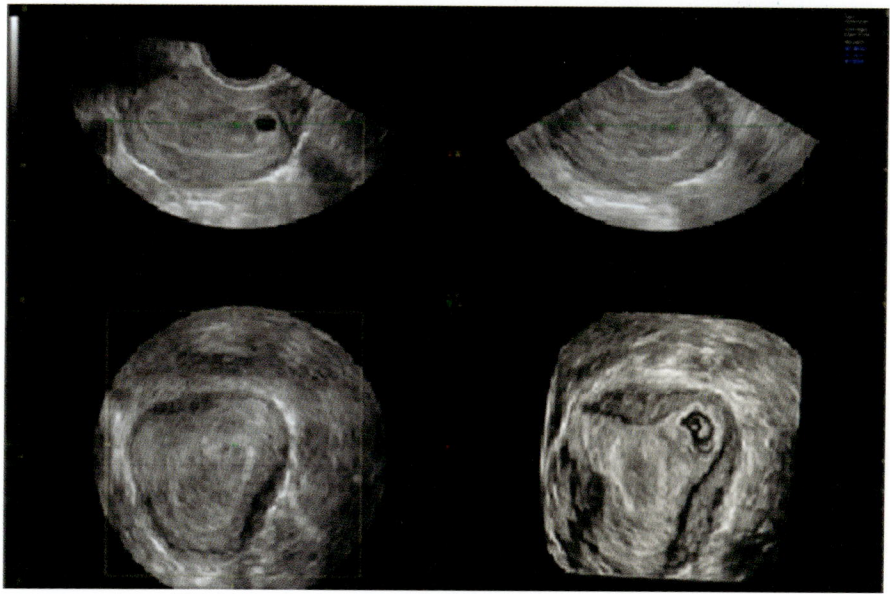

Figure 14.32 Intrauterine pregnancy towards the left cornual region (angular pregnancy), seen clearly on the transverse plane (top left image) and on the 3D coronal plane – rendered view (bottom right image).

Retained Products of Conception

When ruling out retained products of conception following a miscarriage, the endometrial thickness should be measured at the thickest point in the sagittal section. Be sure to pan through the uterus from each lateral wall and in the transverse plane to ensure products of conception (POC) are not missed. A measurement of less than 15 mm, where the endometrium appears smooth and homogeneous, indicates a miscarriage that is complete. Any disruption to the endometrial cavity may indicate POC, which have mixed echogenicity, as these may contain blood, trophoblastic and endometrial tissue (Figure 14.42).

Retained POC (RPOC) (Figure 14.43) can be mistaken for endometrial polyps, but the latter have a bright, regular appearance and contain a feeding blood vessel. Using colour Doppler to assess RPOC is useful to distinguish between RPOC, organized blood clot and an endometrial polyp. As such,

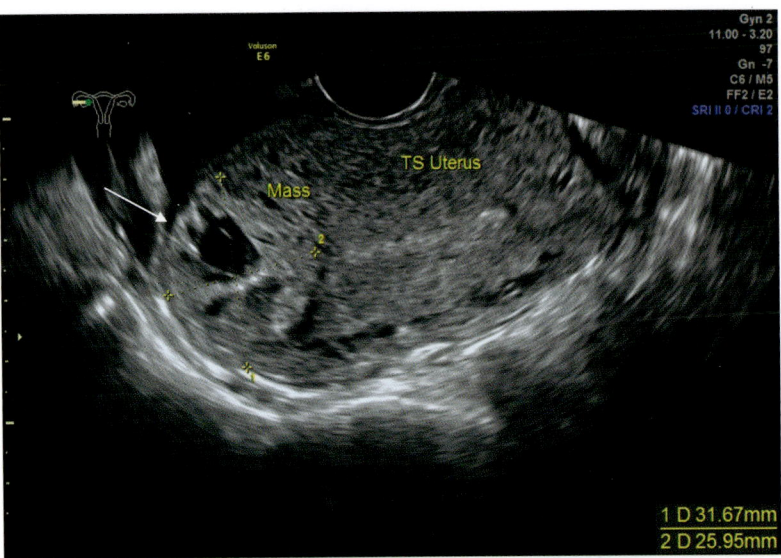

Figure 14.33 Interstitial ectopic pregnancy – transverse view of the uterus. The myometrial rim is almost invisible (arrow). The ectopic pregnancy ('mass') contains a hypoechoic gestation sac within.

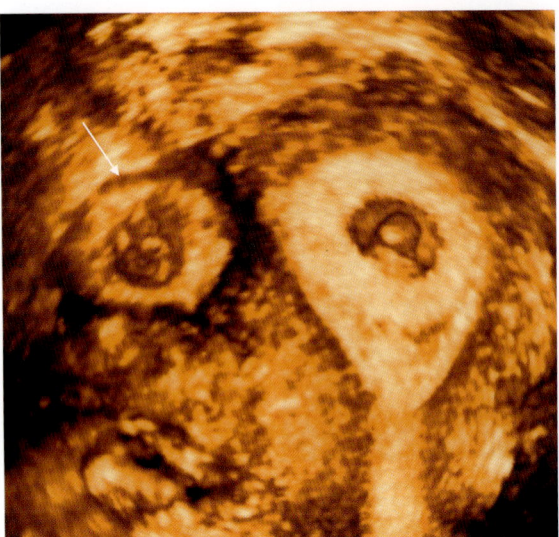

Figure 14.34 Heterotopic pregnancy with an intrauterine and an interstitial ectopic pregnancy – 3D coronal plane. There is a very thin rim of myometrium (arrow) surrounding the ectopic pregnancy. Image courtesy of Dr Amna Malik.

Doppler assessment should be carried out in every case of miscarriage and suggestion of RPOC. Identifying vascularity may also help to exclude an arteriovenous malformation (AVM), which will inform decision-making regarding surgical

intervention. In a complete miscarriage the midline will be intact from the fundus to the cervix and the endometrial echo will be thin and regular. As with every assessment of the uterus, imaging in the sagittal and transverse views with panning through the whole uterus allows excluding RPOC lateral to the midline segment or high up in the endometrial cavity.

Hydatidiform Mole

The classic ultrasound features of a complete molar pregnancy (Figures 14.44 and 14.45) are:

- an enlarged uterine cavity containing multiple cystic areas within a heterogeneous mass;
- the absence of embryonic structures; and
- in 15 per cent of cases, the presence of bilateral *theca lutein* cysts.

Retained products of conception which have undergone hydropic changes may also share similar cystic appearances. A clinical history of heavy bleeding is more indicative of an incomplete miscarriage rather than a molar pregnancy, as patients with a complete molar pregnancy will often have minimal bleeding.

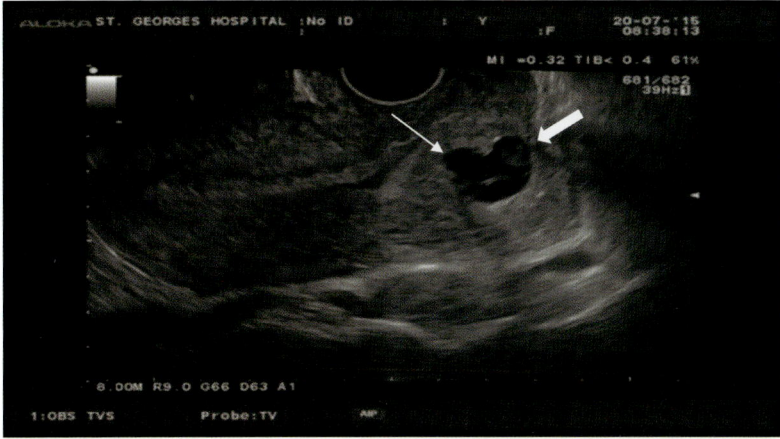

Figure 14.35 Cervical ectopic pregnancy. The gestation sac (thin arrow) is located just above the external cervical os (large arrow) and is invading into the posterior lip of the cervix.

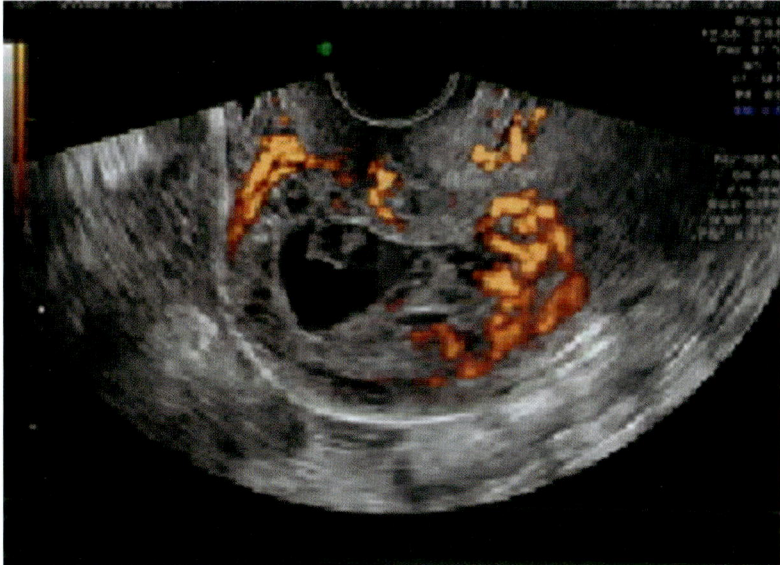

Figure 14.36 Cervical pregnancy with power Doppler on indicating significant vascularity surrounding the pregnancy sac.

'What Will Impede My Views?'

Views will be impeded by:

- high BMI;
- the presence of fibroids, which may distort the cavity. This prevents the visualization of a single plane where the operator can view the continuity of the uterine canal from cervical canal to the gestation sac. It can be difficult to visualize the enlarged fibroid uterus entirely with TVS;
- an axial uterus;
- incomplete emptying of the bladder, causing artefacts to appear and obscure the view of the cavity.

Tips and Tricks

- Find the cervical canal, then follow it into the endometrial cavity and to the gestational sac, thereby confirming an intrauterine pregnancy.
- Don't forget that a transabdominal scan can also be performed to locate intrauterine pregnancy if views of the fundus are limited due to fibroids.
- Adipose tissue can significantly impede views of the adnexa when looking for an extra-uterine ectopic pregnancy.
- Look at the settings on the machine: most now have a 'penetration' function that reduces the frequency of the ultrasound and allows for assessment of the deeper structures in the pelvis.

(a)

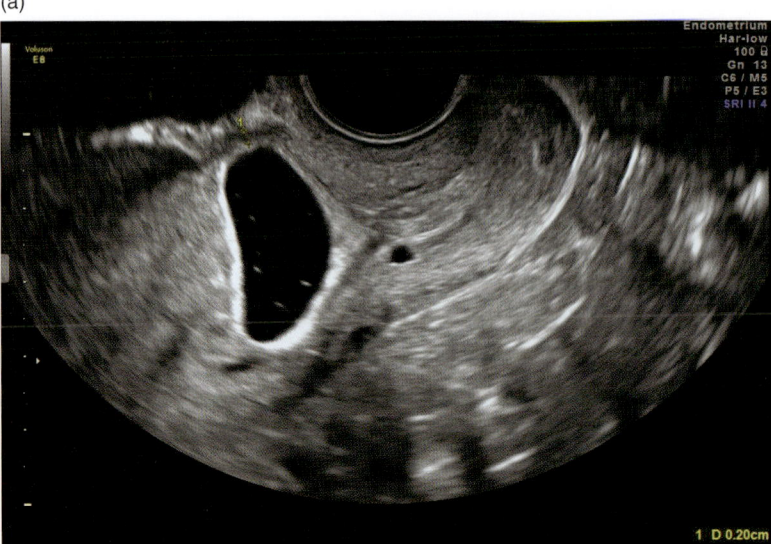

(b)

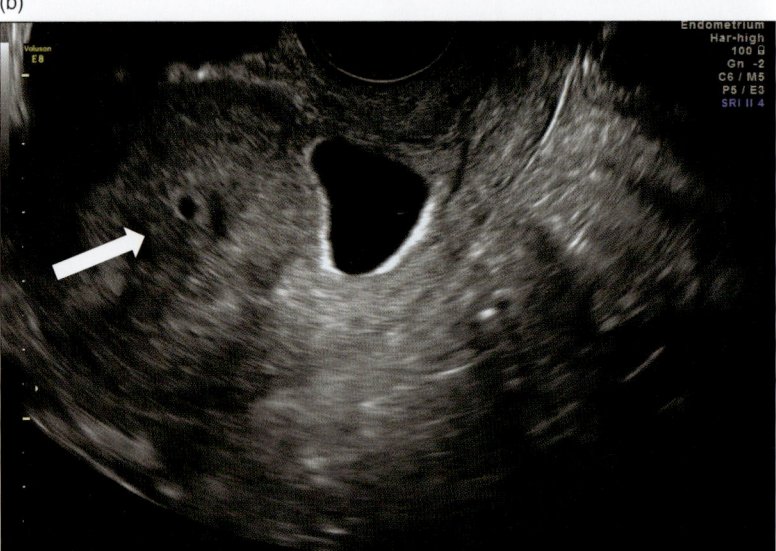

Figure 14.37 Caesarean scar pregnancy. Triangular gestational sac attached to the scar site with myometrial thickness at the scar site of 2 mm (a). Within the endometrial cavity in (b), mixed echogenic material is present, likely representing decidualized endometrium and blood clots (arrow).

References

1. Jurkovic D, Mavrelos D. Catch me if you scan: ultrasound diagnosis of ectopic pregnancy. *Ultrasound Obstet Gynaecol* 2007;**30**:1–7.

2. Jurkovic D, Gruboeck K, Campbell S. Ultrasound features of normal early pregnancy development. *Curr Opin Obstet Gynecol* 1995;**7**(6):493–504.

3. Chudleigh T, Thilaganathan B (eds). *Obstetric Ultrasound: How, Why and When*. 3rd ed. Elsevier Churchill Livingstone, 2004.

4. Alty J, Hoey E. *Practical Ultrasound: An Illustrated Guide*. 2nd ed. CRC Press, 2013.

5. Smith NC, Smith APM. *Obstetric and Gynaecological Ultrasound: Made Easy*. 2nd ed. Elsevier Churchill Livingstone, 2006.

6. Nyberg DA, Filly RA, Mahony BS, et al. Early gestation: correlation of HCG levels and sonographic identification. *Am J Roentgenol* 1985;**144**:951–4.

7. Kirk E (ed.). *Early Pregnancy Ultrasound: A Practical Guide*. Cambridge University Press, 2017.

8. National Institute for Health and Care Excellence (NICE). *Ectopic Pregnancy and Miscarriage*. Evidence Update 71. NICE, 2014.

9. Bottomley C, Bourne T. Diagnosing miscarriage. *Best Prac Res Clin Obstet Gynaecol* 2009;**23**:463–77.

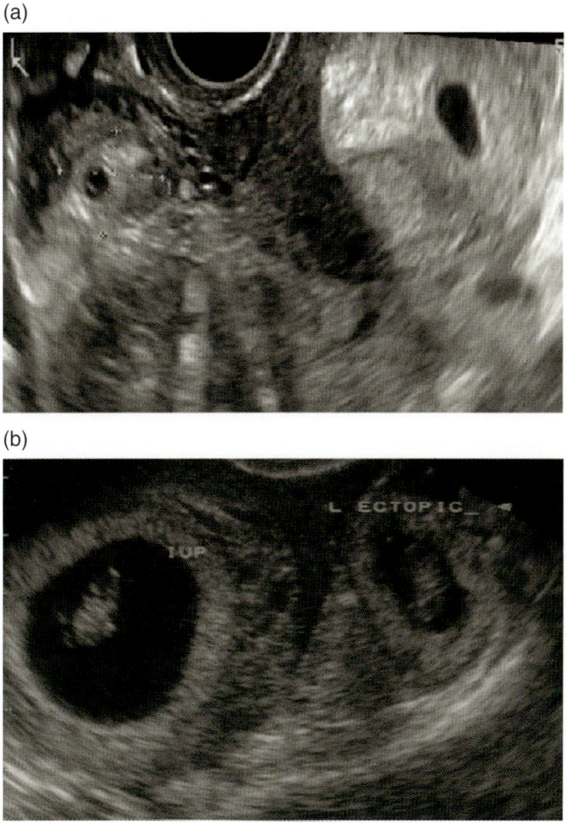

(a)

(a)

(b)

(b)

Figure 14.38 (a) Heterotopic pregnancy of about five weeks' gestation (callipers indicate the tubal ectopic pregnancy). (b) Live heterotopic pregnancy, with foetal hearts seen in both embryos. IUP = intrauterine pregnancy.

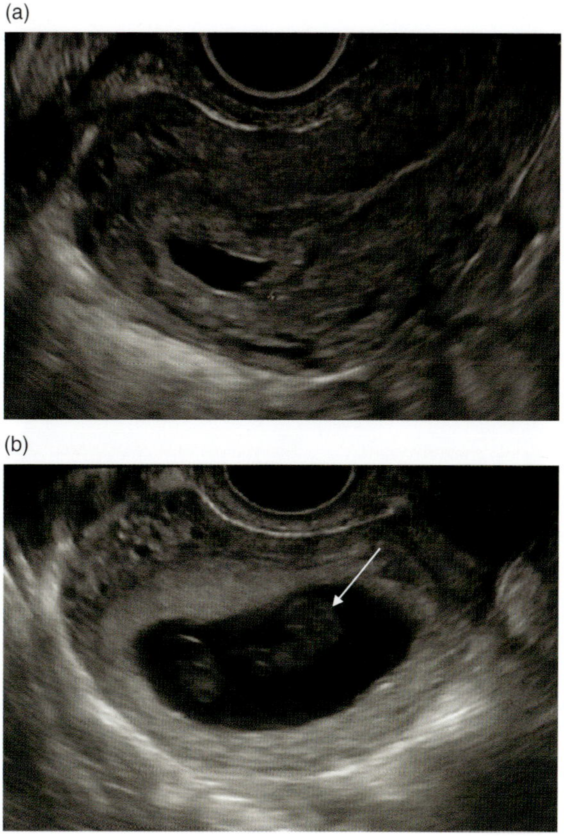

Figure 14.40 The gestational sac is not round and the outline is less echogenic (no bright ring surrounding the sac) than in a normal pregnancy. Note the twin embryos in (b); one appears curled up (sagittal view, arrow) and less echogenic than a live embryo. There is less definition of features than in a normal pregnancy of 8/40.

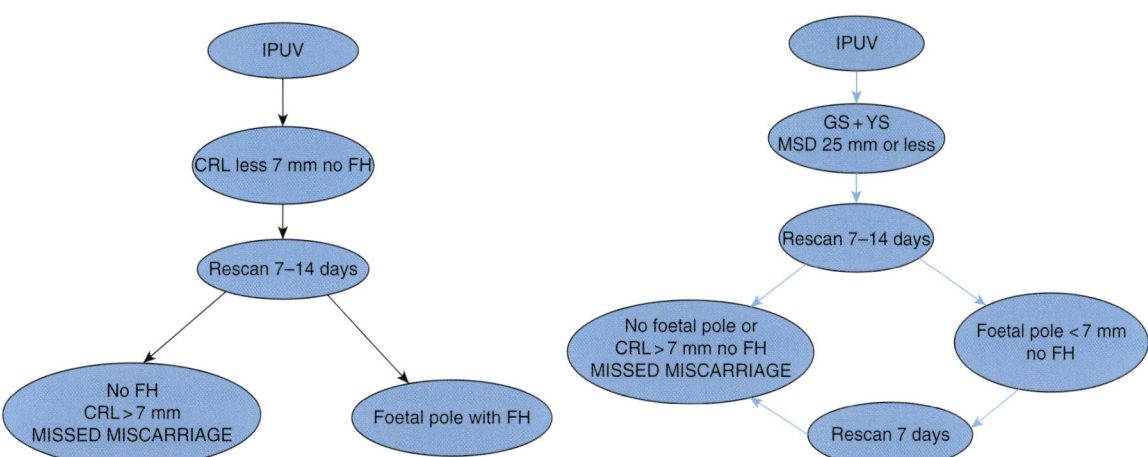

Figure 14.39 Ultrasound diagnosis of miscarriage and intrauterine pregnancies of uncertain viability (IPUV). Follow-up as in keeping with the Royal College of Obstetricians and Gynaecologists (RCOG) and National Institute for Health and Care Excellence (NICE) guidelines.

(a)

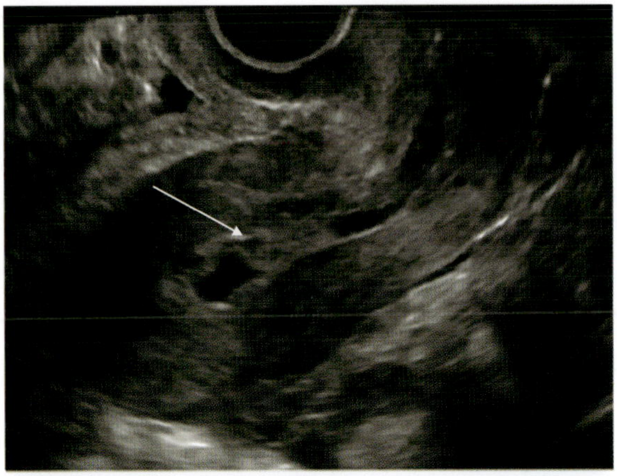

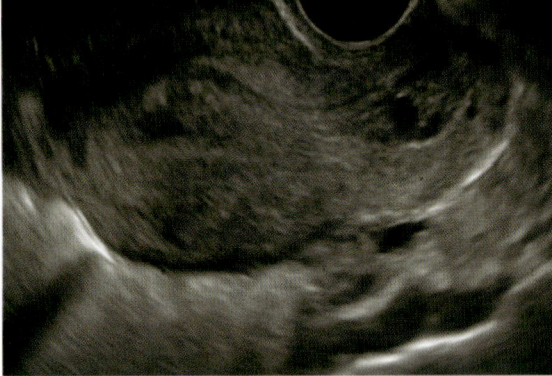

(b)

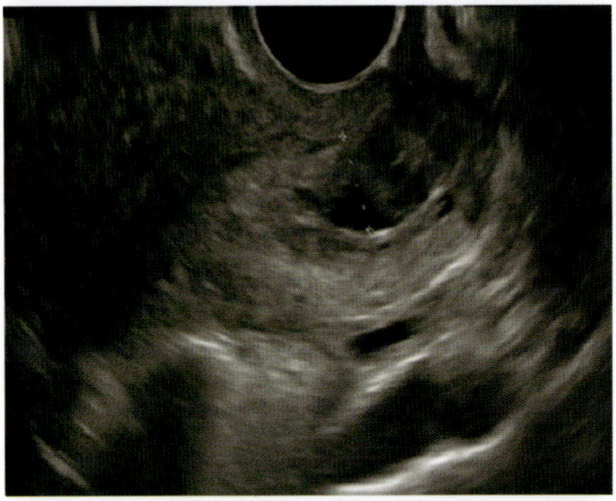

(c)

Figure 14.41 (a) The gestational sac has been passed but there is still tissue within the endometrial cavity (arrow). The internal and external os can be seen to be open in (b) and (c). These are all suggestive of an incomplete miscarriage.

(a)

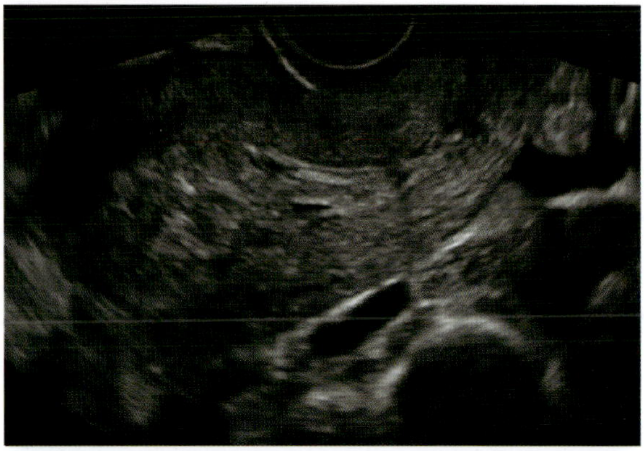

(b)

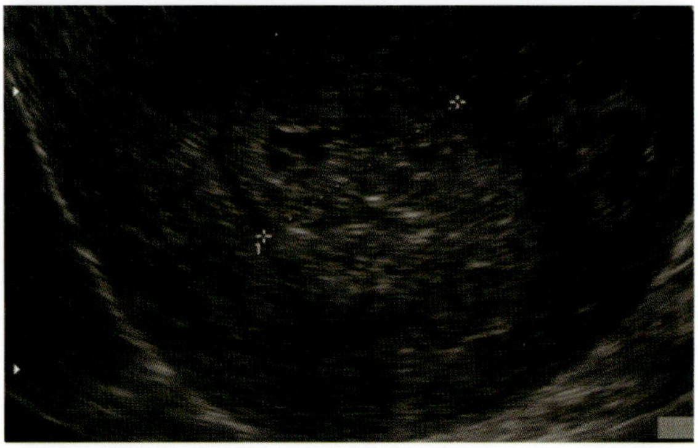

Figure 14.42 The midline can clearly be seen in (a) and there is a more homogeneous area (marked by callipers) of POC. The midline cannot be visualized in (b), but an organized blood clot can clearly be seen.

(a)

(b)

(c)

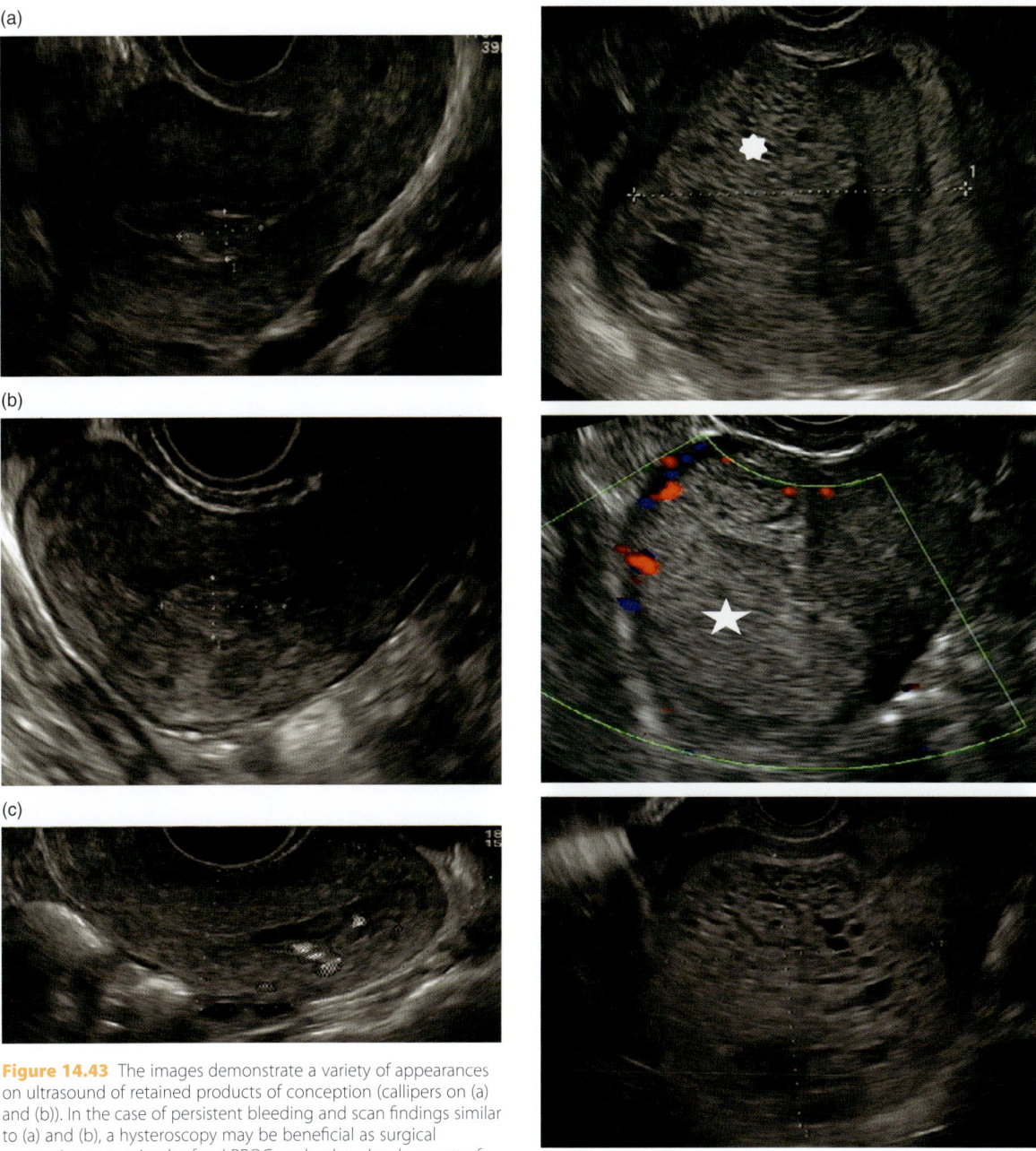

Figure 14.43 The images demonstrate a variety of appearances on ultrasound of retained products of conception (callipers on (a) and (b)). In the case of persistent bleeding and scan findings similar to (a) and (b), a hysteroscopy may be beneficial as surgical evacuation may miss the focal RPOCs or lead to development of intrauterine adhesions in the cases of repeat procedures. Addition of Doppler imaging (c) demonstrates vascularity within the myometrium but not the trophoblastic tissue. There is a high likelihood that this minimal amount of RPOC and blood (echoic fluid) within the cavity will miscarry naturally.

Figure 14.44 Complete molar pregnancy. Note the multiple cystic spaces within the endometrial cavity (dilated villi). The images demonstrate the typical 'snow storm' appearance of the trophoblast (star).

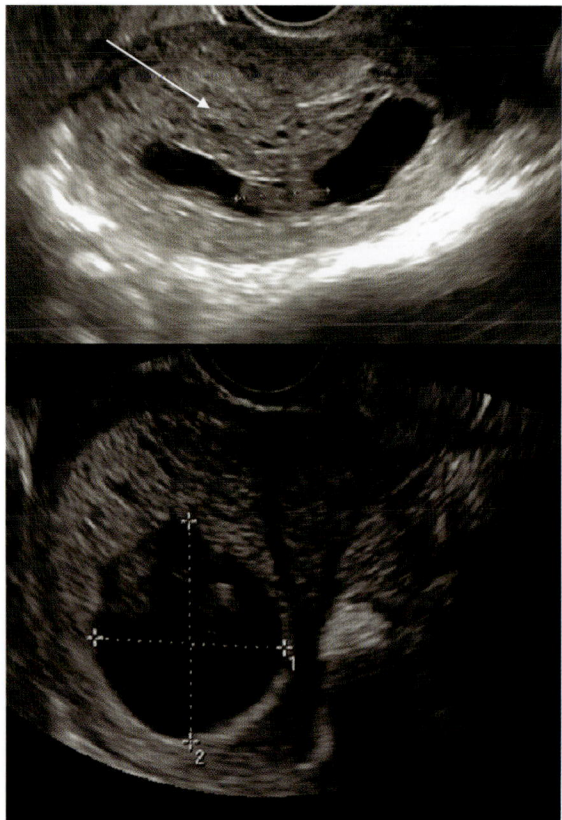

Figure 14.45 Partial molar pregnancy. The embryo (see calliper placement) can be visualized within the sac with cystic-looking trophoblastic tissue (arrow).

Tips and Tricks when Using Ultrasound in a Contraception Clinic

Sheila Radhakrishnan and Shilpa Kolhe

Introduction

Long-acting reversible contraceptives like intrauterine devices (IUDs) and systems (IUSs) and subdermal implants (SDIs) are widely used contraceptive devices in the world today [1]. Intrauterine devices and systems together are referred to as intrauterine contraception (IUC). In the UK, IUCs and SDIs constitute approximately 38 per cent of the contraceptives used by women of reproductive age [2]. Imaging plays an important role in a contraceptive clinic in ensuring IUDs/IUSs are correctly sited, locating them in case of missing threads and aiding in their removal or insertion. Of the imaging methods available, ultrasound is the most commonly used due to ease of availability, lack of exposure to radiation and cost-effectiveness. The transducers used to locate IUCs are usually a transvaginal probe and a curved transabdominal probe. The latter proves to be very useful in performing ultrasound-guided procedures. Other imaging methods such as x-rays are used only when a translocated coil is not seen within the uterine cavity on scan. A plain x-ray of the abdomen and pelvis will then help identify whether the coil is intra-peritoneal and extra-uterine or has been expelled. Magnetic resonance imaging (MRI) or computed tomography (CT) are very rarely used when assessing IUDs, but coils may be seen when these modalities are used for other indications.

Intrauterine Contraception: Types

When performing an ultrasound in a case with an IUC *in situ* it is always best to note the type of coil inserted from the history. Coils in general can be classified into three types.

Inert. These are rarely seen nowadays. It is a historic ring, seen sometimes in patients from China, where it was once quite popular. They are easily seen on ultrasound, lack a thread and are best removed under local anaesthesia as an ultrasound-guided procedure. If this approach fails, a hysteroscopy under general anaesthesia with direct visualization of the device may be the only option for removal of these coils.

Copper coils. These have evolved over the years from a first-generation device, through to the second generation and then to the third-generation coils (T Safe Cu 380A) that we see today. The current third-generation coils used in contraception clinics generally have a straight shaft with a horizontal arm in the shape of a T. The denseness of the shaft along with the copper coil makes it easily identifiable on a scan. The newer versions of the coils also have barium incorporated into them, which makes them easily identifiable on scans and x-rays. On ultrasound, both the horizontal and vertical stems of the copper IUD appear very echogenic (Figures 15.1–15.3).

Hormonal coils. Hormonal coils available in the UK market are the Mirena*, Levosert* or Jaydess*. The Mirena is composed of a T-shaped polyethylene frame with a 32 mm vertical stem and 32 mm horizontal arm containing barium sulphate. The stem has a reservoir containing a mixture of levonorgestrel and silicone covered by a silicone membrane [3]. On ultrasound the appearance of the Mirena IUD is characteristic, with acoustic shadowing between the echogenic proximal and distal ends (Figure 15.4), unlike copper IUDs, which are more or less completely echogenic [4]. While the early versions of the Mirena IUD were very difficult to visualize sonographically, recent versions have an easily identifiable shaft appearance with a slightly less echogenic but readily identifiable string.

Complications of IUCs

It is when complications of IUCs develop that they become radiologically relevant. These include malposition, uterine perforation, pelvic inflammatory disease and pregnancy.

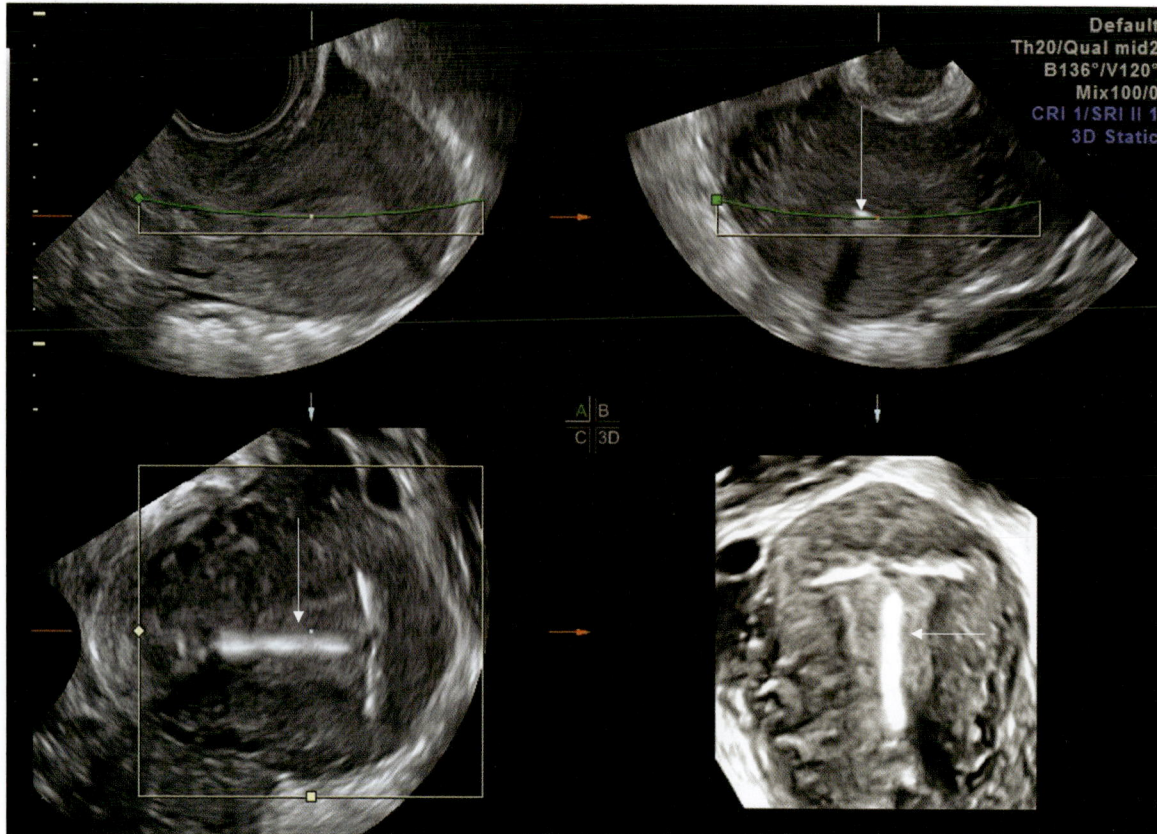

Figure 15.1 Three-dimensional multiplanar and rendered view of a copper IUD (arrows).

Malposition of the IUC

For an IUC to be effective it is expected to be as close to the fundus of the uterus as possible. There is no real consensus as to how much below the fundus the IUC must be before it can be deemed ineffective. For a copper IUD, if it is >3 mm below the fundus it is considered misplaced, with adequate contraceptive protection not guaranteed [5]. In theory, the hormonal coils (e.g. Mirena IUD) may remain effective in low positions. However, the guideline from the Faculty of Sexual and Reproductive Health is that if the IUC is at a distance of 2 cm from the fundus the contraceptive effect cannot be guaranteed [6].

On ultrasound, the malpositioned IUC can be visualized with the tip in the mid or lower uterus or in the cervix. However, for a hormonal IUD, as long as it is completely within the uterine cavity it will continue to be effective, unlike the copper IUD. Malpositioned IUCs can be a cause of pain, especially during intercourse. When positioned low they are also

at risk of expulsion spontaneously, though they are sometimes known to migrate into a normal position 2–3 months later [7]. However, the recommendation is that malpositioned IUCs should be removed and replaced unless it is an IUS that is completely within the uterine cavity. Three-dimensional transvaginal sonography has been shown to be more accurate in identifying the type and location of the IUC than 2D transvaginal sonography [8]. However, in clinical practice this is rarely necessary. Three-dimensional sonography is especially useful in accurate evaluation of misplaced IUCs as, with this type of scanning, structures that are not located in the same plane can be imaged simultaneously, thus giving a much clearer picture of the displacement [9].

There is evidence that in patients with prior uterine surgery it is possible that the IUC will migrate into the scar and be a cause of pain [1]. In patients with previous Caesarean section deliveries there may be extension of the lower end of the IUC into the scar.

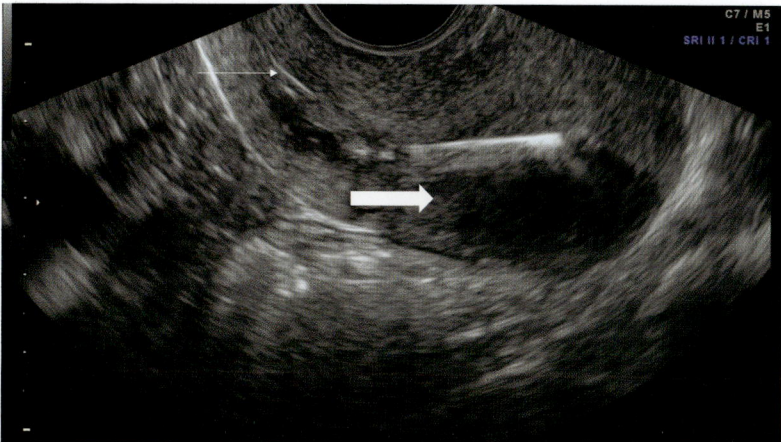

Figure 15.2 Longitudinal view of the uterus with a copper IUD, along with echogenic string seen in the cervical canal (thin arrow). Posterior shadow of the copper IUD is seen (thick arrow).

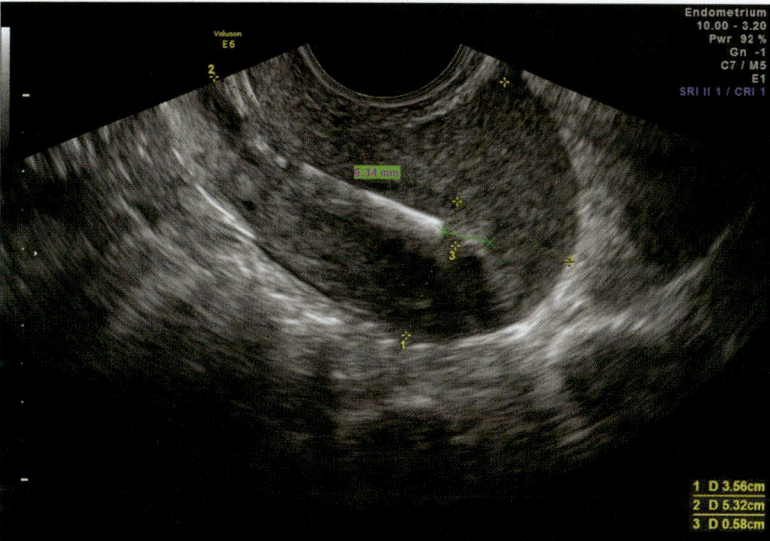

Figure 15.3 Longitudinal view of the uterus with a copper IUD. The IUD is displaced down slightly from the fundus (by 0.58 cm).

While the clinical importance of such migration is uncertain, removal is recommended only in the presence of pain.

Malposition can also occur when the shaft or crossbar of an IUC extends into the myometrium. It could be an incidental finding or the patient may complain of pain. Clues to this diagnosis are when the crossbars are low in the uterus or when they extend in an antero-posterior direction rather than the typical transverse position in the uterine fundus (Figures 15.1 and 15.2). Extension into the myometrium typically occurs at the time of insertion. Therefore, when scanning it is important to assess for extension of the echogenic portion of the IUC outside the endometrium into the myometrium.

Sometimes this can be a subtle finding, seen only on a single image.

Uterine Expulsion

Incidence of this complication is somewhere around 1 in 20 [6] and occurs within the first three months of insertion, especially around menstruation. Clinically the string of the IUC cannot be felt either by the patient or by the clinician. The possibilities are as follows: (1) the IUC has been ejected from the uterus; (2) the IUC is in the uterus (in either a normal or an abnormal location), but the string is broken or misplaced; or (3) the uterus has been perforated, and the IUC has translocated into the uterine cavity. The expulsion

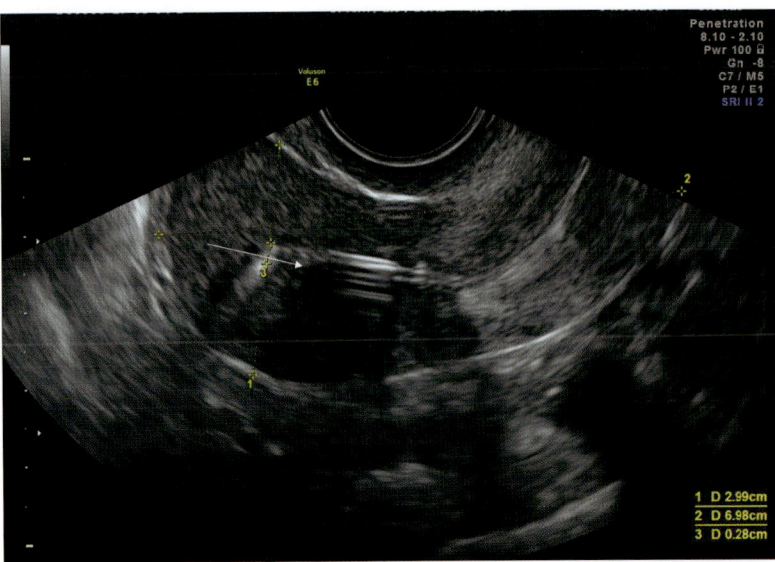

Figure 15.4 Longitudinal view of the uterus with a Mirena IUD. Parallel shadowing with no apparent linear echogenic shadow of the vertical stem seen (arrow).

rate is highest when the IUC is placed in the immediate postpartum period after a vaginal delivery [10].

Uterine Perforation

The perforation rate for IUCs is quoted as less than 1 per 1000 and is increased in the following instances: (1) with placement by inexperienced operators; and (2) when the IUC is placed less than six months postpartum. When the IUD migrates outside the uterus, it can lead to additional complications, such as bowel or bladder perforation. In addition, in a hormone-containing IUC, the serum hormone levels can be up to 10 times higher when the IUC is in a peritoneal location than when it is intrauterine. When an IUC cannot be visualized within the uterine cavity using ultrasound, a plain radiograph of the abdomen and pelvis can help in localizing the IUC.

Pregnancy in Patients with IUCs in Place

When pregnancy occurs with an IUC in the uterus, an ectopic pregnancy will have to be excluded. Therefore, patients with IUCs in place and positive pregnancy test results should be expected to have ectopic pregnancy until proven otherwise. However, intrauterine pregnancy can occur especially if the coil is malpositioned. In patients with IUCs and intrauterine pregnancy, the IUC typically is removed under ultrasound guidance to lessen the risks of infection, miscarriage and preterm premature rupture of membranes and/or delivery, which can occur

if the IUC is left in place. At scan, it is important to note the position of the coil in relation to the sac (Figure 15.5). Provided the coil is below the sac and the threads are easily visualized, removal should be undertaken as early in the pregnancy (within 12 weeks) as possible. Where the sac is below the coil it may not be possible to remove the coil without endangering the pregnancy and the patient will have to be counselled accordingly.

Pelvic Inflammatory Disease

Patients with IUCs are rarely at increased risk of pelvic inflammatory disease, as used to be thought in the past. However, the presence of cervical chlamydial or gonorrhoeal infection at the time of insertion of an IUC increases the risk of infection. Pelvic inflammatory disease can manifest as endometritis, pyosalpinx, or a tubo-ovarian abscess. Removal needs to be considered if there is no improvement in symptoms on review after 72 hours of antibiotic treatment.

Retention and Fragmentation

An IUC left in the uterus for a prolonged period can become encrusted with a fibrous reaction and can be difficult to remove. It may also be a potential site of infection in the postmenopausal period. At times, there can be fragmentation and retention of all or portions of the IUC during removal. Removal in such cases is best undertaken under ultrasound

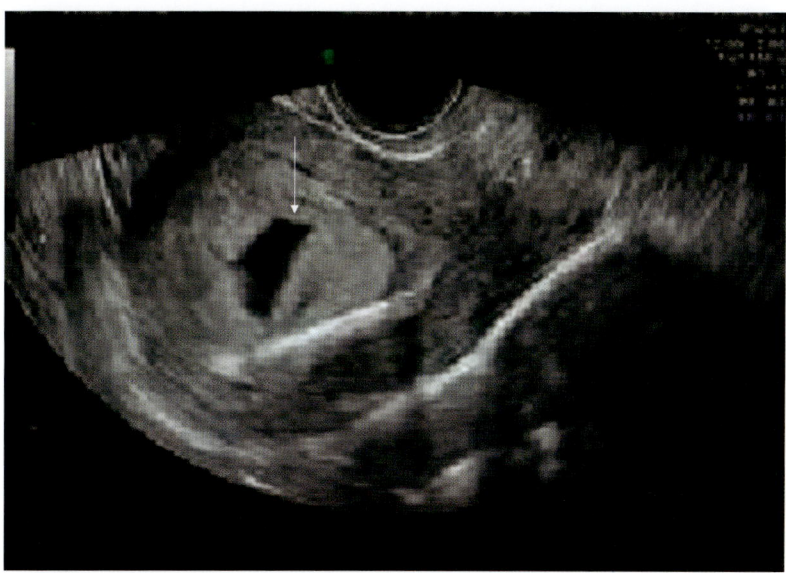

Figure 15.5 Longitudinal view of the uterus with a copper IUD along with an intrauterine gestational sac (pregnancy; arrow).

guidance to ensure complete removal. If all parts cannot quite be removed in this fashion, hysteroscopic-guided removal will have to be undertaken.

Subdermal Implant

The subdermal implant or Nexplanon is a single 4 cm-long rod composed of polyvinyl acetate containing 68 mg of etonorgestrel. It releases etonorgestrel at a rate of 60–70 mcg in the first five weeks of insertion and then slowly decreases to 25–30 mcg at the end of three years.

Use of ultrasound imaging in those using SDIs is usually undertaken when the implants are no longer easily palpable. This occurs when the guidelines for insertion are not followed or when there has been excessive weight gain resulting in an inability to localize the implant. These contraceptive implants are not biodegradable and are meant to be removed after three years or when the patient desires to come off the method. When they are not palpable, removal following the standard technique should not be undertaken.

If it is not palpable, until proved otherwise, it should be assumed that a non-insertion has occurred and investigations to confirm the presence of the implant should be undertaken while the woman is advised on alternative forms of contraception. One should not assume the implant is deeply placed.

Surgery without ascertaining the precise location of the implant also should be avoided [11]. A high-frequency linear array ultrasound is the first-line imaging technique for locating non-palpable or deep implants. If the implant is not easily identified with ultrasound, both arms should be examined for insertion site scars. Barium sulphate has been added to the Implanon/Nexplanon rod to make it radiopaque. This makes it visible on x-ray and CT scans, in addition to ultrasound and MRI. X-ray can therefore be used to investigate the presence/absence of an impalpable Implanon/Nexplanon that cannot be found using ultrasound.

Removal should not be attempted without precise localization and the presence of appropriate operator skills [12]. The linear transducer is best placed on the medial surface of the non-dominant arm (which is the usual site for insertion) at right angles to the length of the arm and moved slowly cranially and then caudally. This would approximately be at right angles to the implant. When present the ultrasound beams will bounce off the implant, giving a picture of a 2 mm hyperechoic structure with a hypoechoic shadow emerging from beneath it to pass into the deeper layers of the arm (Figure 15.6). An attempt is made to note the first 'end-on' appearance of the implant with the acoustic shadow inferiorly. This is marked with a skin pencil and on subsequent scanning when this shadow goes out of sight it is again noted. The distance between the two points should roughly correspond to a length of 4 cm, which is the length of the implant. The image should also give an idea as to the depth from the surface of the skin at which the implant is sited, its proximity to any nearby vessels, etc. Then, with an assistant holding the probe, the

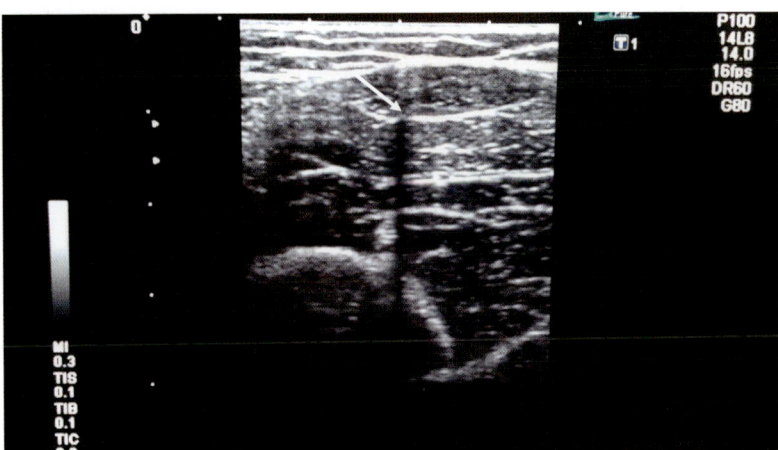

Figure 15.6 End-on appearance of the subdermal implant (arrow) with hypoechoic shadow into the deeper layers of the arm.

implant can be removed under ultrasound guidance using local anaesthetic and a 'modified U technique', with which the physician grasps the implants anywhere along their shaft, not just near the tip.

When implants are impalpable the general consensus is that they must have been placed deeply at the time of insertion, rather than being displaced subsequently through migration [12,13]. Deep insertion may possibly be more likely to occur in thin women [14]. Weight gain subsequent to insertion may make an implant less easy to palpate, and thus more difficult to remove.

Should an implant remain undetectable despite imaging, the manufacturer can send instructions for a blood ENG (etonorgestrel) assay. If ENG is identified in the sample, MRI may be considered for those with a non-radiopaque implant or x-ray for those with a radiopaque implant. With undetectable levels of ENG when the implant is within three years of insertion, it can safely be assumed that there is no implant present in the body.

However, cases of non-insertion have been reported from pharmacovigilance, spontaneous reporting and analysis of medico-legal cases. These cases are associated only with the single-rod implants in which the rod is contained within an applicator. Despite an applicator redesign from Implanon to Nexplanon in 2010, non-insertion [15] has still been reported with the new version and needs to be kept in mind when an implant is not seen on imaging.

Location of Essure Devices

Between 2002 and 2017, hysteroscopic sterilization was offered as an alternative to laparoscopic sterilization for permanent female contraception. The manufacturer estimates that 750,000 women received Essure [16].

With Essure, a coil designed to induce fibrosis and tubal occlusion is placed into each fallopian tube to prevent fertilization. This Essure micro-insert device is inserted hysteroscopically after visualization of tubal ostium and is typically performed as an outpatient procedure. The FDA recommends that three months following this a confirmatory test is done using either a transvaginal ultrasound or a hysterosalpingogram (HSG) to locate correct position of these devices and confirm tubal occlusion.

Unfortunately, Essure has been removed from the market after Bayer stopped distributing it in September 2017. We decided to include the ultrasound technique for confirmation of Essure devices in this chapter as it is relevant to the topic and there are women who have these implants in place. Besides using ultrasound as a reliable confirmatory test post-procedure, the knowledge of imaging of these micro-insert devices will also enable assessment of women who present with a past history of Essure sterilization.

Most centres offering Essure hysteroscopic sterilization used either HSG or transvaginal ultrasound as a standard confirmatory test. Transvaginal ultrasound has been evaluated and has been shown to be a less invasive test compared to HSG [17]. Transvaginal ultrasound is also more acceptable to women, thereby improving patient compliance and patient outcomes by minimizing their chances of unintended pregnancy. An ultrasound scan is unsuitable if the Essure procedure was challenging, if there was difficult placement of either of the two devices or if zero or more than eight coils were seen hysteroscopically at the ostium at the time of insertion.

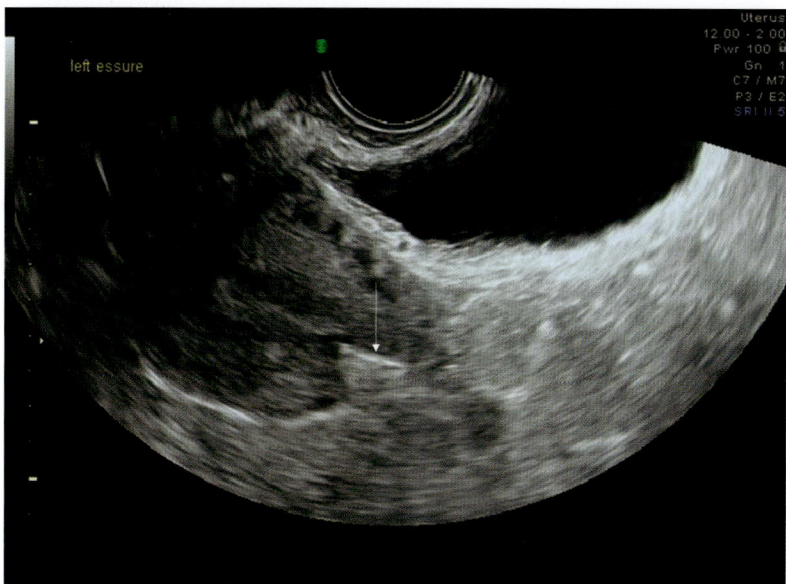

Figure 15.7 Transverse plane showing optimal placement of left Essure micro-insert (arrow) device in contact with the endometrium.

The transvaginal ultrasound should be performed using a high-resolution probe (minimum 6 MHz). A coronal or oblique coronal view showing a portion of each micro-insert in the cornua should be obtained. Sweeping in the sagittal plane, the intramural portion of the micro-insert can be seen in the cross-section. When the endometrium is visualized and the micro-insert is in contact with it, this is regarded as the optimal position of the Essure device (Figure 15.7). If the proximal end of the device is distal to the endometrium, it suggests satisfactory location of the device. This can be seen in the slightly deeply sited device (Figure 15.8). The linear axis of the device is seen within the myometrium in the cornua. The portion of the micro-insert located in the fallopian tube may or may not be seen, depending on the position of the tube. If ultrasound evaluation is unsatisfactory or equivocal, then the woman should be advised to undergo HSG to locate the devices and ensure tubal occlusion.

Conclusion

Imaging, especially ultrasound, has a crucial role in locating IUCs as well as in the management of associated complications. Knowledge of the various types of IUCs and their appearances will aid the sonographer considerably. Currently more and more malpositioned IUCs, IUCs with missing threads and IUCs in enlarged, distorted uterine cavities are being removed as an office procedure under ultrasound guidance.

Similarly, as seen above, despite a great thrust towards training personnel in fitting long-acting reversible contraceptives properly and improvement in applicator design of SDIs, there are still cases with impalpable implants. An additional linear array transducer helps in locating deep implants which can then be removed under local anaesthetic in the clinic. This decreases the need for operative intervention in theatre, thus proving to be a convenient and cost-effective procedure for the patient.

Tips and Tricks

- A systematic approach to scanning with a 2D transducer will allow conformation of correct placement of IUCs. This must be done in the longitudinal and transverse planes of the uterus.
- 3D ultrasound, where available, may help in assessment of IUC placement.
- Good practice suggests an immediate ultrasound scan after placement of the IUC to confirm its initial position. This does not guarantee that the coil will not be expelled.
- Inability to visualize a device does not equate to its expulsion or migration – failed insertions may happen.
- Small parts linear transducers should be used to locate subdermal implants. The site of both ends of the implant should be marked on the skin.

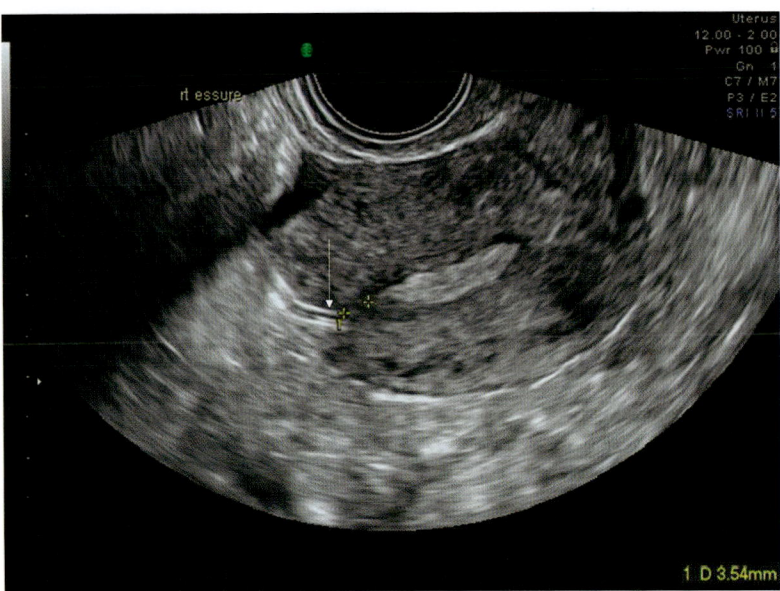

Figure 15.8 Transvaginal ultrasound with satisfactory/slightly deeply sited right Essure device (arrow).

References

1. Peri N, Graham D, Levine D. Imaging of intrauterine contraceptive devices, *J Ultrasound Med* 2007;**26**:1389–401.

2. Health and Social Care Information Centre. *Statistics on Sexual and Reproductive Health Services. England 2015/ 2016.* Health and Social Care Information Centre, 2016.

3. Schering Oy. Mirena [product information], 2006.

4. Zalel Y. Sonographic and Doppler flow characteristics of levonorgestrel and copper-releasing intrauterine devices. *Med Gen Med* 2003;**5**:38.

5. Wildemeersch D, Hasskamp T, Goldstuck ND. Malposition and displacement of intrauterine devices: diagnosis, management and prevention. *Clin Obstet Gynecol Reprod Med* 2016;**2**(3):183–8.

6. Faculty of Sexual and Reproductive Healthcare. Intrauterine contraception: CEU guidance. 2015.

7. Morales-Rosello J. Spontaneous upward movement of lowly placed T-shaped IUDs. *Contraception* 2005;**72**:430–1.

8. Bonilla-Musoles F, Raga F, Osborne NG, Blanes J. Control of intrauterine device insertion with three-dimensional ultrasound: is it the future? *J Clin Ultrasound* 1996;**24**:263–7.

9. Lee A, Eppel W, Sam C, et al. Intrauterine device localization by three-dimensional transvaginal ultrasonography. *Ultrasound Obstet Gynecol* 1997;**10**:289–92.

10. Muller LAL, Ramos LJG, Martins-Costa SH, et al. Transvaginal ultrasonographic assessment of the expulsion rate of intrauterine devices inserted in the immediate postpartum period: a pilot study. *Contraception* 2005;**72**:192–5.

11. Faculty of Sexual and Reproductive Healthcare. Progestogen-only implants, 2014. Available at: www .fsrh.org/pdfs/CEUGuidanceProgestogenOnlyImplant s.pdf.

12. Walling M. How to remove impalpable Implanon® implants. *J Fam Plann Reprod Health Care* 2005;**31** (4):320–1.

13. Singh M, Mansour D, Richardson D. Location and removal of non-palpable Implanon® implants with the aid of ultrasound guidance. *J Fam Plann Reprod Health Care* 2006;**32**(3):153–6.

14. Mansour D, Fraser IS, Walling M, et al. Methods of accurate localisation of non-palpable subdermal contraceptive implants. *J Fam Plann Reprod Health Care* 2008;**34**(1):9–12.

15. Rowlands S, Searle S. Contraceptive Implants: current perspective – a review. *OAJC* 2015;**5**:73–84.

16. Jeirath N, Basinski CM, Hammond MA. Hysteroscopic sterilization device follow-up rate: hysterosalpingogram versus transvaginal ultrasound. *J Minim Invasive Gynaecol* 2017;**25**(5):836–41.

17. Dhruva SS, Ross JS, Gariepy AM. Revisiting Essure – towards safe and effective sterilization. *NEJM* 2015;**373**:e17.

Doppler Ultrasound in Gynaecology

Ligita Jokubkiene, Victor P. Campos, Walter C. Borges and Wellington P. Martins

Introduction

Doppler ultrasound imaging can be used to identify and assess blood vessels by producing a colour-coded map of Doppler shifts superimposed on a B-mode ultrasound image. The effect, first described by the Austrian scientist Christian Doppler in the middle of the nineteenth century, has been used to provide information regarding blood flow in ultrasound's daily practice in the last five to six decades. Blood flow in arteries and veins can be recorded from the surface of the skin, allowing flow analysis in systole and diastole, in both normal and diseased blood vessels. Over time, Doppler techniques became an important technique in diagnostic ultrasound for haemodynamic assessment, replacing some invasive procedures in many clinical situations [1,2].

This chapter aims to describe the use of Doppler ultrasound in gynaecology, the most important Doppler settings in gynaecology and its role in diagnosing normal and pathological findings.

Doppler Settings

Blood flow can be detected and visualized by colour, power and pulse wave Doppler. While pulse wave Doppler is widely used in obstetrics, colour and power Doppler give us essential information in gynaecology. With the help of colour Doppler, colour pixels with Doppler frequency shift are visualized and colour content in a structure can be subjectively assessed. Colour Doppler offers also the possibility to identify the direction of flow. In power Doppler – also referred to as energy Doppler, amplitude Doppler or Doppler angiography – the energy of backscattered ultrasound waves with changed frequency is displayed. It is mandatory to take into account that in order to detect Doppler signals, the correct Doppler settings are essential. In gynaecology, blood vessels with low velocities are examined and assessed – therefore, Doppler settings are different from those used in obstetrics.

In daily practice the ultrasound examiner needs to 'calibrate his/her brain' to the quality of the ultrasound system (Doppler technique sensitivity) and will make many changes to the controls and try different probe positions to optimize the image [3]. Factors affecting Doppler ultrasound image are: Doppler gain, power, frequency, pulse repetition frequency (PRF), wall motion filter (WMF), Doppler persistence, angle of insonation, distance between transducer and the vessels, the size of region of interest and density of red blood corpuscles. These Doppler settings and factors affecting Doppler ultrasound examination have to be taken into account for each patient. Out of these, the three most important Doppler settings are PRF, WMF and gain. In gynaecology, we suggest using low PRF (0.3–0.6 kHz) and low WMF to avoid missing low-velocity flows. For adjusting the gain, we suggest using the sub-noise technique. Briefly, the sub-noise gain is obtained by increasing gain until noise artefacts are visible, then reducing it until the artefacts just disappear [4].

Uterus: Changes through the Menstrual Cycle

Vascularization of the endometrium changes every month because of physiological angiogenesis in women with natural menstrual cycles. In 3D power Doppler ultrasound studies, endometrial vascularization was found to increase during the follicular phase and reach a maximum two or three days before ovulation, and thereafter decrease dramatically 2–5 days after ovulation and then increase progressively during the remaining luteal phase [5,6]. Low vascularization in the endometrium directly after ovulation might be important for endometrial receptivity and angiogenesis. In postmenopausal women, normal endometrium is thin (≤4 mm) and no blood flow in the endometrium is detected using Doppler ultrasound [7].

Infertility

Tubal Patency

Increasing interest has been given to ultrasound evaluation of subfertile women and a thorough investigation of infertility factors is proposed by performing a single ultrasound scan between days 5 and 9 of the menstrual cycle: the 'one-stop shop' approach [8]. As part of this comprehensive strategy, tubal patency status is usually assessed by injecting echogenic contrast media (air + saline in hysterocontrast sono-salpingography (HyCoSy); foam in hystero-salpingo-foam sonography (HyFoSy)) into the uterine cavity [9].

Doppler and 3D ultrasound can be used as complementary tools for investigating tubal patency, enhancing diagnostic accuracy [9]. During 2D/3D ultrasound scan with a vaginal probe, power Doppler is turned on simultaneously with foam injection in a transverse/coronal view of the uterus at the level of the uterine horns; this is the 2D/3D Doppler HyFoSy technique [10] (Figure 16.1). A pervious tube creates a positive flow next to the uterine lateral wall, suggesting free movement of the contrast media along the tubal lumen. A positive flow has been recently described as the 'flaming-tubes' sign [10], and it is

helpful to improve the reliability of tubal patency testing [11].

Endometrial Receptivity for Embryo Transfer

Some reports have suggested that Doppler, particularly 3D power Doppler quantification, could be useful to predict outcomes after embryo transfer as higher pregnancy and lower miscarriage rates would occur in a highly vascular endometrium; in such a scenario, spectral Doppler would help identify an endometrium with lower resistance or higher vascularization indices and select the ideal cycle for embryo transfer [12–16].

However, conflicting results [12,17], high heterogeneity among study designs and variables measured [14], small numbers of patients included [17] and low reproducibility and high dependency on machine settings [18] still represent major limitations, and the evaluation of endometrial vascularization by Doppler ultrasound is still considered a very limited tool for assessing endometrial receptivity [19].

Benign Uterine Pathology

The use of Doppler ultrasound in assessing the endometrium and uterine cavity shows good performance in differentiating benign from malignant endometrial lesions [20,21]. The endometrial pathologies are different in their vascularization, and Doppler ultrasound helps to identify blood vessels in different lesions.

Endometrial Hyperplasia

Endometrial hyperplasia is a condition that might be suspected at ultrasound examination. The morphological appearance of the endometrium with endometrial hyperplasia with and without atypia overlaps. The progression of atypical hyperplasia to endometrial cancer might be observed in up to 28 per cent of cases, which increases the importance of its early detection [22]. When using colour and power Doppler, in the case of endometrial hyperplasia disordered vessels may be seen (Figure 16.2), while the presence of multiple vessels with focal origin may be associated with endometrial cancer.

Multifocal vascularization at the endometrial–myometrial junction is related to non-specific findings,

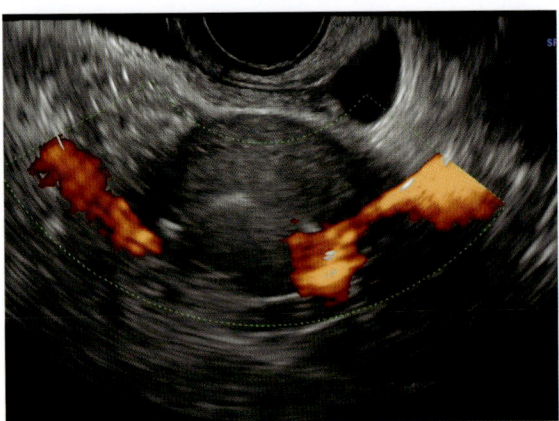

Figure 16.1 Ultrasound examination of tubal patency using the HyFoSy technique: power Doppler is turned on simultaneously with foam injection in a transverse view of the uterus at the level of the uterine horns.

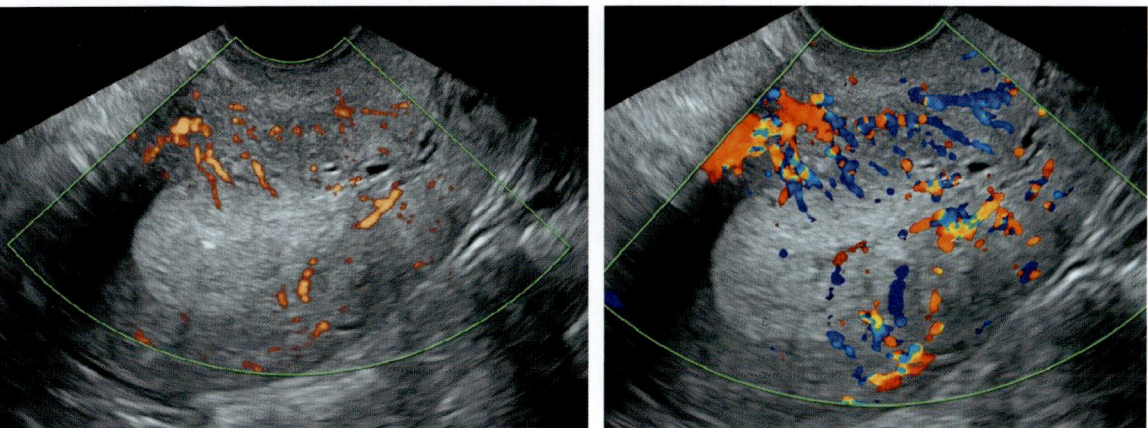

Figure 16.2 Complex endometrial hyperplasia with atypia in a 61-year-old woman with postmenopausal bleeding. Ultrasound examination shows hyperechoic endometrium with multiple vessels of multifocal origin.

(a) (b)

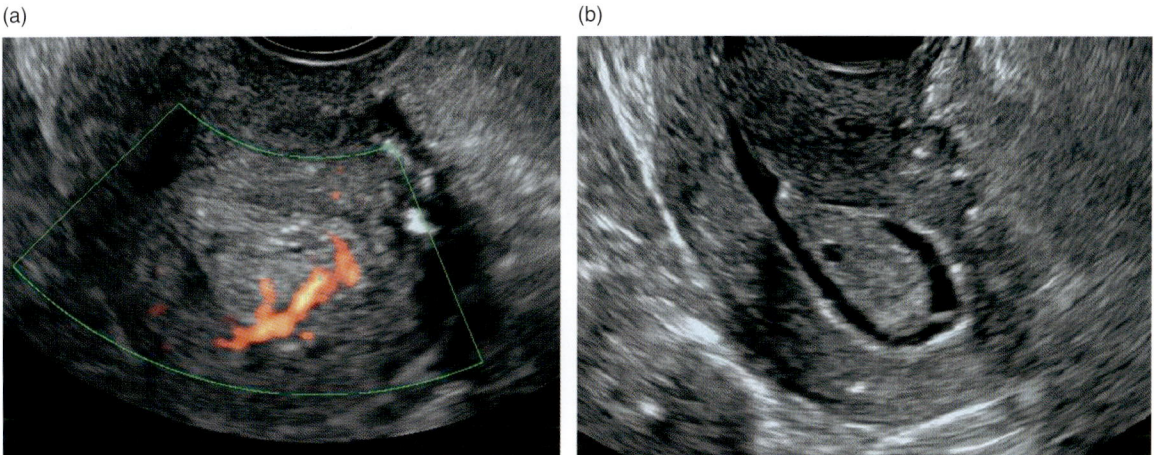

Figure 16.3 Benign endometrial polyp in an 88-year-old woman with postmenopausal bleeding. Ultrasound examination shows (a) retroverted uterus, thick endometrium and 'pedicle artery', endometrial polyp is suspected; (b) intrauterine focal lesion is clearly visible during saline sonohysterography. The histology showed benign endometrial polyp.

including atrophic endometrium, secretory or prolif-erative endometritis.

Endometrial Polyp

Most endometrial polyps are benign; however, 1–4 per cent of polyps may be malignant [23,24]. Several factors are related to the increased risk of endo-metrial cancer, such as age, overweight, diabetes, hypertension, Lynch syndrome and polycystic ovary syndrome. There is a strong relationship between the presence of a feeding vessel (a pedicle artery) and the diagnosis of polyp, with a specificity of 98 per cent and a positive predictive value of 96 per cent [25] (Figure 16.3). The presence of a single dominant vessel, a 'pedicle artery', with or without branching, in the Doppler study decreases the risk of malignant lesion. However, pedicle artery is observed in only 24 per cent of the polyps in postmenopausal women [7].

Myoma

Uterine myoma is a common benign gynaecological condition, affecting about 25 per cent of women. Myomas are usually well-defined lesions [26]. A typical myoma has a circumferential or intralesional blood flow

221

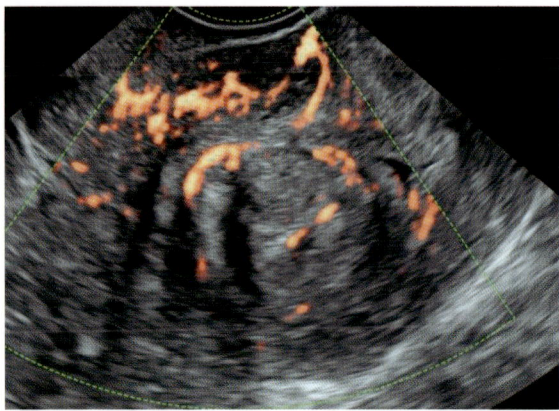

Figure 16.4 Benign uterine myoma. Circumferential and intralesional blood flow is commonly seen on Doppler ultrasound

pattern [27,28] (Figure 16.4). The vascular patterns of myomas and focal adenomyosis (adenomyomas) are different and colour and power Doppler ultrasound may help in discriminating these pathologies.

Adenomyosis

Adenomyosis can be diagnosed using greyscale ultrasound [28–30]; however, histological examination of the uterus specimen is still the gold standard. Focal adenomyosis (adenomyoma) might simulate a myoma on greyscale ultrasound examination. In the case of focal adenomyosis, the lesion is ill-defined and has translesional flow, i.e. blood vessels are perpendicular to the uterine cavity/serosa crossing the lesion [28].

Malignant Uterine Pathology

Endometrial Cancer

Transvaginal ultrasound examination helps to discriminate between benign and malignant endometrial lesions. Irregular echogenicity of the endometrium at greyscale ultrasound examination gives us a suspicion of malignancy. Irregular echogenicity together with higher vascularization of endometrium at colour and power Doppler ultrasound, irregular branching of blood vessels, dense areas of the vessels and colour splashes increase risk of endometrial malignancy [31–33] (Figure 16.5).

Uterine Sarcoma

Uterine sarcoma is usually a single, large tumour. It may mimic a benign myoma or in some cases appear

as a large tumour with irregular vascularization and sometimes necrotic areas [34,35] (Figure 16.6). There is very scarce information on the role of greyscale and Doppler ultrasound in differentiating benign myomas from sarcomas and most of the studies are small, retrospective case series.

Ovary

Normal Ovary

Ovarian angiogenesis is a required condition for the early stages of folliculogenesis and growth of the *corpus luteum*. Vascular supply in the ovary may play an important role in the growth and differentiation of the follicles and in the selection of the dominant follicle [36,37]. In premenopausal women with natural menstrual cycles, vascularization of the dominant ovary and dominant follicle increases during the follicular phase and continues to increase after ovulation, being higher during the luteal than follicular phase, while no changes in vascularization occur in the non-dominant ovary [38]. At the end of the luteal phase, vascularization of the *corpus luteum* decreases physiologically.

Colour and power Doppler ultrasound can help in identifying *corpus luteum* as this physiological lesion typically presents abundant peripheral blood vessels, surrounding it as a thin rim: the 'ring of fire' sign [39] (Figure 16.7). Colour and power Doppler ultrasound allow for differentiating the *corpus luteum* from other adnexal masses, i.e. endometriomas, and helps to confirm ovulation in infertility patients monitored by serial transvaginal sonography in natural or stimulated cycles [40].

It has been suggested that blood flow in the *corpus luteum* is closely related to its function, and significant changes are observed during the menstrual cycle [41,42] and pregnancy [43]. However, the diagnostic role of spectral Doppler is no longer considered useful [44]. Ovaries in postmenopausal women are small; the size of the ovaries is similar regardless of the number of years in menopause, and colour Doppler signals may be detected in only about two-thirds of ovaries [45].

Ovarian Torsion

Ovarian torsion is one of the reasons for acute pelvic pain. Signs of ovarian torsion at transvaginal greyscale ultrasound examination are enlarged ovary, oedematous stroma, loss of follicular content or peripheral cysts, solid appearance or abnormal position of the

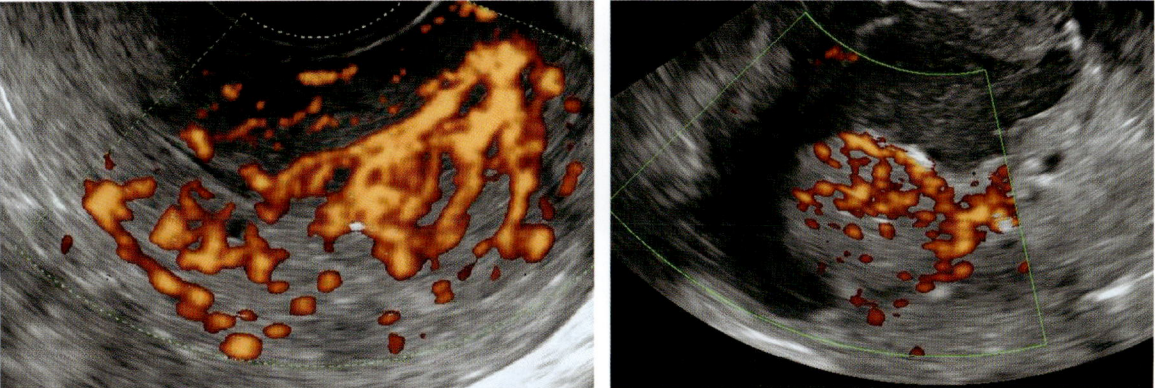

Figure 16.5 Two cases of endometrial adenocarcinoma in women with postmenopausal bleeding. Ultrasound examination shows heterogeneous highly vascularized endometrium with irregular branching vessels and colour splashes.

(a)   (b)   (c)

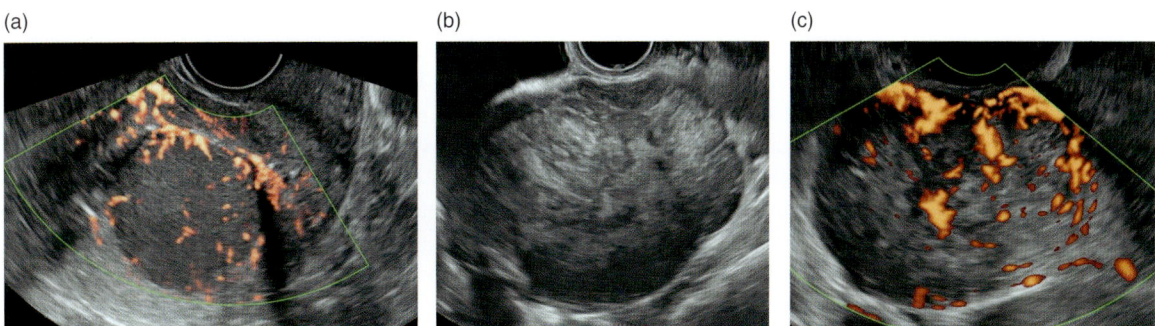

Figure 16.6 Two cases of sarcoma. (a) Endometrial sarcoma – 30-year-old woman with menometrorrhagia. Ultrasound shows a rounded lesion in the uterine cavity with multifocal vessels. Diagnosis was made after hysteroscopy and resection. (b,c) Leiomyosarcoma: a 45-year-old woman with irregular bleeding. Ultrasound shows a heterogeneous single large mass with increased vascularization.

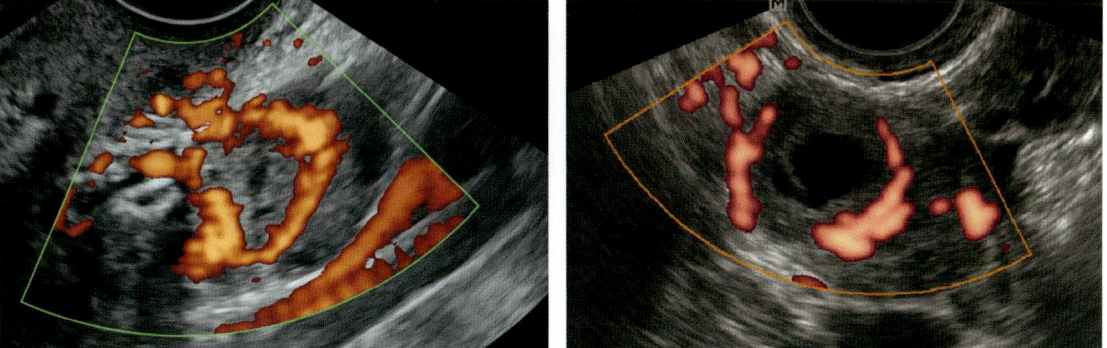

Figure 16.7 Typical appearance of the *corpus luteum* with surrounding vessels – the 'ring of fire' sign.

ovary. When using colour and power Doppler, a twisted ovarian pedicle ('whirlpool sign') may be seen. There may be reduced or absent arterial flow; however, normal Doppler findings do not exclude ovarian torsion (Figure 16.8).

Benign Ovarian Pathology

New vessel formation is essential in growth of benign ovarian cysts, malignant tissue growth and metastasis to the ovaries. Tumour vascular

(a) (b)

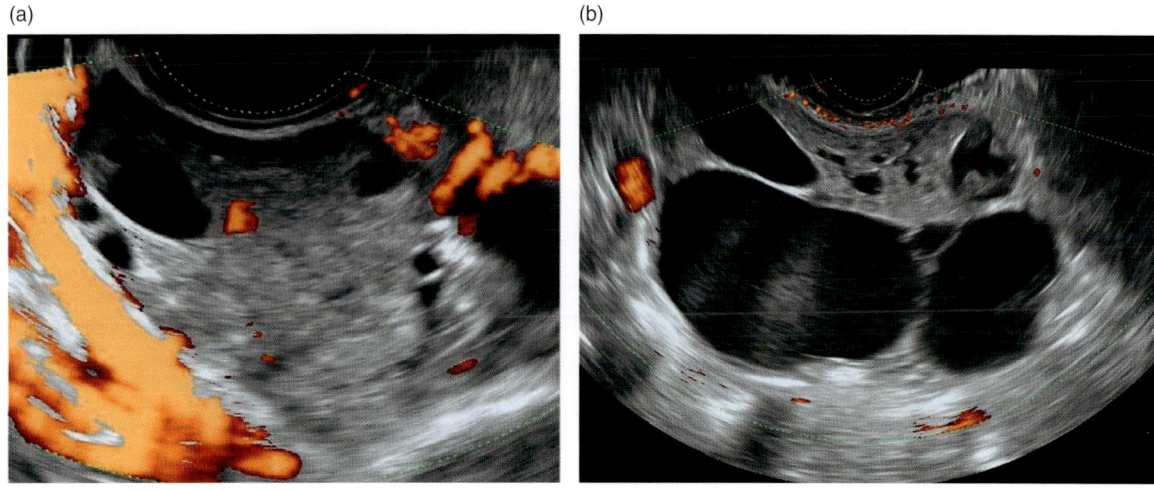

Figure 16.8 Two cases of ovarian torsion confirmed at laparoscopy. Ultrasound examination shows (a) enlarged ovary, oedematous stroma and peripheral cysts – only minimal Doppler signals are visible; (b) enlarged ovary with cystic lesions, no visible Doppler signals.

morphology and biological behaviour differ from normal vasculature [46]. Vascularization of ovarian pathology can be assessed using colour and power Doppler ultrasound. Colour content in the tissue can be estimated subjectively or objectively. The International Ovarian Tumor Analysis (IOTA) group suggested colour score in estimating vascularization in the lesion: colour score 1 = no vascularization; colour score 2 = only minimal flow detected; colour score 3 = moderate flow present; colour score 4 = richly vascularized lesion [47]. Good intra- and interobserver agreement for the colour score has been observed [3]. Objective quantification of blood flow using spectral Doppler has been shown to fail in discriminating between benign and malignant ovarian lesions. 3D power Doppler ultrasound vascular indices have been found to add little to a correct diagnosis of malignancy in the ordinary tumour population [48].

Specific ultrasound diagnosis in the majority of ovarian cysts can be made by using pattern recognition on greyscale ultrasound and subjective assessment of the colour content in the lesion contributes little to the specific diagnosis [49,50]. High diagnostic accuracy of transvaginal ultrasound is described in diagnosing endometriomas with sensitivity and specificity of over 90 per cent, particularly among women aged up to 35 years [51]. Similarly, a cystic ovarian mass with detectable flow within an internal papillary projection is seen in only 2.5 per cent of histologically confirmed

endometriomas and in 30 per cent of confirmed malignant ovarian masses [52,53]. However, vascularization in endometriomas may vary widely, from absent detectable blood flow to moderate or abundant vascularization; therefore, Doppler ultrasound adds little in confirming the diagnosis of endometriomas [52] (Figure 16.9).

Malignant Ovarian Pathology

Ovarian cancer is a lethal disease and early detection is important. Furthermore, correct assessment of an adnexal lesion helps to decide the correct management and operative approach [54]. Different types of ovarian malignancies have been shown to have different clinical and ultrasound characteristics [55]. However, the diagnostic accuracy of ultrasound has been shown to be dependent on the experience of the examiner [56]. The IOTA group created Simple Rules and mathematical models that can be used in discriminating benign ovarian lesions from malignant ones [57,58]. The Simple Rules report 10 different features, five benign and five malignant, to be described when assessing ovarian tumours in order to classify the tumour as benign or malignant [58]. The Simple Rules have been proven to be highly sensitive and specific in differentiating between benign and malignant ovarian masses with similar or superior diagnostic performance when compared to other prediction models [57]. They incorporate colour score 1 as a benign feature and colour score 4 as a malignant

(a)   (b)

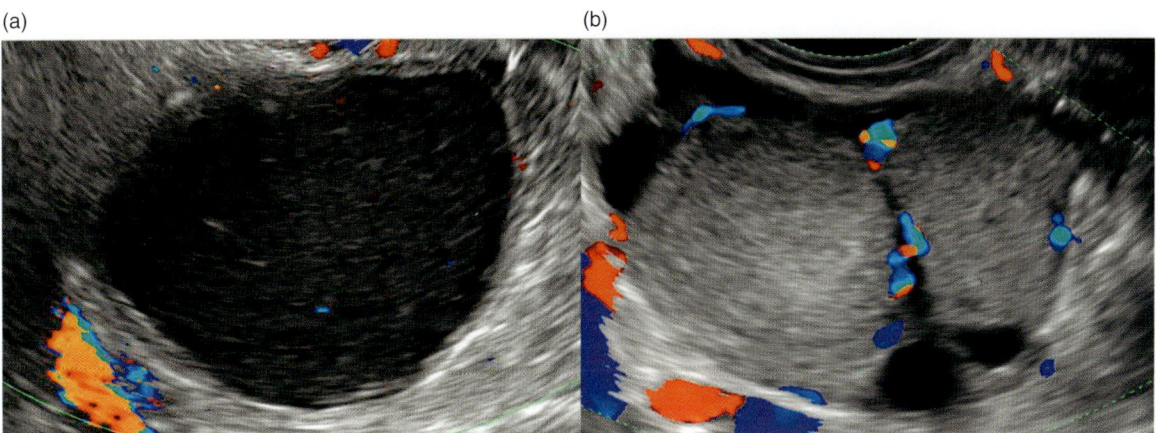

Figure 16.9 Two cases of ovarian endometriomas: (a) typical endometrioma – unilocular cyst with ground glass echogenicity; (b) bilocular endometrioma with ground glass echogenicity. Vascularization in endometriomas may vary from no visible Doppler signals, colour score 1 (a) to moderate vascularization, colour score 3 (b) or abundant vascularization.

(a)   (b)

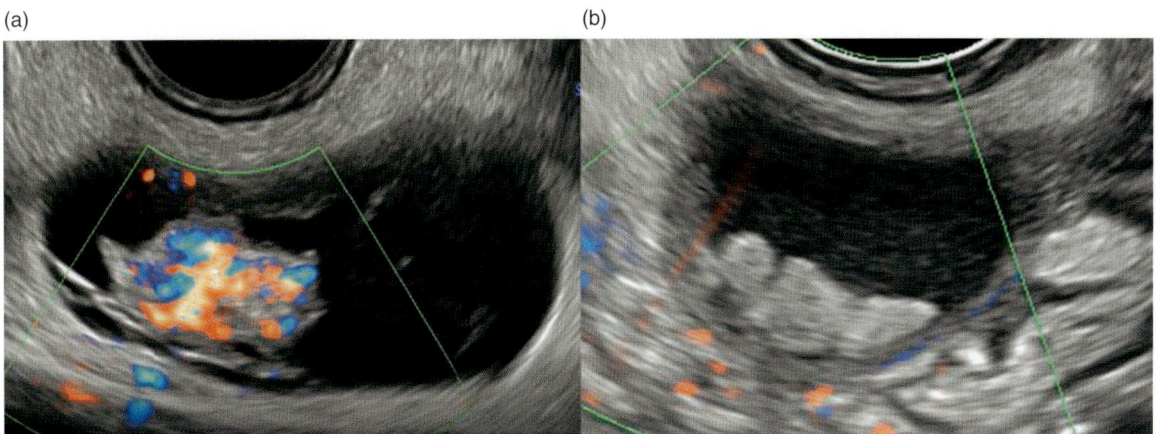

Figure 16.10 Differentiation between true solid component and a blood clot. (a) Unilocular-solid lesion with highly vascularized papillary projection. Malignancy was suspected and histology showed serous cystadenocarcinoma; (b) unilocular cyst with tissue protruding into the cyst cavity – the tissue is not a solid component and there are no Doppler signals.

feature. Colour scores 2 and 3 should be considered as inconclusive [58], but might increase the risk of malignancy in inconclusive lesions, when neither benign nor malignant features are found in the tumour [47,59].

A prediction model for individual ovarian cancer risk estimation using the IOTA Simple Rules was recently published [59]. Although Doppler must be used along with other greyscale ultrasound features for ultimate risk estimation, when assessed solely a colour score 1 is as rare as 3–4 per cent in malignant tumours, while colour score 4 has a general prevalence of 28–31 per cent in malignancies, suggesting that masses with absent flow are most likely benign [59].

While assessing an echogenic mass within a cystic cavity, Doppler can also help to differentiate between solid and non-solid components (such as a clot), additional information that can be helpful in estimating malignancy risk [59] (Figure 16.10). Any detectable flow within the mass is conclusive of a solid component; when blood flow is absent, other sonographic features should be addressed to make such a distinction [47].

To select appropriate management of the patient it is also important to differentiate primary and metastatic ovarian malignancy. 'Lead vessels' is a sonographic Doppler feature in solid ovarian metastasis, present in about one-third of metastatic ovarian tumours [60] (Figure 16.11).

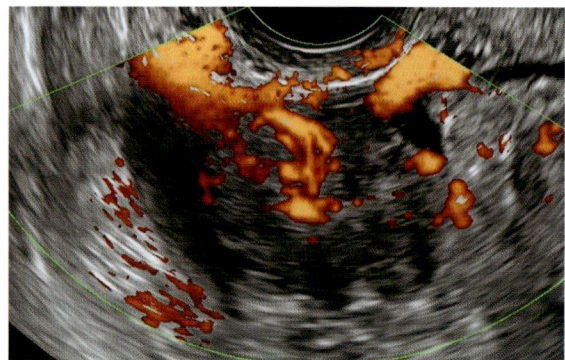

Figure 16.11 Metastatic ovarian cancer in a 40-year-old patient with primary breast cancer. Doppler ultrasound examination shows 'lead vessels' that can be found in about one-third of solid metastases to the ovary.

Pelvic Venous Congestion Syndrome and Hydrosalpinx

Women with chronic pelvic pain should undergo a transvaginal ultrasound examination at least once during the clinical investigation in order to assist in making a correct diagnosis and detection of pelvic venous congestion syndrome. The main type of dilation of the parametrial veins is represented as long tubal retort-like structures of different diameters, which do not show pulsation, and most cases are due to organic pathologies. Based on the diameter and location of the veins, ultrasound is useful for diagnosis and has correlation with symptoms (pain) [63,64]. The typical finding of an elongated mass with incomplete septa may lead to

(a)   (b)

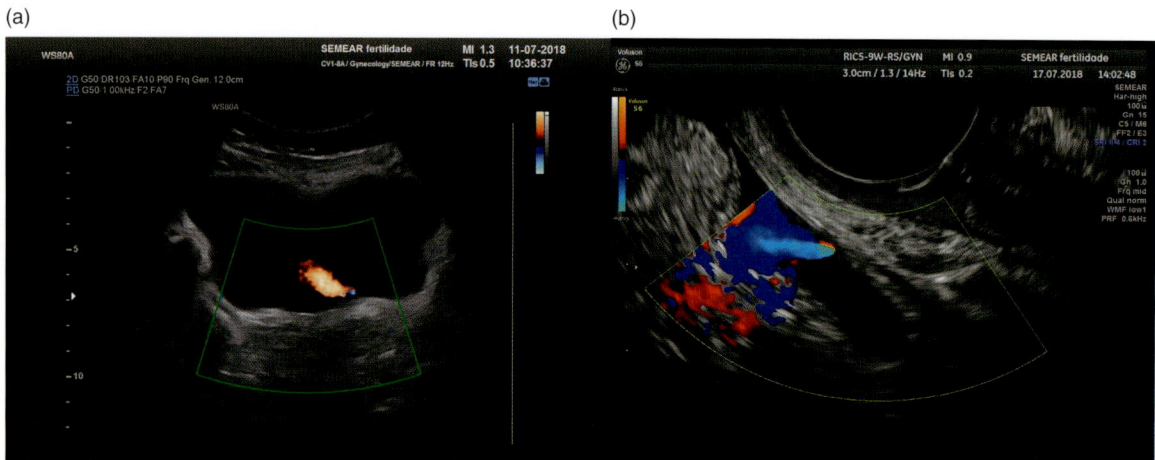

Figure 16.12 Demonstration of the urinary flow from the ureter into the bladder by Doppler ultrasound using transabdominal (a) and transvaginal (b) ultrasound scan.

Other Conditions

Ureteral Function

Doppler can be used to identify ureteric jets through the bladder's internal ostia (Figure 16.12). Such evaluation provides indirect information on ureteral patency and function, as a significant reduction in ureteral flow (subjectively compared to the contralateral ureter) suggests an ongoing obstruction that might occur before the onset of hydronephrosis [61].

Additionally, Doppler can be used along with 3D ultrasound scan of the bladder for precise location of endometriotic lesions close to the trigone – presurgical information that can help define the best operative approach [62].

the diagnosis of hydrosalpinx, where B-mode ultrasound is sufficient for making a diagnosis. Doppler transvaginal examination allows for differentiation between these two pathologies in inconclusive cases, where Doppler signal is present within the lesion in a blood vessel and occasional Doppler signal within the wall of the dilated tube [65].

Conclusion

Use of Doppler assessment during 2D and 3D transvaginal ultrasound scan may add information and help in evaluation of the female reproductive tract. Colour and power Doppler ultrasound are helpful in differential diagnosis between benign and malignant lesions; predicting endometrial and ovarian malignancy; and analysing ureteral function and tubal patency. Based on the large amount of data available, colour and power Doppler ultrasound can be recommended to be used in order to enhance evidence-based gynaecological care.

Tips and Tricks

- Various Doppler modalities should be used routinely in assessment of the female pelvis.
- Various ultrasound machine settings may affect the Doppler output; the suggested settings are: PRF (0.3 or 0.6 kHz), low wall motion filter and use of the sub-noise technique gain setting.
- Doppler signals undergo changes throughout the menstrual cycle, within both the endometrium and the ovary.
- Addition of colour Doppler to HyCoSy or HyFoSy improves the reliability of tubal patency testing.
- A single blood vessel (pedicle artery) is pathognomonic for an endometrial polyp.
- Circumferential blood flow pattern with sporadic signal within a lesion is characteristic of a myoma.
- Perpendicular blood vessels crossing a 'focal' myometrial lesion may suggest an adenomyoma.
- Irregular, branching blood vessels, dense areas of the vessels and colour splashes when detected in an endometrial lesion increase risk of malignancy.
- The presence of blood flow within an ovary does not exclude torsion.
- IOTA's Simple Rules incorporate colour score 1 as a benign feature and colour score 4 as a malignant feature.
- In an ovarian mass, any detectable Doppler signal within the mass or solid component is conclusive of a solid structure, rather than a blood clot.
- Doppler may aid in diagnosing ureteric patency.

References

1. Bhide A, Acharya G, Bilardo CM, et al. ISUOG practice guidelines: use of Doppler ultrasonography in obstetrics. *Ultrasound Obstet Gynecol* 2013;**41**:233–9.

2. Naguib NN, Nour-Eldin NE, Serag-Eldin F, et al. Role of uterine artery Doppler in the management of uterine leiomyoma by arterial embolization. *Ultrasound Obstet Gynecol* 2012;**40**:452–8.

3. Zannoni L, Savelli L, Jokubkiene L, et al. Intra- and interobserver reproducibility of assessment of Doppler ultrasound findings in adnexal masses. *Ultrasound Obstet Gynecol* 2013;**42**:93–101.

4. Collins SL, Stevenson GN, Noble JA, Impey L, Welsh AW. Influence of power Doppler gain setting on Virtual Organ Computer-aided AnaLysis indices in vivo: can use of the individual sub-noise gain level optimize information? *Ultrasound Obstet Gynecol* 2012;**40**:75–80.

5. Jokubkiene L, Sladkevicius P, Rovas L, Valentin L. Assessment of changes in endometrial and subendometrial volume and vascularity during the normal menstrual cycle using three-dimensional power Doppler ultrasound. *Ultrasound Obstet Gynecol* 2006;**27**:672–9.

6. Raine-Fenning NJ, Campbell BK, Kendall NR, Clewes JS, Johnson IR. Quantifying the changes in endometrial vascularity throughout the normal menstrual cycle with three-dimensional power Doppler angiography. *Hum Reprod* 2004;**19**:330–8.

7. Jokubkiene L, Sladkevicius P, Valentin L. Transvaginal ultrasound examination of the endometrium in postmenopausal women without vaginal bleeding. *Ultrasound Obstet Gynecol* 2016;**48**:390–6.

8. Groszmann YS, Benacerraf BR. Complete evaluation of anatomy and morphology of the infertile patient in a single visit; the modern infertility pelvic ultrasound examination. *Fertil Steril* 2016;**105**:1381–93.

9. Ludwin I, Martins WP, Nastri CO, Ludwin A. Pain intensity during ultrasound assessment of uterine cavity and tubal patency with and without painkillers: prospective observational study. *J Minim Invasive Gynecol* 2017;**24**:599–608.

10. Ludwin A, Nastri CO, Ludwin I, Martins WP. Hysterosalpingo-lidocaine-foam sonography combined with power Doppler imaging (HyLiFoSy-PD) in tubal patency assessment: 'flaming tube' sign. *Ultrasound Obstet Gynecol* 2017;**50**:808–10.

11. Ludwin I, Ludwin A, Nastri CO, et al. Inter-rater reliability of air/saline HyCoSy, HyFoSy and HyFoSy combined with power Doppler for screening tubal patency. *Ultraschall Med* 2019; **40**;47–54.

12. Khan MS, Shaikh A, Ratnani R. Ultrasonography and Doppler study to predict uterine receptivity in infertile patients undergoing embryo transfer. *J Obstet Gynaecol India* 2016;**66**:377–82.

13. Koo HS, Park CW, Cha SH, Yang KM. Serial evaluation of endometrial blood flow for prediction of pregnancy outcomes in patients who underwent controlled ovarian hyperstimulation and in vitro fertilization and embryo transfer. *J Ultrasound Med* 2018;**37**:851–7.

14. Wang J, Xia F, Zhou Y, et al. Association between endometrial/subendometrial vasculature and embryo transfer outcome: a meta-analysis and subgroup analysis. *J Ultrasound Med* 2018;**37**:149–63.

15. Polanski LT, Baumgarten MN, Brosens J, et al. Endometrial spatio-temporal image correlation (STIC) and prediction of outcome following assisted reproductive treatment. *Eur J Obstet Gynecol Reprod Biol* 2016;**203**:320–5.

16. Nandi A, Martins WP, Jayaprakasan K, et al. Assessment of endometrial and subendometrial blood flow in women undergoing frozen embryo transfer cycles. *Reprod Biomed Online* 2014;**28**:343–51.

17. Hoozemans DA, Schats R, Lambalk NB, Homburg R, Hompes PG. Serial uterine artery Doppler velocity parameters and human uterine receptivity in IVF/ICSI cycles. *Ultrasound Obstet Gynecol* 2008;**31**:432–8.

18. Martins WP, Welsh AW, Lima JC, Nastri CO, Raine-Fenning NJ. The 'volumetric' pulsatility index as evaluated by spatiotemporal imaging correlation (STIC): a preliminary description of a novel technique, its application to the endometrium and an evaluation of its reproducibility. *Ultrasound Med Biol* 2011;**37**:2160–8.

19. Nastri CO, Ferriani RA, Raine-Fenning N, Martins WP. Endometrial scratching performed in the non-transfer cycle and outcome of assisted reproduction: a randomized controlled trial. *Ultrasound Obstet Gynecol* 2013;**42**:375–82.

20. El-Sharkawy M, El-Mazny A, Ramadan W, et al. Three-dimensional ultrasonography and power Doppler for discrimination between benign and malignant endometrium in premenopausal women with abnormal uterine bleeding. *BMC Women's Health* 2016;**16**:18.

21. Sladkevicius P, Opolskiene G, Valentin L. Prospective temporal validation of mathematical models to calculate risk of endometrial malignancy in patients with postmenopausal bleeding. *Ultrasound Obstet Gynecol* 2017;**49**:649–56.

22. Lacey JV, Jr., Sherman ME, Rush BB, et al. Absolute risk of endometrial carcinoma during 20-year follow-up among women with endometrial hyperplasia. *J Clin Oncol* 2010;**28**:788–92.

23. Van den Bosch T, Van Schoubroeck D, Ameye L, et al. Ultrasound assessment of endometrial thickness and endometrial polyps in women on hormonal replacement therapy. *Am J Obstet Gynecol* 2003;**188**:1249–53.

24. Lee SC, Kaunitz AM, Sanchez-Ramos L, Rhatigan RM. The oncogenic potential of endometrial polyps: a systematic review and meta-analysis. *Obstet Gynecol* 2010;**116**:1197–205.

25. Timmerman D, Verguts J, Konstantinovic ML, et al. The pedicle artery sign based on sonography with color Doppler imaging can replace second-stage tests in women with abnormal vaginal bleeding. *Ultrasound Obstet Gynecol* 2003;**22**:166–71.

26. McLucas B. Diagnosis imaging and anatomical classification of uterine fibroids. *Best Pract Res Clin Obstet Gynaecol* 2008;**22**:627–42.

27. Epstein E, Valentin L. Gray-scale ultrasound morphology in the presence or absence of intrauterine fluid and vascularity as assessed by color Doppler for discrimination between benign and malignant endometrium in women with postmenopausal bleeding. *Ultrasound Obstet Gynecol* 2006;**28**:89–95.

28. Van den Bosch T, Dueholm M, Leone FP, et al. Terms, definitions and measurements to describe sonographic features of myometrium and uterine masses: a consensus opinion from the Morphological Uterus Sonographic Assessment (MUSA) group. *Ultrasound Obstet Gynecol* 2015;**46**:284–98.

29. Van den Bosch T, de Bruijn AM, de Leeuw RA, et al. Sonographic classification and reporting system for diagnosing adenomyosis. *Ultrasound Obstet Gynecol* 2019;**53**:576–82.

30. Munro MG, Critchley HO, Broder MS, Fraser IS. FIGO classification system (PALM-COEIN) for causes of abnormal uterine bleeding in nongravid women of reproductive age. *Int J Gynaecol Obstet* 2011;**113**:3–13.

31. Epstein E, Skoog L, Isberg PE, et al. An algorithm including results of gray-scale and power Doppler ultrasound examination to predict endometrial malignancy in women with postmenopausal bleeding. *Ultrasound Obstet Gynecol* 2002;**20**:370–6.

32. Opolskiene G, Sladkevicius P, Valentin L. Ultrasound assessment of endometrial morphology and vascularity to predict endometrial malignancy in women with postmenopausal bleeding and sonographic endometrial thickness >or= 4.5 mm. *Ultrasound Obstet Gynecol* 2007;**30**:332–40.

33. Opolskiene G, Sladkevicius P, Valentin L. Prediction of endometrial malignancy in women with postmenopausal bleeding and sonographic endometrial thickness >/= 4.5 mm. *Ultrasound Obstet Gynecol* 2011;**37**:232–40.

34. Exacoustos C, Romanini ME, Amadio A, et al. Can gray-scale and color Doppler sonography differentiate between uterine leiomyosarcoma and leiomyoma? *J Clin Ultrasound* 2007;**35**:449–57.

35. Aviram R, Ochshorn Y, Markovitch O, et al. Uterine sarcomas versus leiomyomas: gray-scale and Doppler sonographic findings. *J Clin Ultrasound* 2005;**33**:10–13.

36. Richards JS. Maturation of ovarian follicles: actions and interactions of pituitary and ovarian hormones on follicular cell differentiation. *Physiol Rev* 1980;**60**:51–89.

37. Zeleznik AJ, Schuler HM, Reichert LE, Jr. Gonadotropin-binding sites in the rhesus monkey ovary: role of the vasculature in the selective

distribution of human chorionic gonadotropin to the preovulatory follicle. *Endocrinology* 1981;**109**:356–62.

38. Jokubkiene L, Sladkevicius P, Rovas L, Valentin L. Assessment of changes in volume and vascularity of the ovaries during the normal menstrual cycle using three-dimensional power Doppler ultrasound. *Hum Reprod* 2006;**21**:2661–8.

39. Brezinka C. 3D ultrasound imaging of the human corpus luteum. *Reprod Biol* 2014;**14**:110–14.

40. Baerwald AR, Adams GP, Pierson RA. Form and function of the corpus luteum during the human menstrual cycle. *Ultrasound Obstet Gynecol* 2005;**25**:498–507.

41. Tamura H, Takasaki A, Taniguchi K, et al. Changes in blood-flow impedance of the human corpus luteum throughout the luteal phase and during early pregnancy. *Fertil Steril* 2008;**90**:2334–9.

42. Miyazaki T, Tanaka M, Miyakoshi K, et al. Power and colour Doppler ultrasonography for the evaluation of the vasculature of the human corpus luteum. *Hum Reprod* 1998;**13**:2836–41.

43. Valentin L, Sladkevicius P, Laurini R, Soderberg H, Marsal K. Uteroplacental and luteal circulation in normal first-trimester pregnancies: Doppler ultrasonographic and morphologic study. *Am J Obstet Gynecol* 1996;**174**:768–75.

44. Dal J, Vural B, Caliskan E, Ozkan S, Yucesoy I. Power Doppler ultrasound studies of ovarian, uterine, and endometrial blood flow in regularly menstruating women with respect to luteal phase defects. *Fertil Steril* 2005;**84**:224–7.

45. Sladkevicius P, Valentin L, Marsal K. Transvaginal gray-scale and Doppler ultrasound examinations of the uterus and ovaries in healthy postmenopausal women. *Ultrasound Obstet Gynecol* 1995;**6**:81–90.

46. Folkman J. Tumor angiogenesis. *Adv Cancer Res* 1985;**43**:175–203.

47. Timmerman D, Valentin L, Bourne TH, et al. Terms, definitions and measurements to describe the sonographic features of adnexal tumors: a consensus opinion from the International Ovarian Tumor Analysis (IOTA) Group. *Ultrasound Obstet Gynecol* 2000;**16**:500–5.

48. Jokubkiene L, Sladkevicius P, Valentin L. Does three-dimensional power Doppler ultrasound help in discrimination between benign and malignant ovarian masses? *Ultrasound Obstet Gynecol* 2007;**29**:215–25.

49. Valentin L. Pattern recognition of pelvic masses by gray-scale ultrasound imaging: the contribution of Doppler ultrasound. *Ultrasound Obstet Gynecol* 1999;**14**:338–47.

50. Valentin L, Hagen B, Tingulstad S, Eik-Nes S. Comparison of 'pattern recognition' and logistic regression models for discrimination between benign and malignant pelvic masses: a prospective cross validation. *Ultrasound Obstet Gynecol* 2001;**18**:357–65.

51. Guerriero S, Van Calster B, Somigliana E, et al. Age-related differences in the sonographic characteristics of endometriomas. *Hum Reprod* 2016;**31**:1723–31.

52. Van Holsbeke C, Van Calster B, Guerriero S, et al. Endometriomas: their ultrasound characteristics. *Ultrasound Obstet Gynecol* 2010;**35**:730–40.

53. Guerriero S, Ajossa S, Mais V, et al. The diagnosis of endometriomas using colour Doppler energy imaging. *Hum Reprod* 1998;**13**:1691–5.

54. Woo YL, Kyrgiou M, Bryant A, Everett T, Dickinson HO. Centralisation of services for gynaecological cancer. *Cochrane Database Syst Rev* 2012;**2012**:CD007945.

55. Valentin L, Ameye L, Jurkovic D, et al. Which extrauterine pelvic masses are difficult to correctly classify as benign or malignant on the basis of ultrasound findings and is there a way of making a correct diagnosis? *Ultrasound Obstet Gynecol* 2006;**27**:438–44.

56. Timmerman D, Schwarzler P, Collins WP, et al. Subjective assessment of adnexal masses with the use of ultrasonography: an analysis of interobserver variability and experience. *Ultrasound Obstet Gynecol* 1999;**13**:11–16.

57. Kaijser J, Sayasneh A, Van Hoorde K, et al. Presurgical diagnosis of adnexal tumours using mathematical models and scoring systems: a systematic review and meta-analysis. *Hum Reprod Update* 2014;**20**:449–62.

58. Timmerman D, Testa AC, Bourne T, et al. Simple ultrasound-based rules for the diagnosis of ovarian cancer. *Ultrasound Obstet Gynecol* 2008;**31**:681–90.

59. Timmerman D, Van Calster B, Testa A, et al. Predicting the risk of malignancy in adnexal masses based on the Simple Rules from the International Ovarian Tumor Analysis group. *Am J Obstet Gynecol* 2016;**214**:424–37.

60. Testa AC, Mancari R, Di Legge A, et al. The 'lead vessel': a vascular ultrasound feature of metastasis in the ovaries. *Ultrasound Obstet Gynecol* 2008;**31**:218–21.

61. Pepe F, Pepe P. Color Doppler ultrasound (CDU) in the diagnosis of obstructive hydronephrosis in pregnant women. *Arch Gynecol Obstet* 2013;**288**:489–93.

62. Thonnon C, Philip CA, Fassi-Fehri H, et al. Three-dimensional ultrasound in the management of bladder endometriosis. *J Minim Invasive Gynecol* 2015;**22**:403–9.

63. Labropoulos N, Jasinski PT, Adrahtas D, Gasparis AP, Meissner MH. A standardized ultrasound approach to pelvic congestion syndrome. *Phlebology* 2017;**32**:608–19.

64. Malgor RD, Adrahtas D, Spentzouris G, et al. The role of duplex ultrasound in the workup of pelvic congestion syndrome. *J Vasc Surg Venous Lymphat Disord* 2014;**2**:34–8.

65. Guerriero S, Ajossa S, Lai MP, et al. Transvaginal ultrasonography associated with colour Doppler energy in the diagnosis of hydrosalpinx. *Hum Reprod* 2000;**15**:1568–72.

Index